REVISED EDITION

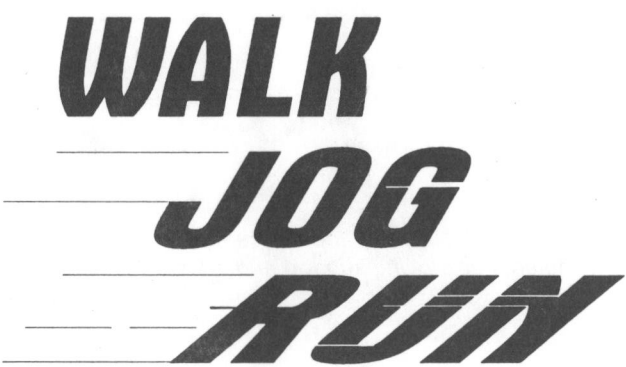

FOR WELLNESS
EVERYONE

Patricia A. Floyd, Ph.D.
Alabama State University

Janet E. Parke, Ed.D.
Broward Community College

⊞ Hunter Textbooks Inc.

Dedicated to my daughter and son, Courtney J. Floyd Zinke
and Matthew H. Zinke with love, respect, appreciation and
admiration.

Patricia Alford Floyd

Dedicated to my parents, Joseph and Margaret Prock,
and friends who provided loving support and encouragement.

Janet E. Parke

Cover design by Hugh West
Photographs by Victor Farran

Copyright 1998 by Hunter Textbooks Inc.

ISBN 0-88725-252-4

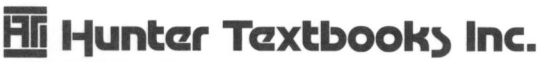 **Hunter Textbooks Inc.**

823 Reynolda Road
Winston-Salem, North Carolina 27104

PREFACE

The purpose of this book is to serve as a resource for people of all ages who are interested in walking, jogging and/or running as a means to achieve aerobic fitness. It can be used as a textbook for secondary school, college/university and community activity classes or groups, and as a guide for anyone interested in the three aerobic activities of walking, jogging and running. It is helpful to anyone starting a program of walking, jogging or running since it provides information on preparation, training principles and suggested programs to follow. The book also contains helpful information for individuals currently involved in a walking, jogging or running program who want to improve or progress to a higher level in their aerobic activity. In addition, those who wish to race as a runner or racewalker will find training information and programs that can improve racing performance.

The uniqueness of this book is that it provides information on three of the most popular aerobic activities under one cover. Not only does it discuss walking, jogging and running as individual exercise activities, but it provides information on how one may progress from walking to jogging to running; from walking to racewalking; and also from jogging to running and racing. The mechanics of each are compared and programs are suggested which help a person improve in aerobic fitness by changing from walking to jogging and then running, or from walking to racewalking.

Currently a number of excellent books have been published which deal with only one of the three aerobic activities of walking, jogging or running. Many people plan to progress from one of the three activities to another at a higher level or may find that once they begin a program they wish to progress to one of the other two aerobic activities that is more strenuous. Also, many schools offer classes that are designed to provide an option of any of the three activities. It is more convenient and useful to have a book that covers all three activities of walking, jogging and running. Therefore, since no book has been published at this time that involves walking, jogging and running, this unique publication serves a valuable purpose.

Information in this book reflects the most current research, theories and trends regarding walking, jogging and running. It helps an individual evaluate his/her aerobic fitness level and, based upon the evaluation, provides suggestions and sample programs on how to improve aerobic fitness by means of walking, jogging or running.

Since total wellness cannot be achieved through aerobic fitness alone, additional information has been presented to assist the reader in becoming optimally fit. Sections have been included that discuss flexibility and strength training needed to enhance the walking, jogging or running programs and to complete the fitness triangle. Also, help is provided in preparing for exercise and in preventing and caring for injuries sustained during exercise.

This book provides up-to-date information about the vital role of nutrition in achieving wellness. Detailed facts on nutrients, analysis and planning of food intake, and weight control are discussed in two important chapters. The final chapter discusses stress — the causes, signs and symptoms — and stress management techniques to reduce, eliminate or cope with stress.

ACKNOWLEDGEMENTS

The authors wish to thank those who so graciously donated their time and efforts to make this book possible: Doug Adkins, Cynthia Barnard, David Bowden, Aliece Bristol, Tom Drum ('fraid Knots), Victor Farran, Bob Fine, Carol Findley, Courtney Floyd Zinke, Jerry Floyd, Kathy Johnson, Henry Laskau, Janet Levins, Mark Rifkin, Meg Sarakas (Running Wild, Inc.), Bonnie Stein, Jean A. Thompson, and Helena Toner.

Contents

One: Lifetime Fitness Through Walking, Jogging, or Running 1
Fitness and Wellness, *2;* Walking, Jogging, and Running, *4*

Two: Preparation 7
Physical Examination, *7;* Essential Clothing and Equipment, *8;*
Optional Clothing and Equipment, *19;* Safety and Environmental
Concerns, *20;* Additional Hazards, *22;* Exercise in Hot Weather, *23;*
Exercise in Cold Weather, *25;* Safety Guidelines, *28;* Summary, *29*

Three: Training Principles 30
Mechanics for Walking and Racewalking, *30;* Mechanics of Jogging
and Running, *37;* Physiology, *44;* Psychology, *48;* Training
Principles—FITT, *52;* Conclusion, *59;* Summary, *59*

Four: Training Programs 60
Determining the Starting Level, *60;* Walking, Jogging, and Running
Programs, *69;* Running and Racewalking Programs for Race Com-
petitors, *82;* Walking/Jogging/Running During Pregnancy, *102;*
Program Execution, *104;* Wheelchair Workouts/Racing, *104;* Additional
Exercise Program and Race Procedures, *104;* Summary, *110*

Five: Fitness Enhancing Programs 111
Flexibility, *111;* Strength, *121;* Plyometrics, *138;* Cross Training,
141; Summary, *145*

Six: Common Injuries: Prevention and Care 146
Prevention, *146;* Injuries, *147;* Care, *155;* R.I.C.E.S. Formula, *156;*
Heat Application, *158;* Summary, *158*

Seven: Nutrition 160
Nutrients, *160;* Food Guide Pyramid, *162;* Basic Nutrients, *165;*
Caffeine and Alcohol, *196;* Airplane Foods, *197;* Fast Foods, *197;*
Supermarket Shopping, *199;* Dietary Guidelines for Americans, *200;*
Nutrition Labels, *201;* Summary, *205*

Eight: Weight Management 206
Theories of Obesity, *206;* Health Problems, *209;* Desirable Body
Weight, *211;* Assessing Body Fatness, *214;* Weight Loss, *222;*
Weight Maintenance, *232;* Weight Gain, *234;* Summary, *234*

Nine: Stress Management 236
What is Stress? *236;* Managing Stress, *237;* Recognizing Signs
and Symptoms of Stress, *238;* Identifying or Removing the Stressor,
238; Stress Management Techniques, *240;* Stress Management
Guidelines, *247;* Summary, *249*

Appendixes 251
A: References and Suggested Readings, *252;* B: Muscles of the
Body, *260;* C: Chapter Evaluations, *262;* D: Laboratories, *281*

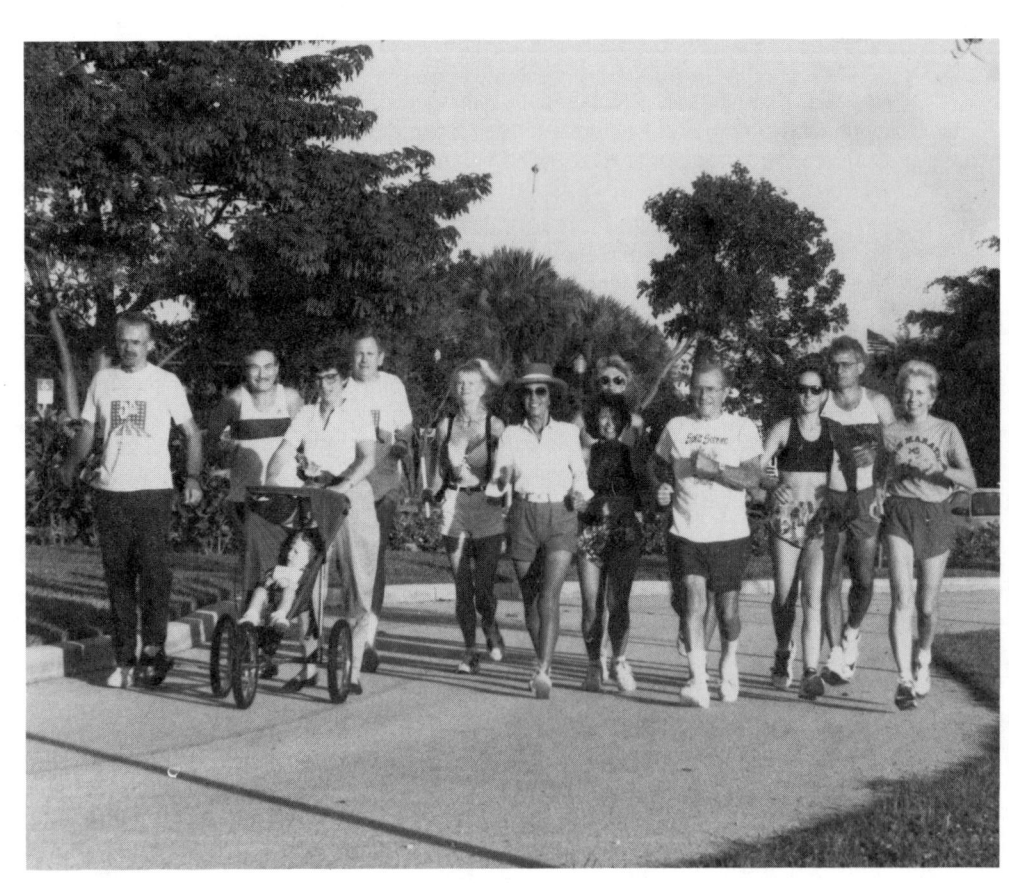

CHAPTER ONE

Lifetime Fitness Through Walking, Jogging, or Running

During the past two decades, fitness and more recently wellness have increased in importance. Why? Lifetime fitness and/or wellness promotes a healthier, happier and a more productive life for those individuals involved in a fitness/wellness lifestyle. Studies have shown that physical inactivity and negative habits are a serious threat to one's health. Individuals are meant to be active in order for the body to grow, develop and improve. In essence, muscles must move for the body to improve. Medical advances have eliminated most of the causes of infectious diseases while there is a significant increase in lifestyle diseases (inactivity) which are the leading causes of death in America. Inactivity leads to diseases of hypertension, adult onset diabetes, obesity, high cholesterol, coronary heart disease, and stroke.

Today many individuals are making the right choices and are doing something to improve their fitness and wellness, therefore maximizing their chances for enjoyment of life. However, many individuals have embarked on fitness or total wellness programs with little guidance or knowledge. This book provides the necessary guidance and information in assisting an individual in establishing a sound base for lifetime participation in fitness/wellness activities such as walking, jogging, and/or running. Through these activities an individual may achieve an active way of living and accomplish positive lifestyle habits which could last a lifetime. Through regular participation in aerobic workouts and the establishment of good nutritional habits and stress management, individuals cannot only prolong their life but improve the quality of their life.

It is much cheaper and more effective to maintain good health than it is to regain it once it is lost. — Kenneth H. Cooper, M.D.

FITNESS AND WELLNESS

It appears there is a strong base of support for fitness and wellness in America. Former President John F. Kennedy ranked physical fitness along with mental, moral, and spiritual fitness as essential to the nation's strength. Every year, America celebrates National Physical Fitness Day on May 1. On this special day, all Americans are encouraged to become physically fit and active in their daily activities.

Physical fitness is only one component of wellness. The American Medical Association defines fitness as the general capacity to adapt and respond favorably to physical effort. In essence, individuals are fit when daily activities can be safely and effectively carried on with energy left over for leisure and recreational activities.

Physical fitness is classified into two components: health-related fitness and skill-related or motor fitness. Health-related components of fitness are those qualities which are more important to a person's health while skill-related or motor components are those qualities which enable a person to perform motor tasks. Most experts agree that to achieve overall fitness in walking, jogging, and running, an individual must participate in specific programs to develop each one of the five basic health-related components:

1. Cardiorespiratory fitness: The ability of the heart, lungs, and blood vessels to supply oxygen and nutrients to the muscles to provide sufficient energy to sustain aerobic exercise for prolonged periods of time.
2. Muscular strength: The ability of a muscle group to contract against a resistance or force.
3. Muscular endurance: The ability of muscles to repeatedly contract themselves for prolonged periods of time.
4. Flexibility: The ability of a joint to move freely through a normal range of motion.
5. Body composition: The analysis of the body into two primary components, lean body mass and body fat. Body mass is composed mostly of muscle and bone tissue.

The skill-related components of fitness are associated with motor skills or sports/athletics. In addition to the health-related components, the skill-related components consist of agility, balance, coordination, power, reaction time and speed. While these components are necessary to achieve success in motor skills or sports, they are not crucial for development of better health. Therefore, only the health-related components of fitness are discussed in the book related to walking, jogging, and running.

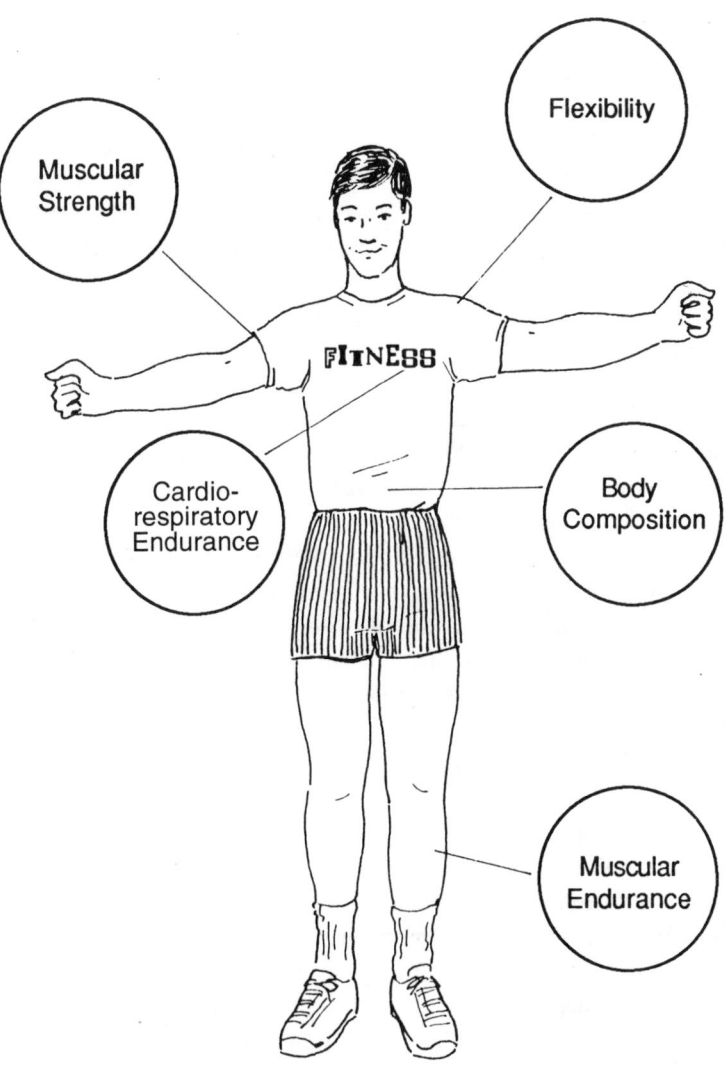

Health-Related Components of Fitness

Wellness is a continuous effort to stay healthy and achieve the highest potential for well-being. It is an approach to optimal health where the individual has the responsibility for his or her own well-being. In addition, the emphasis on prevention in promoting wellness is reflected in the Healthy People 2000: National Health Promotion and Disease Prevention Objectives, and the most recent 1996 Surgeon General's Report on Physical Activity and Health. In prevention the individual must change in attitude and stop demanding medication, surgery, or hospitalization for every ache and pain. The choices made by an individual influence the health and well-being of the individual. No one is going to demand that the individual walk, jog, run, stretch, eat proper foods, and practice relaxation techniques. Physicians, government, and society are not responsible for individuals. Each individual has his/her own responsibility. In addition to physical fitness, the wellness component includes nutrition, smoking cessation, stress management, sexuality, substance abuse control, cancer prevention, spirituality, cardiovascular risk reduction, safety, diet/weight management, physical examination, health education and environmental support. Wellness is a way of life, an ongoing process.

The best fitness and wellness programs accommodate each individual's lifestyle. The choices made influence the state of health and well-being. Practicing seven simple lifestyle habits can significantly increase longevity. These include:
1. Sleep six to eight hours each night.
2. Eat breakfast every morning.
3. Select snacks predominantly from grain, fruit and vegetable groups.
4. Maintain ideal body weight.
5. Exercise regularly.
6. Consume moderate (or no) alcohol.
7. Never start to smoke cigarettes.

This book, *Walk, Jog, Run for Wellness Everyone*, is a positive approach to fitness and/or wellness. Its emphasis is on what to do to enhance the quality of life through fitness activities such as walking, jogging, or running and to achieve wellness for a lifetime of health.

WALKING, JOGGING, AND RUNNING

Walking, jogging, and running have increased in popularity as choices for aerobic activity. During most mornings, evenings, and lunch hours, walkers, joggers, and runners can be found exercising throughout local neighborhoods, downtown areas, and parks. Accessibility and minimal equipment needs have been contributing reasons for selecting walking, jogging, and running to obtain aerobic benefits.

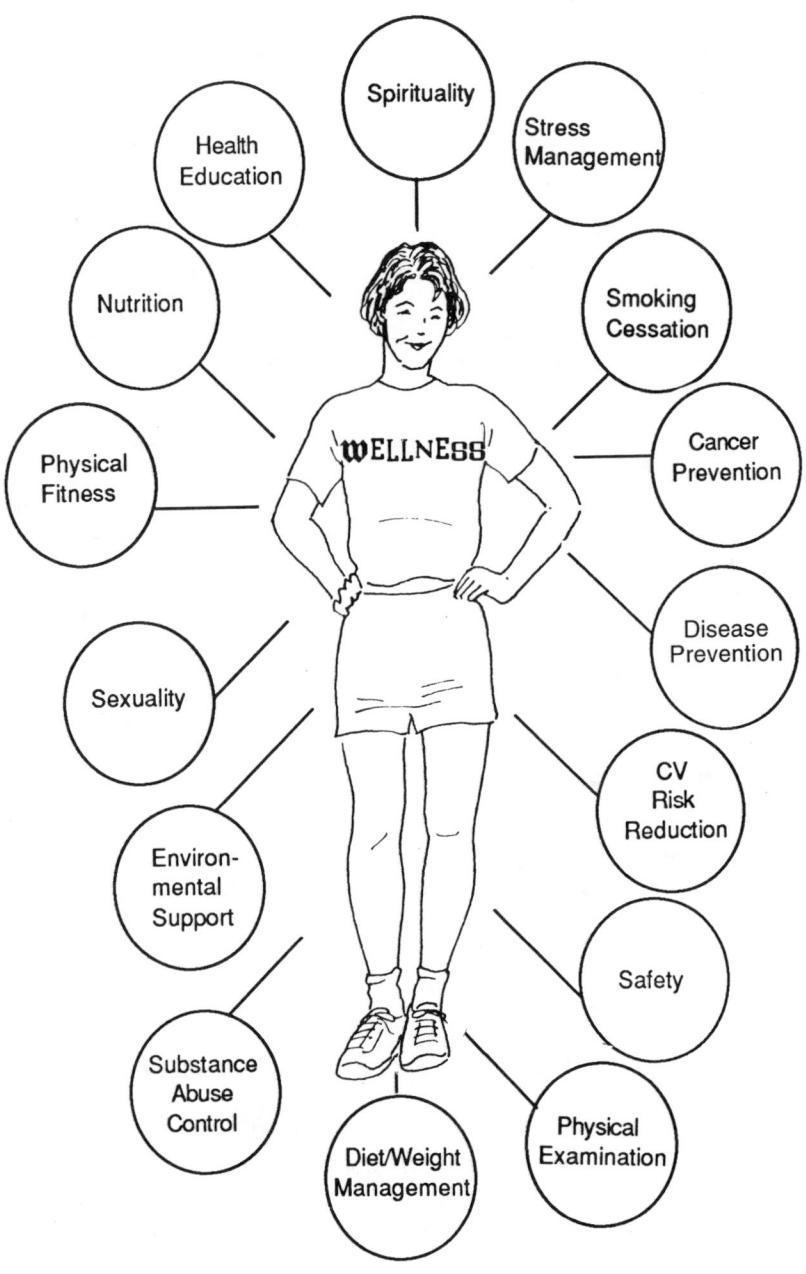

The Components of Wellness

Walking, jogging and running provide both physiological and psychological benefits. The primary physiological benefits are the improvement of the cardiorespiratory system and the reduction of heart attack risk. Psychologically, walkers, joggers, and runners improve their ability to adapt and cope with stress and improve their powers of concentration.

Many people begin a brisk walking program because it imparts less stress to the body than jogging or running. Often individuals jog or run because they enjoy moving faster than a brisk walking pace. Jogging is slower than running. A jogging pace is generally five to six miles per hour and a running pace is generally seven miles per hour or more. Often aerobic exercisers begin as walkers and progress to jogging, then running.

As an individual undertakes a walking, jogging, or running program for wellness, it's important to understand proper preparation procedures. Next it is essential to understand the training principles which guide an aerobic program. Once the principles are comprehended, it is important to learn how to set up or select an aerobic exercise program for walking, jogging, or running. Program starting levels can be determined by participation in simple aerobic tests.

By adding flexibility and strength exercise to the workout program, well rounded fitness can be achieved. Also, it is essential that participants in fitness programs have an understanding of potential injuries and the procedures needed for injury prevention and care.

To complement a fitness program and contribute to total wellness, an individual must learn and apply information on good nutrition and weight management. If a person follows a stringent fitness program but eats poorly and has difficulty managing his/her weight, the fitness benefits are diminished. Also, it is important to learn how to manage stress, since unmanaged stress can cause devastating physiological and psychological damage. Therefore, a total wellness program should include aerobic exercise such as walking, jogging or running, flexibility and strength exercises, good nutritional habits, weight control, and stress management.

By reading and participating in the selected activities in this book it is our desire to encourage each individual to be persistent and committed to this program because it is left up to each individual to take control of his/her own lifestyle and thereby reap the benefits of wellness.

CHAPTER TWO

Preparation

When beginning a regular physical activity such as a walking, jogging or running program, it is important to be adequately prepared. Exercise is a lifetime commitment, and preparation for exercise should become a normal routine in life.

PHYSICAL EXAMINATION

Having a physical exam is important to make certain that an individual is ready to participate in a walk, jog, or run program. **Anyone doubtful about his/her state of health, regardless of age, should seek medical consultation prior to beginning or altering an exercise program.**

The American College of Sports Medicine, in its guidelines for evaluating health status for exercise participation, recommends a pre-exercise test (EKG-monitored graded test during exercise) for individuals age 45 and over, regardless of health status, and for those individuals 35 years and over who have symptoms of heart disease, higher than normal risk of heart disease, and for all individuals with known disease, regardless of age. Risk factors include high blood pressure, high cholesterol, cigarette smoking, diabetes, overweight, and family history of coronary heart disease prior to age 50. Healthy individuals under 45 may not need to have a pre-exercise exam but if an individual has not had a medical examination during the past two years, is returning to an exercise program after extended layoff or illness or injury, or has questions concerning his/her health status, then a physician should be consulted prior to beginning an exercise program.

The authors recommend consultation with a physician before beginning an exercise program if the person has not had a medical examination within the previous two years.

ESSENTIAL CLOTHING AND EQUIPMENT

Walking, jogging or running do not require expensive clothing and equipment, but in order to prevent irritations and injuries to the body, basic information is needed. Participants in all three activities can use the same clothing and equipment except shoes. **Walkers and joggers may use running shoes, but joggers and runners should not use walking shoes.**

SHOES

The first concern in an exercise program is the selection of the proper pair of shoes. With the proper shoes, an individual will be able to walk, jog or run more miles, more comfortably, and with less chance of injury (i.e., Achilles tendon strain, heel bruises, blisters). When shopping for shoes, allow extra time to shop for good quality and a proper fit. Before you shop for your walking or jogging/running shoes, check out the shoe reviews in *Runner's World.* They usually have fall and spring comprehensive shoe reviews to assist any exerciser. Be prepared to visit several stores, trying on several brands or styles, and it is advisable to jog or walk in the store before making the selection of shoes. To find the correct shoe, the shape of the foot, body type, degree of pronation or no pronation, training or racing patterns, and surfaces should be considered. Proper shoes are the most important investment. A myriad of muscular skeletal problems can arise from incorrect or poor quality shoes.

Some or all of the following general guidelines may be used in selecting a walking, jogging or running shoe:

1. Walking, jogging or running shoes are specialty shoes designed specifically for walking, jogging or running. Assuming the individual may walk some days and jog other days, select different shoes. If planning to walk or jog during a workout, select a jogging shoe.
2. Jogging and running shoes have nylon or mesh uppers which are cooler and therefore allow the feet to breathe. If an all-leather shoe is preferred for walking, the ventilation holes should be on the top and sides of the shoe. Extra design leather or suede along the ball-edge of the foot area (toes) provide for a longer shoe life.
3. Good quality shoes can help prevent foot and leg problems that make exercise ineffective and unenjoyable. Shoes should have a good fit, stability, motion control and durability, therefore offering comfort and protection from injury. Special running and walking shoes are designed to take the stress of repeated shock off the hips, knees, lower legs, ankles, and feet.

4. **Shoes may fit as normal shoe size or may fit one-half size larger than regular shoes.** Consult the salesperson about the manufacturer's recommendation. Toes should be able to move freely. When purchasing shoes, try on the shoes with two pairs of socks if planning to wear the extra pair of socks when walking or jogging. Choose a pair of well conditioned shoes that fits both feet while standing. Each foot may be different—one foot may be a different size. Be fitted for shoes in the middle of the day when feet have expanded, rather than the morning or evening when they may be smaller.

5. **Break in new shoes gradually.** Replace them when the recommended mileage for the shoe has been reached or the inside of the shoe deteriorates. A breakdown of the shoe's support and shock absorption occurs when the recommended mileage is reached. Injury may result from further usage. Do not gauge buying shoes by how the rubber on the sole wears.

6. **Buy shoes at a reputable walking/running shoe store.** They may cost slightly more than they would at a large sporting goods or department store, but the service is usually by a knowledgeable salesperson who is probably a walker or runner. Be fitted by an expert or go to another store.

7. **For special problems such as flat feet, unusual widths, rigid, high arch feet, excess body weight, pronation, and toe shape, ask for special assistance in selecting the proper shoe.** Special shoes are designed to alleviate these problems; however, some problems require that a podiatrist make adjustments to the shoes.

8. **Ask to test the shoes on a non-carpeted surface or even take a test walk/run around the block rather than simply jumping around the store.** Testing the shoes on a hard surface rather than the padded carpet commonly found in shoe stores will help determine the amount of comfort and cushion of the shoe.

9: **Expect to pay for a good pair or a high quality pair of shoes.** However, the most expensive does not necessarily mean it is the best shoe for every individual. The shoe industry is changing rapidly. New technology in shoes is described in fairly objective evaluations found in special issues of walking and running magazines.

To find the right shoe for you, it is necessary to consider your personal walking/running characteristics, including (1) your body size and weight; (2) shape of your foot; (3) the number of miles you walk or run per week and the type of training you do; (4) the surface on which you walk, jog or run; (5) if you overpronate, have a stable foot, or underpronate; and (6) if you wear orthotics.

Walking Shoes

1. The outer soles should be reasonably soft and made of durable material and should have a bounce. A good walking shoe has a rocker-shaped sole which helps the foot rock forward from heel to toe.
2. The shoe should have a double- or triple-layered heel to absorb the impact of each step and a treaded sole and heel for adequate traction, when the heel strikes the walking surface and also for pushing off with the toes. The tread is not as deep as is found on running shoes.
3. The inner sole should include an arch support and a heel cup. It may also provide additional air or gel cushioning. The inner sole can be removed from any good quality walking shoes so it can air out between workouts and be replaced when it wears out. A podiatrist or orthopedic doctor can make an inner sole that perfectly fits the foot.
4. Many walking shoes feature a reflective material as a safety measure for those walking at night.

When purchasing a walking shoe, consider the function of the shoe rather than the fashion. The shoe should fit snugly at the heel and instep and conform to the natural outline of the foot. It should be well cushioned since the heel takes the largest force on impact. Women land with more force on their heels per body weight than men at any walking speed; therefore, it is important for women to purchase a shoe which is specifically designed for women. The heel should be elevated one-half to three-fourths inch higher than the sole in order to relieve the strain placed on the back of the leg.

The heel and sole should have an inner padding which should be spongy and soft to absorb the impact during walking. The outer sole should be soft and should have some bounce in it. The sole of a walking shoe should be less flexible than that of a running shoe because it provides more support since the transfer of weight is slower in walking than it is in running. Foot muscle fatigue occurs when there is too much flexibility in the outer sole.

The upper construction of a walking shoe may consist of leather or a combination of leather and fabric. This type of construction allows for support in the shoe and breathability, both of which are necessary to minimize leg and foot fatigue of the muscles.

Lightweight shoes will allow the person to walk longer and with less effort than is required with heavier shoes. Lightweight materials and shoes specially designed for walking provide better support and motion control.

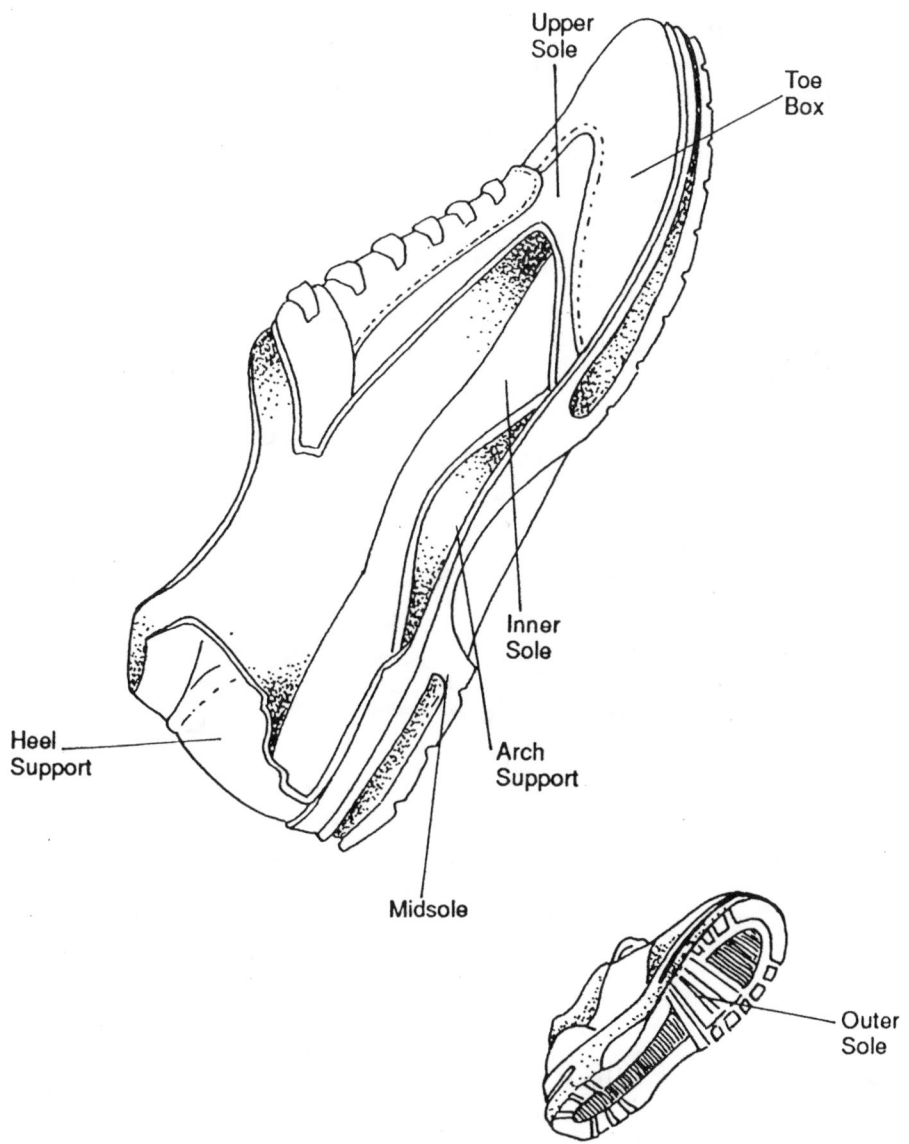

Figure 2-1. Important components of a quality walking shoe.

Running Shoes

1. The back of the shoe should be high to support the Achilles tendon.
2. The heel should be elevated, wide, and cushioned with a heel counter for motion control. Each shoe manufacturer has a special means by which to provide the much-needed shock absorption in the heel area.
3. The exterior of the heel should be rounded and the exterior sole should be made with durable tread material which is typically dimpled or rippled.
4. The interior should be cushioned and provide good arch support.

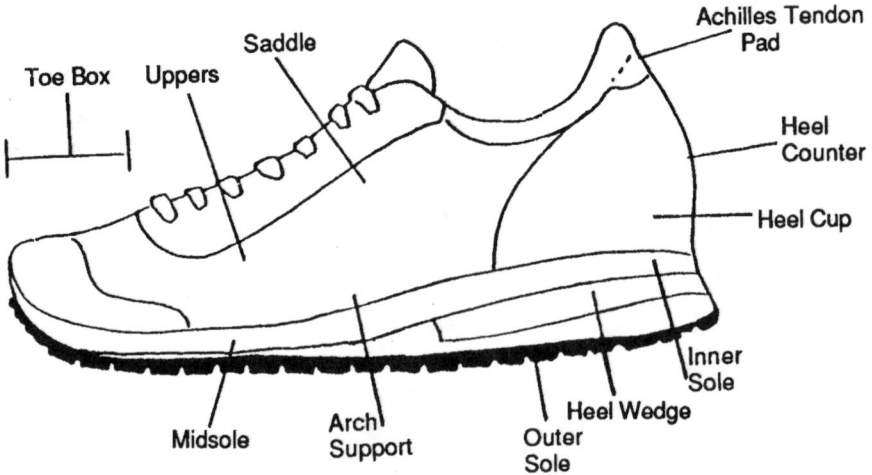

Figure 2-2. Construction of a running shoe.

Choosing the Right Shoe

Four categories of training shoes include motion-control, stability, cushioned and lightweight training. The first step to finding the right shoe is to match your biomechanical and running needs, including the surface (road, trail, track, treadmill, etc.) you most often run. Refer to Appendix E for more information about training shoe types.

Determine Your Foot Type

When you have determined the right kind of shoe you should be wearing, the next step is to determine your foot type. This will ensure that you buy a shoe which fits the characteristics that match your feet and your biomechanical needs. Determining the shape of the foot is necessary to determine whether to purchase a shoe that is straight shaped, slightly curved, semicurved or curved. To determine your foot shape, take the "wet test." Wet your foot and make a footprint on a piece of paper which rests on a flat surface. See Figure 2.3.

Trace the shape of the foot and take it along when purchasing shoes in order to match the feet to the shoes. Read Appendix E for more information about the three foot types. Refer to Lab 2.1, Foot Evaluation, to record results.

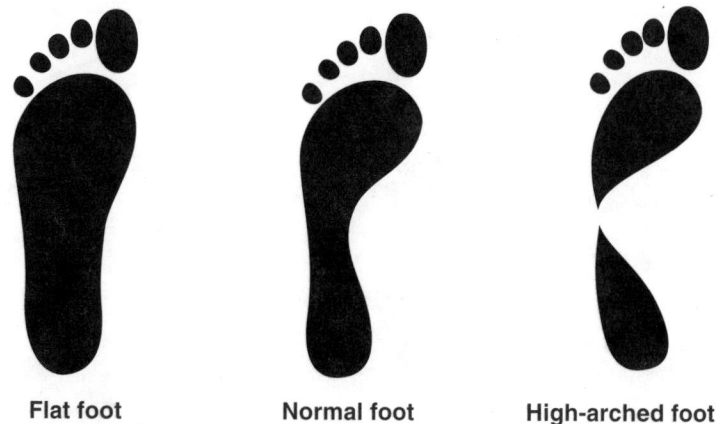

| **Flat foot** | **Normal foot** | **High-arched foot** |
| You probably overpronate. | You pronate normally. | You probably underpronate. |

Figure 2-3. The wet test.

Shoe Construction

Knowledge of shoe construction is also important when buying running shoes. The method of construction may be **board lasted, slip lasted,** or **combination lasted.**

A **board lasted** shoe is different since fiberglass is inserted in the shoe between the foot and midsole material. A **slip lasted** shoe is more flexible and is characterized by a nylon upper which is stitched inside the shoe like a moccasin and attached directly to the midsole. A **combination lasted** shoe is moderately flexible and is typically board lasted in the rear foot area and slip lasted in the forefoot area. Currently most running shoe manufacturers produces slip or combination lasted shoes and very few board lasted models.

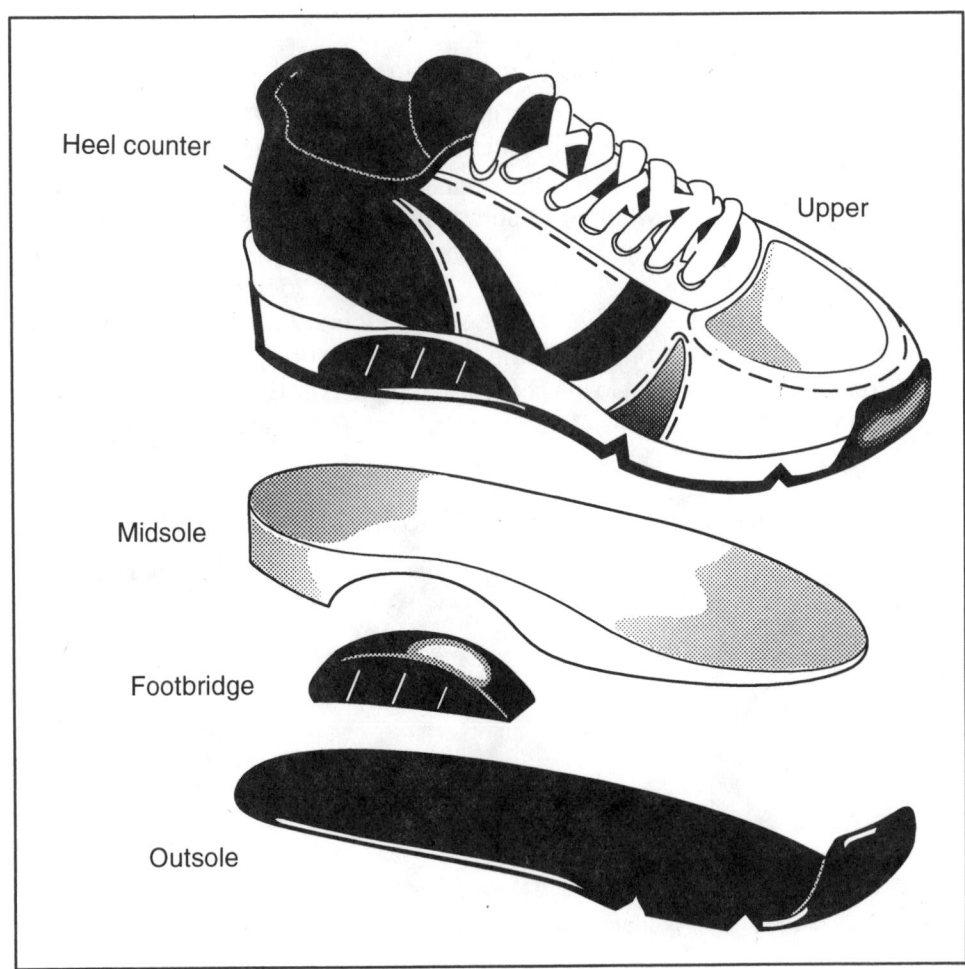

Heel counter

Upper

Midsole

Footbridge

Outsole

Figure 2-4. Parts of a running shoe.

The shape of running shoe construction is significant. A shoe may be curved, moderately curved, or straight lasted. Type of feet and movement of the feet while running should be considered when selecting a running shoe. A person who is flat-footed, overpronates (rolls excessively to the inside of the foot while running and shows excessive shoe wear on the inside heel and/or the inside of the forefoot), or has floppy feet (feet move side to side easily) should be concerned with stability and select a straight lasted shoe which is also board or combination lasted.

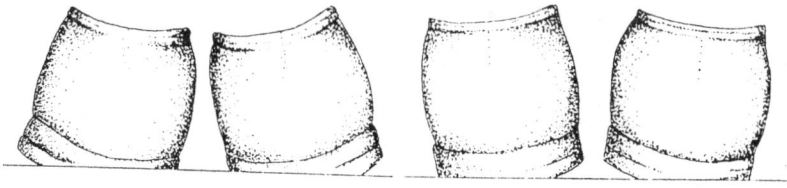

Overpronation   **Oversupination**

The average runner with average foot stability and arch should generally select a shoe with a moderately curved, slip or combination lasted. A runner who has a high arch, supinates (rolls to the outside of the foot and shoes show wear on the outside of the sole), or has rigid feet (feet move forward and backward easily with a strong forefoot push-off) should select a combination lasted.

The purpose of the running shoe is important. For fitness or training, running or jogging, a training shoe should be selected as described above. For races, a racing flat is generally used, particularly by the faster runners. It is lightweight, less supportive, and curve lasted, since most racers use more of the forefoot and supinate.

A running shoe should be replaced when the shock absorption has diminished in the midsole even though the sole and upper shoe are not worn out. Most shoes are made for 350-750 miles of running or jogging. However replacement should occur every six months regardless of mileage, since perspiration and temperature can break down the support and shock absorption of a shoe. To reduce the risk of injury, a new pair of running shoes twice a year is important.

For further information about individual selection of a running shoe, a salesperson who specializes in running shoes should be consulted. This person should also have the latest information on running shoe technology. Refer to Lab 2.2, Shoe Selection, to record results.

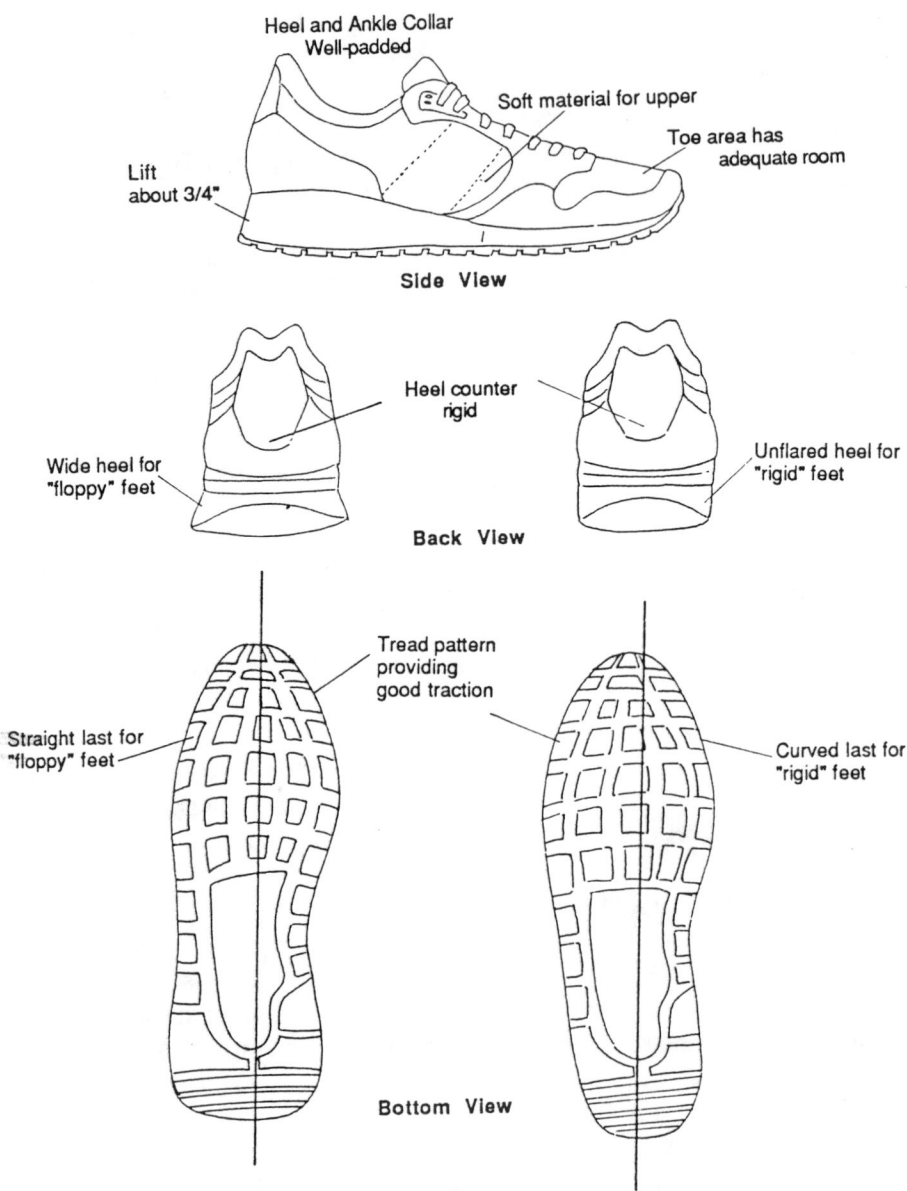

Figure 2-5. Components of a quality running shoe.

CLOTHING

It is important to dress properly for the environment while exercising. Comfort, safety, loose-fitting and lightweight clothing are the keys for a walking, jogging, or running program.

Cold Weather. The first precaution in cold weather is not to overdress. Exercise raises body temperature; a moderate workout can make the body feel that it may be 20° warmer than the actual temperature. When walking, jogging or running on a 25° day, dress for about 45°. Wearing several layers of loose-fitting, thin clothing helps to insulate and trap the heat that is generated by the body. Several layers of clothing are recommended since it is advisable to remove layers of clothing as body heat increases.

The **first layer** should be underwear made of fabric which draws sweat away from the skin (polypropylene, Capilene, Thermax). Cotton holds moisture next to the skin, making the body feel cold and clammy; wet clothes draw heat away from the body. For the **middle layers**, wear a synthetic turtleneck, wool sweater, and/or pile jacket. For the legs, wear sweat pants or tights. For the **outer layer**, wear a windbreaker/windpants which are waterproof and/or wind resistant. A porous jacket will keep the body from getting cool and, at the same time, release body heat. Synthetics (such as Gore-tex) and, for a short workout in dry weather, a windbreaker may be sufficient.

Zippers allow clothes to be adaptable; unzip them halfway to allow air when the body is getting too hot. It is best to remove layers of clothing by opening zippers as soon as sweating begins. When exercising in cold weather, tie a loop of fabric or string to each zipper to open it without having to take off mittens.

Warm Weather. Clothing should be lightweight and minimal. The clothing worn should be specifically for that exercise and should not restrict movement in any way. Shirts made of coolmax, preferably in white or light color, are recommended. Coolmax wicks the perspiration away from the body and has a cooling effect. Shorts should be lightweight nylon, lycra, coolmax or with coolmax liner. Avoid long, loose clothing, since it catches under the feet, and tight-fitting garments which restrict motion. Keep clothing to a comfortable minimum (wear as little as possible), especially when the temperature and relative humidity are high.

If clothing rubs or chafes the body, use some petroleum jelly on the skin before beginning the exercise to stop the irritation. Comfort in exercise is more important than looks in any physical activity.

Wet Weather. Continue exercising during wet weather. If the weather is cool, wet, icy and/or snowy, wear rain-repelling clothing that is breathable. During icy, wet or snowy weather it may be advisable to jog inside due to slippery surfaces. If not, walk, jog, run at a slower pace and plant feet securely. A cap or visor may be necessary to keep water out of the face.

Hat and Mittens/Gloves

During hot and cold weather, a hat should be included in the exercise attire. In warm weather, a hat will allow air circulation around the head, and the brim of the hat will protect the forehead and eyes from sun rays. A wool or synthetic cap or hood is recommended for cold weather, and helps hold in body heat. As much as 30 to 40 percent of body heat can be lost if the head is left uncovered.

Mittens are preferred to gloves because mittens keep the fingers together, therefore having less surface area from which heat can escape. In cold weather, the warmth from the mittens is worth the loss in dexterity. In addition, inner liners made of polypropylene or other materials which draw moisture from the skin may be used.

Athletic Bra and Supporter

To eliminate soreness of the breast due to walking or jogging-type movements, women should wear a tight bra (or jogging bra). A good supportive bra will do much to keep the breasts from being sore and possibly prevent early sagging due to continuous movement. A bra should be comfortable and supportive.

Men may need an athletic supporter. Wearing a pair of cotton or nylon briefs under the athletic shorts may provide a firm support, thus making the exercise activity more comfortable. Most athletic shorts are made with built-in linings.

Socks

To prevent blisters and foot irritation, wear special walking/running socks. These socks may be a little more expensive but may help to prevent blisters and reduce friction better than regular socks. Double layer socks or socks made of coolmax are suggested. It is important when purchasing shoes to wear your preferred socks when trying on shoes. Some socks contain extra cushioning in the forefoot and heel areas.

Tights or nylon hosiery are sometimes worn during cold weather to retain the body heat. In warm weather the legs must be allowed to sweat freely by exposing the skin directly to air; therefore, tights or hosiery are not recommended.

Workout Watches

Most sporting goods or department stores carry sports watches. A digital chronograph, also called a "runner's watch," includes functions such as standard and elapsed time, multi-lap or split times, a countdown timer, light, calendar, and alarm. Many watches are waterproof and offer special features such as temperature gauges, telephone number memories, calculators and depth meters. A simple timepiece with a sweep second hand may be all that is necessary to monitor heart rate, length of workout and pace of workout while walking, jogging or running. Expect to pay a higher price for a quality watch, depending on the features.

OPTIONAL CLOTHING AND EQUIPMENT

Because of diverse interests, the following suggestions will assist the individual in making wise choices in the selection of optional clothing and equipment when developing a personal walk, jog, or running program.

Body, Sauna, or Rubberized Suits

Body suits conform to the shape of the body and do not restrict movement. **Sauna or rubber suits are dangerous** and should not be worn while walking, jogging or running because the extra body heat generated while exercising is trapped inside the clothing and the air and moisture cannot pass through. The body temperature is raised causing an increase in sweating, which may lead to heat-related disorders such as heat exhaustion, heat cramps, and heatstroke. In cold weather, these suits may be potentially dangerous since chilling can result due to lack of sweat evaporation.

Reflective Materials

Many people walk, jog or run after dark. This is dangerous unless reflective materials are added to the clothing or shoes. Reflective vests and head, wrist and ankle bands are also available. When reflective materials are not used, wear light-colored clothing since it can be seen easily in the dark or early/late hours of the day.

Hand or Wrist Weights

Hand weights are sometimes used during walking to increase muscular effort, oxygen demand, energy expenditure, and heart rate. **Beginners should not use hand or wrist weights.** The additional weights may be harmful for the unconditioned person. Weights are not recommended for jogging or running because they can aggravate the shoulder and elbow joints. In addition, weights disrupt timing and coordination of the arms and legs. If advanced exercisers are determined to use hand weights, they should use only light weights of between one to three pounds. Refer to Chapter Three for additional information on the use of hand or wrist weights.

Monitors (Heart Rate)

Quality pulse monitors are expensive but many serious walkers/ runners regularly use them to ensure working out at the level that will produce the best fitness benefits. In addition, these monitors serve as a safety device for the beginner with or without medical conditions. The best heart rate monitors use a chest-strap or wrist-watch combination. Recent tests show that such models provide significantly more accurate readings than models that use earlobes or fingertips sensors.

Pedometers

Pedometers are devices which measure the distance of walking, jogging or running. The pedometer counts the number of steps taken and is a great way to provide feedback and motivation during the exercise activity.

Sunglasses and Sunscreens

Protecting eyes from harmful sun rays is essential during exercise activity. The best sunglasses provide ultraviolet (UV) protection. Temporary loss of vision, headaches, or dizziness may be experienced when the eyes are not protected from direct sunlight. It is important to always wear sunscreen to protect the skin when exercising outdoors. The recommended sunscreen has the following qualities: SPF (sun protection factor) of at least 15, waterproof or sweatproof so it doesn't rub off, fragrance-free and PABA-free so it doesn't irritate, non-gritty and non-greasy. An SPF 15 sunscreen allows you to stay in the sun 15 times longer than without it. Several companies make disposable sport towelettes saturated with SPF 15 sunscreen. Sunscreen can protect skin from the sun's harmful rays and help prevent skin cancer. To be safer, outdoor exercise should be limited to hours of the day when a person's shadow is shorter than his or her body height.

SAFETY AND ENVIRONMENTAL CONCERNS

Often walkers, joggers, or runners don't think of safety when they are getting in shape. Exercising without taking the proper precautions may not cause any problems. However, serious injury and/or even death may result when exercisers are not aware of the following safety and environmental concerns.

Drugs

There is no place in a fitness program for the use of recreational drugs. When prescription drugs are required, consult a physician before starting an exercise program, since the exercise program may alter the effects of the medicine being taken. Ask a physician about particular drugs and possible side effects during exercise.

Anabolic Steroids

Anabolic steroids are a synthetic version of testosterone and were developed in the 1960s by Dr. John B. Ziegler. Anabolic steroids stimulate the development of muscle, bone, skin, and hair growth, as well as emotional responses. The body produces 2.5 to 10 milligrams of testosterone a day in an adult male; some weight lifters are known to take many times that amount per day. When the body gets too much testosterone, it may shut down skeletal growth mechanisms, lower sperm counts, cause acne, sexual function problems, rashes, uncontrollable "roid rages," baldness, liver tumors and heart disease. Women produce a small amount of the hormone; therefore when using steroids they may experience menstrual irregularities, deepening of the voice, and masculine characteristics.

Steroids are not prescribed often, so athletes use the black market to acquire them. Black market steroids often come from underground laboratories or foreign countries and are of very questionable quality and purity. Often they may not even be steroids.

Most people who use steroids are aware of the possible side effects, but are not concerned with the future. However, many of the side effects or adverse reactions are immediate consequences. **Anabolic steroids have no place in an exercise plan**.

Pollution

Lack of clean air during exercise is a concern in today's society. The atmosphere contains many pollutants which can irritate the lungs and cause respiratory conditions (bronchitis and asthma).

Automobile exhaust fumes (hydrocarbon) are serious for the walker, jogger or runner. Particulate matter and fumes (pollen, ozone, carbon monoxide) can increase resistance to air flow to the lungs and result in less efficiency, headaches, eye irritation, and coughing, therefore decreasing physical performance. Also, the long-term toxic effects on the lungs and circulatory system are well documented in research literature. When the levels are high, avoid exercising in polluted areas close to factories, smoke stacks, and streets with heavy traffic.

In addition, problems may occur because of noise on congested streets, shopping malls, and large airports. Exercise activities should be planned indoors, in quiet neighborhoods, trails, country roads, running tracks (secondary schools, colleges, universities), or in other quiet, safe locations. Whenever possible, enjoy the outdoors and natural surroundings away from automobiles.

Altitude Sickness

The feelings of drowsiness, insomnia, headaches, nausea, vomiting, lung congestion and loss of appetite are symptoms of **altitude sickness**. Exercise with caution and avoid rigorous exercises at high altitudes unless living at that altitude has caused the body to adapt. Moderately descending to lower altitudes will minimize the symptoms. With gradual exposure to high altitudes, the body will improve in performance. However, performance ability at high altitudes is usually less than exercising at sea level. A diet high in carbohydrates and low in fat can reduce the severity of altitude sickness. It requires a minimum of **two weeks (14 days)** and in some cases, months to become acclimated to high altitudes.

ADDITIONAL HAZARDS

Animals. Walking or jogging with an animal may or may not be a safety factor. Most dogs just bark and do not bite, but there are exceptions. Many dogs are territorial so avoid property lines. Check the exercise route by car before taking to the road the first time. Carry Mace or a long stick the first couple of times when exercising on a new course.

Attackers. Female exercisers should be alert at all times to dangerous situations. Exercising with others, not exercising outside at night, and ignoring taunts are recommended ways of avoiding attacks.

Bicycles/Automobiles. Bicycle riders should be on the same side of the road and travel in the same direction as automobiles. Defensively, walk, jog and/or run on the side of the road facing the oncoming traffic. As a bicycle approaches, look directly into the rider's eyes to determine if seen.

Surfaces. Feet placement is of utmost importance when walking, jogging, or running. Be familiar with the surface which will be used when walking, jogging or running. Stay alert, shorten the stride, and slow down for dangerous surfaces.

When exercising on pavement, watch for cracks, holes (dirt roads), gravel, grass, and differences in firmness. **Softer surfaces** are recommended to reduce impact and stress on the body. When walking indoors, watch for slippery spots and obstacles. Always be alert and place feet securely on the various surfaces.

EXERCISE IN HOT WEATHER

The skin must breathe during physical activity. The normal body temperature is 98.6°. Exercising in hot weather, there is an increased need for an excess blood flow to the working muscles and to the skin in order to maintain body temperature. Drinking plenty of water and wearing light clothing allows for a large skin surface and sweat evaporation. Only 30 to 40 percent of the energy produced in the body is used for movement or mechanical work. The other 60 to 70 percent is converted to heat. If this heat can not leave the body because it is too hot or relative humidity is too high, the temperature of the body will increase and death may result in some cases.

The heat required to raise the body temperature by one degree Centigrade is 0.38 calories per pound of body weight per one degree Centigrade (0.38 cal/lb/C). If body heat is not lost, a 150-pound person would only need to burn 57 calories (approximately three miles running) without any heat loss, inner body temperature would increase by 5.3 degrees Centigrade, or the equivalent of going from 98.6 to 108.1 degrees Fahrenheit. If the relative humidity is too high, the body heat cannot be lost through evaporation because of water vapor saturation in the atmosphere. **Exercise with caution when the temperature exceeds 82.4° F and the humidity rises above 60 percent.**

Walkers, joggers and runners lose liquid in sweat and more water is needed than the average requirement. During exercising a loss of 1 to 2 percent body water will result in a decrease in performance. It is possible to lose 1 percent body water in a 45-60 minute workout. Every pound of weight loss represents approximately a pint of water. Avoid dehydration by replacing lost fluids, 6-8 oz. of cool water every 15-20 minutes. (The body absorbs cool fluids faster.) Refer to Chapter Four for additional information on fluid intake during hot weather.

Individuals exercising in hot temperatures can suffer from heat cramps, heat exhaustion, and heatstrokes.

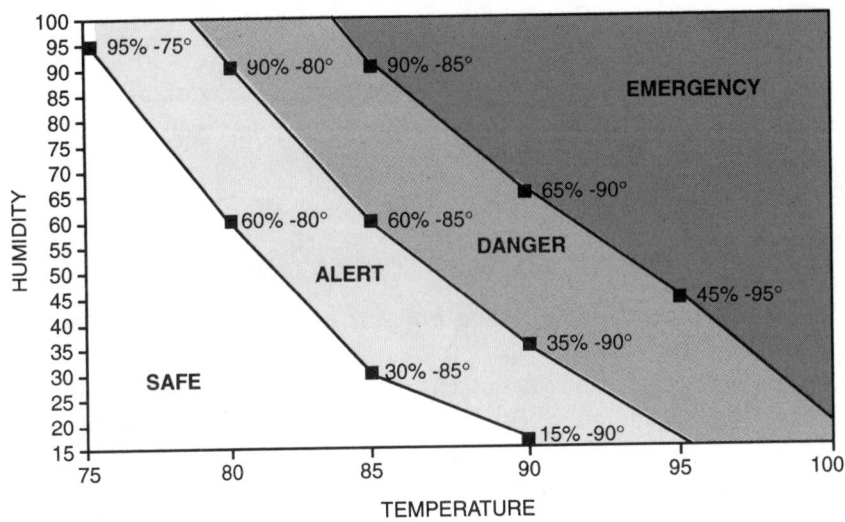

Figure 2.6. Heat-Safety Index.

"Safe" temperature-humidity readings generally allow for normal activity; "alert" conditions require caution during long, hard activity, and "danger" levels may demand a reduction of training. Strenuous exercise is not recommended during "emergency' conditions.

Heat Cramps

Heat Cramps are muscular pains and spasms due to heavy exertion. These cramps usually occur in the legs and abdominal muscles and may be related to the tightness of the muscles, fatigue, or fluid, salt, and potassium imbalance. Drinking plenty of water and stretching before exercising is recommended. First aid includes massaging the area and drinking fluids. Heat cramps are the least severe of the heat-related injuries.

Heat Exhaustion

Heat exhaustion occurs when exercising vigorously in a humid, warm place when body fluids are depleted through heavy sweating; it is not an imminent threat to life. The blood flow decreases in the vital organs resulting in the loss of fluids. Symptoms of heat exhaustion include cold, pale, and moist skin, heavy sweating, dilated pupils, headache, dizziness, cramping, hyperventilation, and nausea or vomiting. Body temperature will be nearly normal. The individual should be moved to a cooler location, placed on the back (feet up), given cool fluids, and cold packs should be applied to the skin.

Heatstroke

Heatstroke is the most severe of the heat-induced illnesses. The person's temperature-control system, which produces sweating to cool the body, stops working. The temperature of the body can rise so high that brain damage and death may result if the body is not cooled quickly. The symptoms of heatstroke includes hot, red and/or dry skin, disorientation, diarrhea, very small pupils, rapid pulse, unconsciousness, and a very high body temperature (106° F or higher). Treatment includes cooling the person rapidly, immersing the person in cool water, or wrapping wet sheets or ice packs around the body (emphasize the head, torso, joints). Fluids should not be given. Since heatstroke is life-threatening, the person should immediately be taken to the hospital.

EXERCISE IN COLD WEATHER

Exercising on cold days with low temperatures, high humidity and winds, **can be dangerous** due to the **loss of body heat**. It is advisable to wear several layers of light clothing rather than one single thick layer, since warm air is trapped between the layers, therefore allowing greater heat conservation. Exercisers exposed to sever cold can suffer from **frostbite, hypothermia** (abnormally low body temperature), and **hyperthermia** (abnormally high body temperature).

A **20° rule** applies to exercisers who are jogging or running in cold weather. The rule states that the temperature seems to automatically rise by that amount in the course of the activity. A very cold 15° day may become a tolerable 35°, or a cool 40° may become a pleasant afternoon of 60°. The feeling of comfort at the start of jogging or running may soon change to warm, hot and even uncomfortable.

Frostbite

Frostbite is the most common injury caused by exposure to cold. It occurs when ice crystals form in body tissues (nose, chin, ears, cheeks, fingers, or toes). Blood flow is restricted to the injured parts. The effect is worse if the frostbitten parts are thawed and then refrozen. Frostbite can lead to permanent circulatory damage and gangrene may result from the loss of blood supply to the area. The frozen body parts should be placed in warm water, not hot. **Do not rub or massage the area**. Loosely cover or bandage the injured parts. Seek medical help immediately.

Prevention includes protecting areas such as fingers, toes, nose, ears, and facial skin and covering head, hands, and wrist. The head and neck can lose from 30-40 percent body heat. Gloves (mittens) should be worn to protect the hands and fingers. A toboggan type hat or stocking should be worn to prevent heat loss through the bare head. Materials made from wool or polypropylene are excellent. Ski masks, surgical masks, and scarves are recommended in very cold environments to keep the inhaled air warm and moist and the facial skin protected. Exposed areas of the body should be protected from frostbite when the temperature is very low and the windchill factor is high. Humidity may make exercising in the summer unsafe while in the winter months, the wind may present problems. The wind-chill factor makes temperatures feel colder. For each mile per hour of wind, the temperature drops approximately 1 degree.

Wind-chills below minus 20° result in "increased danger" of frostbite while those below minus 70° result in "great danger." See Figure 2-7.

Hypothermia

Abnormally low body temperature, **hypothermia**, occurs when body heat is lost faster than it can be produced. Symptoms include shivering, dizziness, confusion, numbness, weakness, impaired judgment, drowsiness, and impaired vision. Exposure to cold temperatures, pain, wind chill and muscle fatigue can cause a loss of heat from the body. Dry clothing should be placed on the person. The body should be warmed slowly and the individual should not be given anything to eat or drink unless fully conscious. Immediately seek medical attention.

Hyperthermia

Abnormally high body temperature, **hyperthermia**, can result when exercising in cold weather. These cases occur when too much clothing is worn. To prevent hyperthermia, dress in several layers of light clothing when exercising and remove clothing as the body temperature increases. Also, retention of heat causes excessive sweating, even in freezing weather. When the skin surface is covered by heavy clothing, sweat cannot evaporate efficiently and cool the body; therefore, the body temperature rises further, and large amount of sweat permeates socks and underclothing. When exercising is stopped, the sweat-soaked clothing may chill the person.

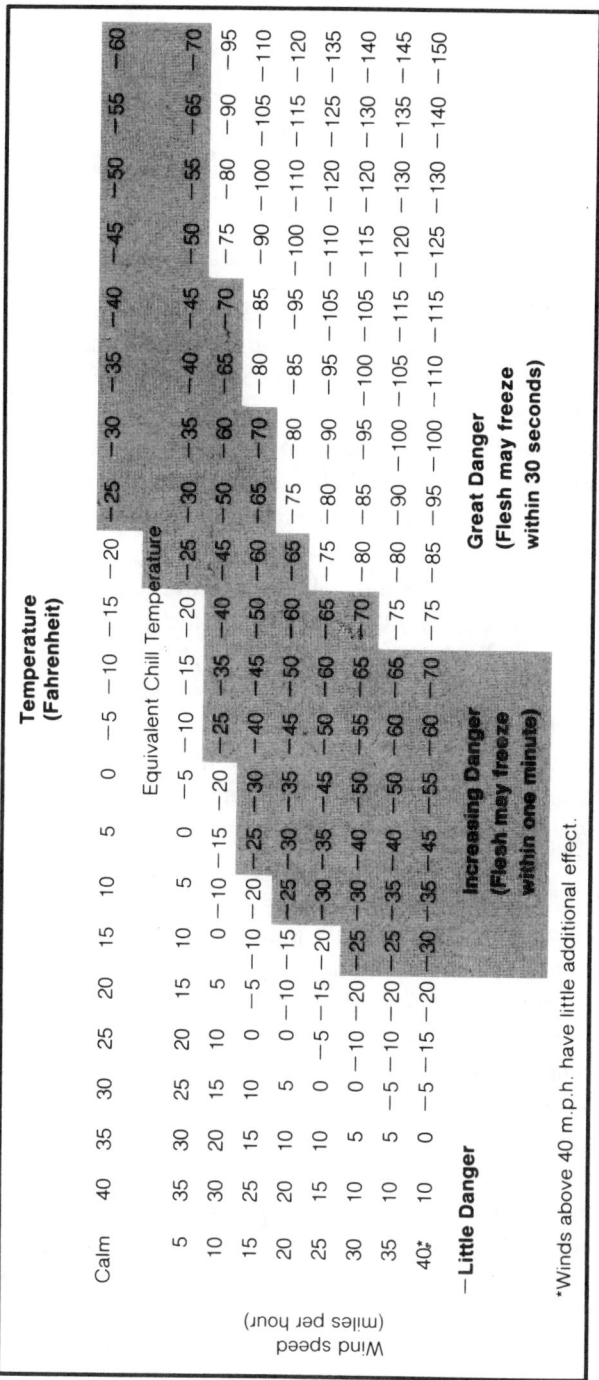

Figure 2-7. Wind-Chill Readings.

SAFETY GUIDELINES

The following guidelines may be helpful for all individuals while exercising during the day or evening hours. However, some of these suggested rules may be more applicable to female than male walkers, joggers or runners.

The suggested rules of the road and trails are:

1. Use reflective gear or light-colored clothing at night.
2. Walk or run toward traffic and look out for objects thrown from vehicles.
3. Cars should always have the right-of-way. Avoid exercising in polluted air. If exercising in those areas, walk, jog or run on the side of the road where the wind is blowing the automobile pollutants away from the body.
4. Avoid exercising in areas with severe smog; pollutants (ozone and nitrogen oxides) may be damaging to the lungs.
5. When using headphones lower the volume so that traffic can be heard. Headphones are not recommended for streets—only trails and paths.
6. Never walk, jog or run alone especially at night. Most attacks occur in the dark. Even if the road is lighted, don't chance it. Retire early and walk, job or run in early morning. Enjoy the event with several friends.
7. Vary exercise routines; change routes frequently and begin at different times each day. Most attacks are by a person who knows the route and usual workout time. Begin at different times each day. Be alert for danger signs such as the appearance of the same person or car on successive days. If something is different, change routes immediately and go to a populated area.
8. Tell someone the exercise destination and approximately when returning. Stick to the predicted arrival time. Carry identification. Tuck a small business card into the exercise attire or wear an identification bracelet. Also carry the name of the person to contact in case of an emergency. Females may want to consider carrying a protective warning device such as a can of Mace or a whistle.
9. Dress conservatively. Wear basic sweatsuit, shorts or no-frills attire unless jogging with others. Call the police if harassed. Alert other walkers, joggers, or runners.
10. Dress appropriately during hot and cold temperatures when exercising.

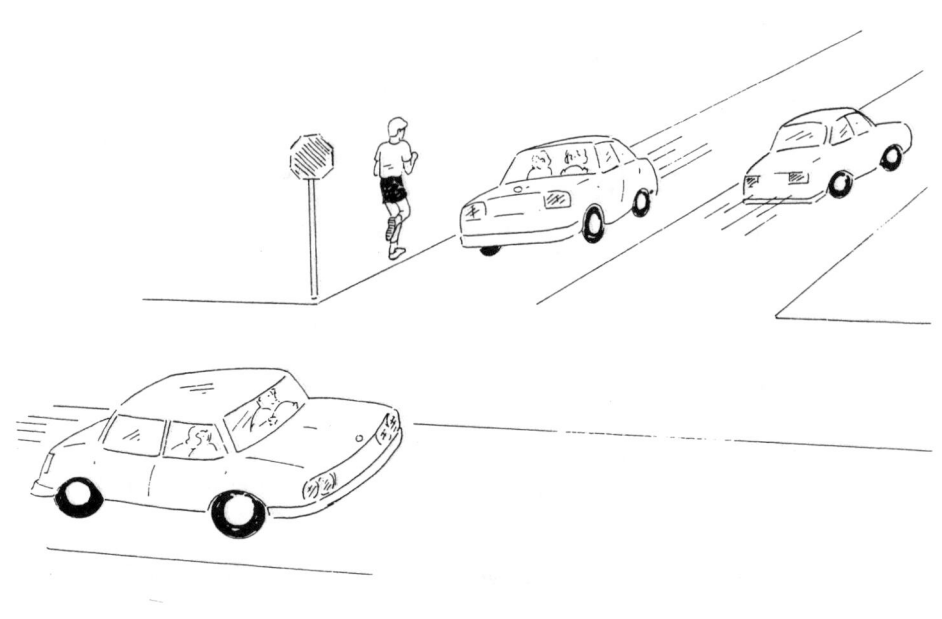

CHAPTER SUMMARY

Being adequately prepared is essential to a walking, jogging or running program while exercising on the streets, trails, or indoors. Sufficient preparation includes a physical examination, proper clothing, equipment and safety and environmental guidelines. Everyone who is adequately prepared will reap the desired benefits of lifetime fitness and wellness. Being diligent and taking control of the exercise situation can help each individual implement a safe and effective exercise program. By preparing and beginning the exercise program today one can journey into a happier, healthier and more productive life.

"You cannot build a reputation on what you are going to do."
—Henry Ford, American Industrialist (1863-1947)

CHAPTER THREE

Training Principles

MECHANICS FOR WALKING AND RACEWALKING

Strolling or easy walking is 3 mph with the arms swinging loosely. **Brisk fitness walking** is 4 mph with faster leg speed and energetic arm action. **Racewalking** is 5+ mph with quicker steps, greater hip action, and arms pumping harder. As the walking progresses from easy to racewalking, the heart rate during the exercise increases.

Fitness buffs may choose walking as a lead-up to jogging and running. Walking or racewalking, on the other hand, may be selected as an alternative to jogging or running. Running imparts a tremendous shock to the body. Since both feet are off the ground during running, the impact on landing with each plant of the foot is 3-4 times a person's body weight. Since walking involves one foot always being in contact with the ground, the impact on landing with each plant of the foot is only 1.25 times a person's body weight. Lesser impact minimizes stress to the ankle, knee and hip joints. However, the technique involved in racewalking increases stress to the back. Therefore, each individual must decide which aerobic activity he or she prefers.

FITNESS WALKING

Mechanics

Good posture and natural movement are essential to fitness walking. Standing posture should be examined to determine if a straight line can be drawn between the ear, mid-shoulder, mid-hip, mid-knee, and the front of the ankle. It is important that the pelvis does not tilt forward causing a distortion in spinal alignment and that the head and shoulders do not hunch forward. (See Fig. 3-1.)

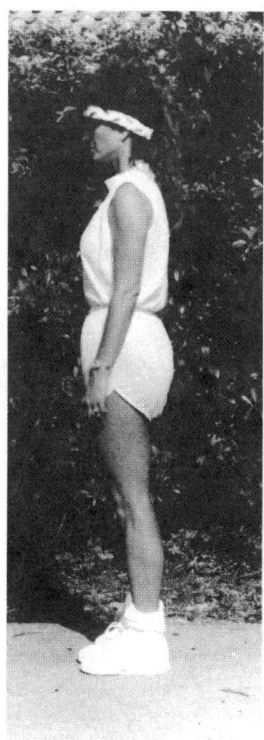 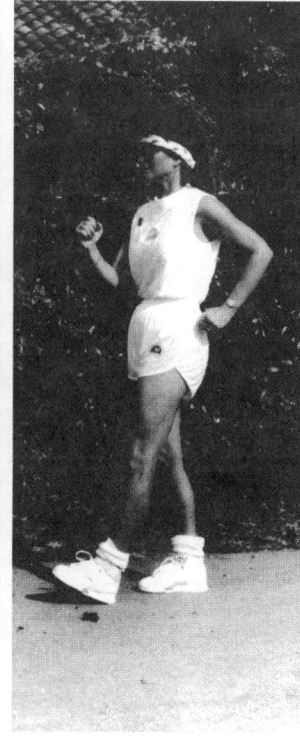 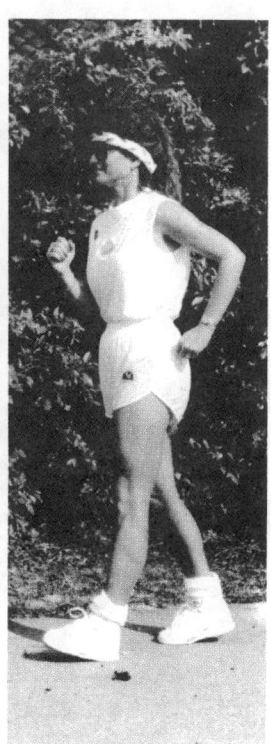

Figure 3-1. Good standing posture.

Figure 3-2. Arms at 90°
angle; opposite arm and
leg.

Figure 3-3. The
body leans from the
ankles.

The arms are held at a 90° angle with relaxed, slightly-clenched fists. The swinging motion is higher than jogging, with the hands raising up to chest height and even up to shoulder height as the pace increases. (In the early stages of a walking program, people often swing straight arms loosely at their sides.) The opposite arm swings forward as the opposite foot reaches forward in its stride. (See Fig. 3-2.)

In order to stride, the body leans forward from the ankles. When the body is off balance, the walker steps forward to catch the body and prevent falling. The Rockport walking program, developed by the Rockport Shoe Company, describes walking as a series of falls. The leg is brought straight forward from the hips with toes pointing forward. (See Fig. 3-3.)

One should stride as if following a three-inch wide line. (See Fig. 3-4.) The foot should land with the inside of the shoe on the outer edge of that line. Impact is on the outer edge of the heel with the foot positioned at a 40°

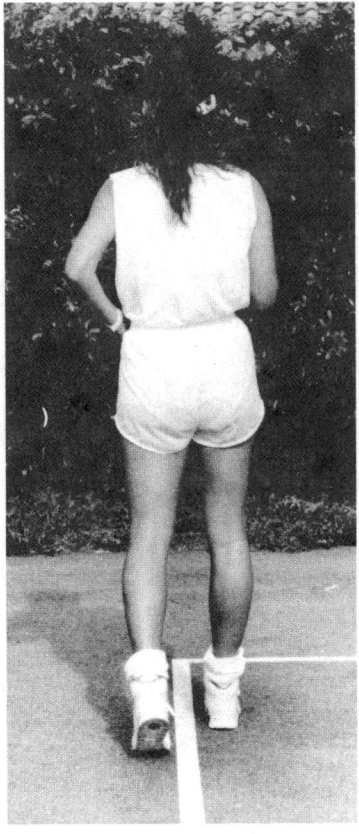

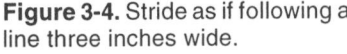

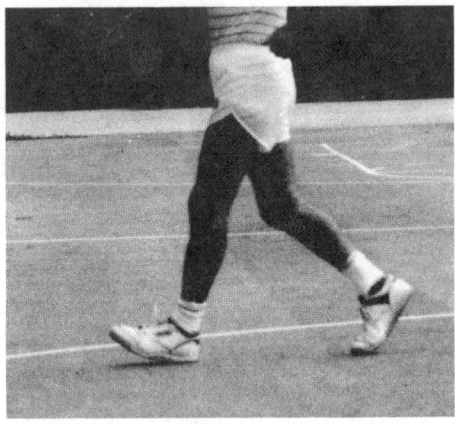

Figure 3-4. Stride as if following a line three inches wide.

Figure 3-5. A strong toe push-off prevents bouncing.

angle to the surface. The knee should be slightly bent at that time. The foot rolls forward on the outer edge onto the ball of the foot and pushes off with the toes. A strong toe push-off is essential to prevent bouncing. It is important to have the foot contacting the surface as long as possible. (See Fig. 3-5.)

To increase walking speed, arms move faster and stride length increases. A turn of the hips will allow a longer stride. Speed will also increase if the back foot remains on the ground longer to enable the leg to fully extend and the toes to push off with more force. Power and speed will be added if the leg is extended straighter, but not locked, as it reaches forward to stride. Also, during the support phase, if the knee is kept straight as the body passes over the leg and remains straight through push-off, the walker should feel a vaulting effect and obtain added power and speed.

Practice Suggestions

1. Watch a videotape showing fitness walking mechanics. Stop or pause the tape, observing posture and mechanical aspects such as arm position, arm position related to leg position, stride length, position of knee and foot at impact, foot plant and push-away, leg reaching forward and leg pushing off. Watching the movement in slow motion is suggested.

2. Walk, concentrating, one at a time, on posture and each phase of the mechanics mentioned above. Ask a friend or workout partner, who watched the tape with you, to observe and critique you as you practice each phase. Keep practicing until the proper posture and mechanics flow naturally.

3. Ask someone to videotape you from all angles as you walk. Then play back the video, stopping it as you did earlier with the professional videotape. Critique yourself using Lab 3.1.

4. If you have more work to do, repeat 2 and 3 concentrating on areas which need improvement.

Breathing

Breathing should be natural. There is no set pattern recommended. However, breathing exercises suggested in the jogging/running section may be helpful.

Increasing Workout Intensity

To increase the intensity of a walking workout, walking with weights, hill walking, stair walking, or sand walking may be selected. Walking while holding and swinging 1-3 pound weights can increase the heart rate 7-13 beats per minute, according to the *Reebok Walking Instructors Manual*. To prepare for using weights, the walker should practice walking with exaggerated arm movements. Once the body adjusts to a normal walking arm swing with weights, intensity of the workout can be increased in three ways: (1) overemphasize the normal arm swings (Fig. 3-6); (2) move arms alternately at shoulder level, holding one at the chest while the other extends to the side at shoulder height (Fig. 3-7); (3) move weights alternately forward at shoulder level using a sustained punching motion (Fig 3-8). **Caution: Individuals with high blood pressure or heart disease should refrain from using hand weights.**

Using specially designed ski poles can provide additional calorie consumption if used vigorously by planting and using a strong push-back with each walking stride. Another device that necessitates greater effort

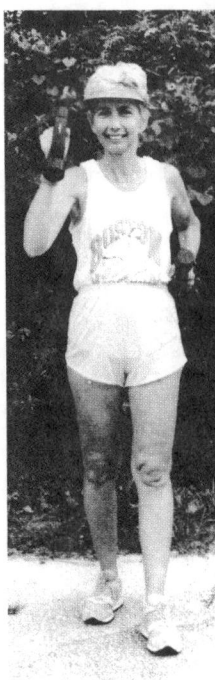 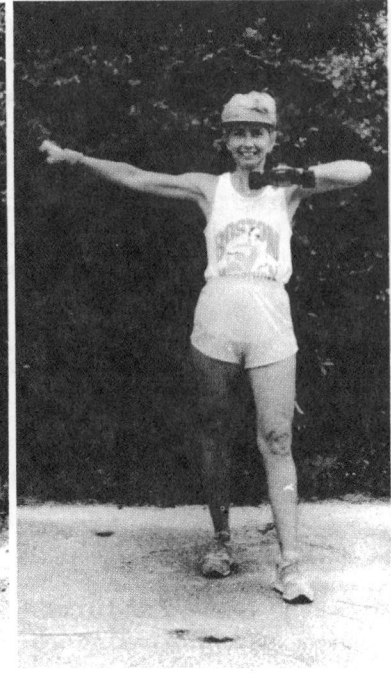 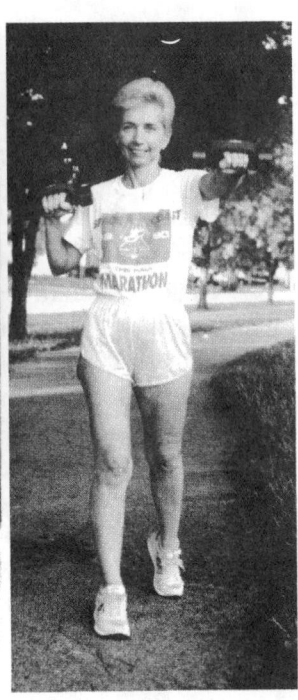

Figure 3-6. Over-emphasize the arm swing.

Figure 3-7. Move arms alternately at shoulder level.

Figure 3-8. Move weights using punching motion.

while walking is the use of resistance chords. Resistance chords are attached to each wrist and a special belt. As the walker swings his/her arms, the movement is resisted by the chord.

Walking up hills and stairs is a more intense activity than walking on a flat surface. The body should lean slightly forward while attempting to walk uphill. Walking downhill and down the stairs provides a break in intensity and utilizes different muscles. However, this activity is more impacting on the joints and may cause muscle soreness. An alternate to hills and stairs is to walk on the ramps in a multilevel parking garage. Caution should be used when walking in softer packed sand; although this type of walking is more intense than walking on a flat surface, it does put a strain on the knees, ankles, and Achilles tendons. Walking backward is another alternative which offers the additional benefit of strengthening the back and abdominal muscles as well as the hamstrings and quadriceps. It also assists in the rehabilitation of ankle and leg injuries. However, one cannot achieve the same pace and workout benefits as forward walking. Therefore, backward walking is used as a portion of a walking workout and often at the end.

RACEWALKING

For walkers who wish to further increase the intensity of their walk workout and/or enter races, racewalking techniques must be learned and employed. Practice is essential for these techniques to become efficient, natural, and comfortable.

Mechanics

Good standing posture is the foundation for racewalking. The body should lean forward from the heels approximately 5° rather than bending from the waist. The arms should be held as in fitness walking; however, the driving motion is lower in racewalking. Shoulders drive the arms as they are held in the 90° angle position. Arms and shoulders should be relaxed and swing back until the hands reach the crest of the hip and forward no more than six inches in front of the chest. Hands never cross the midline of the body or raise higher than chest level. It is important that the arm swing and stride length coordinate and that the arms, shoulders, and torso work as a unit. (See Fig. 3.9.) Upper arms and shoulders should swing naturally with the arm motion. Eyes should focus ahead 12 feet rather than looking downward.

Hips play a greater role in the stride of racewalking. (See Fig. 3-10.) The hip drops vertically as the leg moves forward. The lowest drop of the hip on the side of the swinging leg occurs when the driving foot is under the opposite hip in the support phase and the swinging foot passes the driving

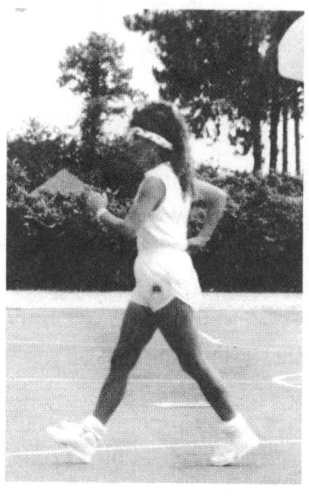
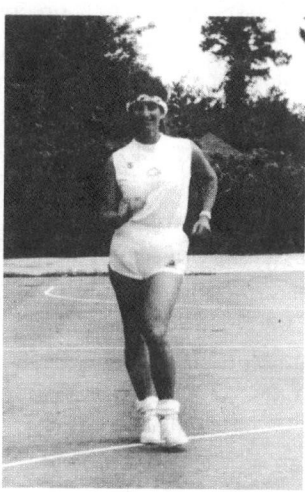

Figure 3-9. Strong arm swing and stride work as a unit.

Figure 3-10. Hip action plays a greater role in racewalking.

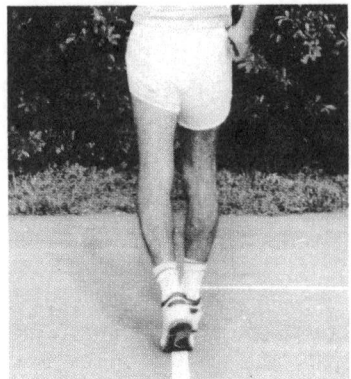 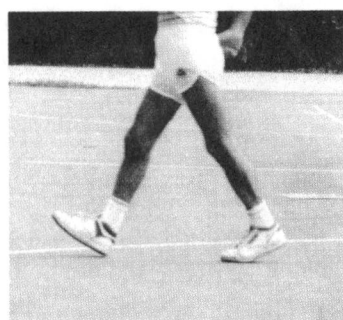

Figure 3-11. A. Foot plant should be as if walking on a straight line.
B. Position planting foot at 90° angle and use straight leg push-off.

leg. Hip rotation is front to back with a feel of smoothly moving up and down. The buttocks should be pulled in and the racewalker should feel as if the bottom of the buttocks is pushing forward and down as the leg swings forward. The driving leg should be straight, but not locked, in the support phase. The forward push occurs after the center of gravity passes over the support/driving foot. This straight position must be maintained for as long as possible to provide maximum forward thrust. This helps to achieve the vaulting action discussed earlier. Stride length will increase with more hip action; however, overstriding should be avoided.

The foot plant for racewalking should be as if walking on straight line. (See Fig. 3-11A.) It is important that the planting foot be positioned at approximately a 90° angle to the shin when the heel strikes the ground. (See Fig. 3-11B.) This helps to straighten the knee as the foot plants. The toes of the rear foot must remain on the ground until the heel of the front foot plants. The final push is from the second through fifth toes, since pushing from the big toe may cause a loss of power.

Judges at racewalking events look for one foot always contacting the ground and straight legs during the support phase to determine correctness of technique. If the knees are bent during the support phase or both feet are off the ground simultaneously, the racewalker will be warned, then disqualified. (See Fig. 3-12.)

Once the racewalker has established good technique, pace will be increased as leg speed increases. Also, more hip action contributes to greater speed.

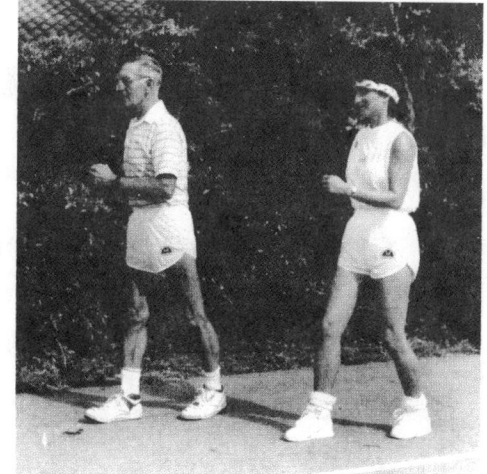

Figure 3-12. Comparison of straight leg during support phase (male walker) and bent knee or creeping (female walker).

Practice Suggestions

A suggested practice progression would be first to attempt walking on the heels with toes up. Next, walk casually while concentrating on a heel plant with toes up. Then experiment by leaning forward and backward while walking until a feeling of push-off is established with the forward lean. To achieve the 5° angle of lean, stand relaxed and lean forward from the heel until it is necessary to step forward to prevent from falling. Walk using that same angle of lean. Add proper arm swing and then concentrate on keeping the legs straight during the support phase. Finally, increase the pace by using more hip action.

For additional practice of the racewalking technique, refer to the suggested practice and analysis outlined in the fitness walking section. Racewalking mechanics should be substituted for fitness walking in the practice plan. Use Lab 3.2, Race Walking Mechanical Analysis, to critique mechanics. Racewalkers may also attend a racewalking event and seek advice from the judges or coaches at that event.

MECHANICS OF JOGGING AND RUNNING

Progression from Walking to Jogging and Running

If a person wishes to progress from fitness walking to jogging and running rather than racewalking, programs suggested in the next chapter may be utilized. In order to understand the change in mechanics, this

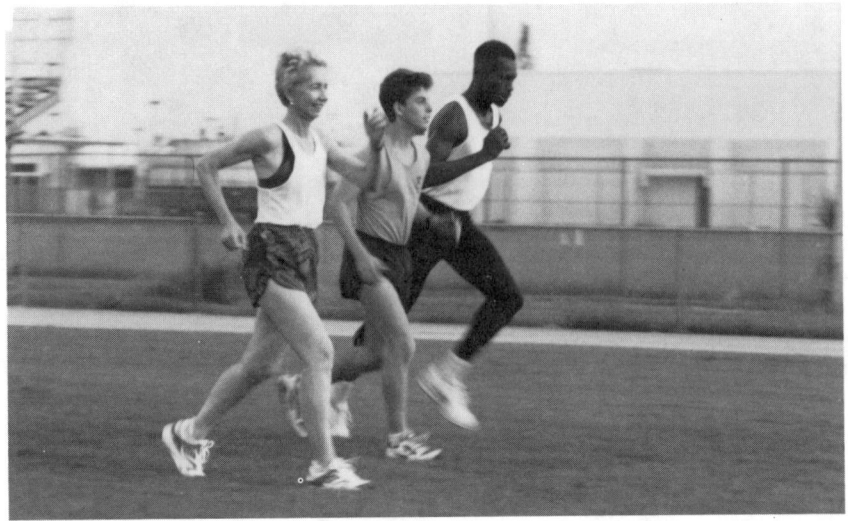

Figure 3-13. Walking, jogging, and running.

section on jogging/running mechanics should be studied and practice techniques employed. The mechanical transition will basically involve a higher, quicker movement during the leg swing, a longer stride, and a stronger push-off to achieve the airborne phase when both feet are off the ground. The arm swing will be less exaggerated, but quicker, to work effectively with the increased leg speed. As a person progresses from fitness walking to jogging and then from jogging to running, the heart rate during the workout will increase due to the increased intensity of the workout.

For a point of clarification, **jogging** will be defined as slower-paced **running**. A jogger is usually motivated by a desire to improve health or appearance but is not interested in speed. In general, a runner loves to run and enjoys pushing for a faster pace. Most runners participate in distance races to challenge their running abilities. In the discussion that follows, adjustments in form will be made as the pace increases.

Mechanics

Running experts agree that form should be relaxed and natural. Form is affected by individual body structure; for example, a taller person will have a longer stride. However, good posture and proper body mechanics are most important. If a person lacks proper posture and sound body mechanics ("doing what comes naturally"), then sound mechanics should be practiced until they become natural.

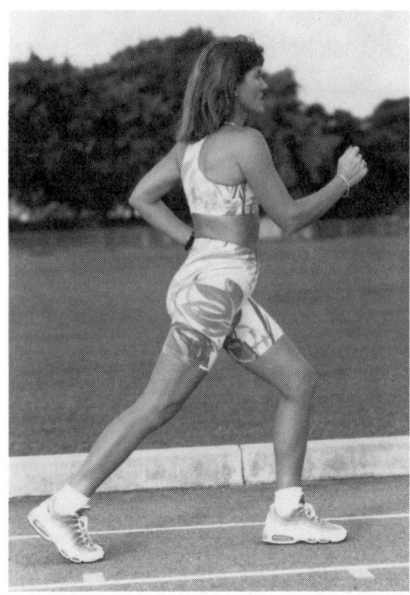

Figure 3-14. Good running/jogging posture.

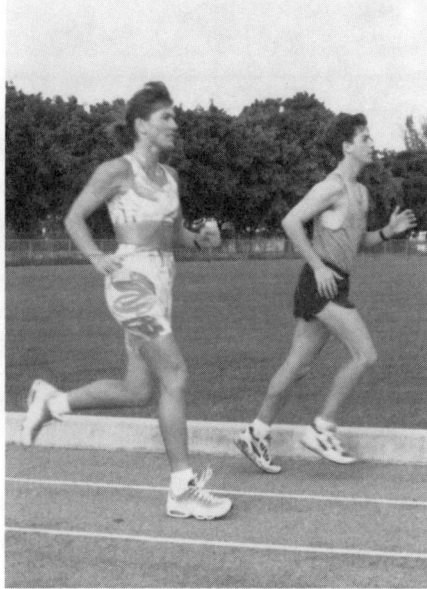

Figure 3-15. Arms are held at 90° angle not crossing the midline of the body.

Proper jogging/running form begins with good postural alignment. Standing posture should be examined following the description in the section on fitness walking mechanics. The basis for good jogging/running posture involves proper standing posture or "standing tall" but relaxed. The head is held erect and looking toward the horizon with jaw open and loose (Fig. 3-14).

Arms are relaxed and held at a 90° angle, with hands and elbows the same distance from the running surface. Joggers may hold hands slightly lower than elbows to help relax the shoulder and neck. Racers will bring hands higher. Hands are slightly cupped with fingers touching and thumb resting on the forefinger. As the arms move, they work in opposition to the legs with the left arm and right leg moving forward simultaneously. As the arms swing rhythmically, the elbows move in a straight line and the hands may cross in front of the body, but not across the midline (Fig. 3-15). As the pace increases, the arms move faster and more powerfully.

A natural stride length is most efficient, according to *Running Research News* (September/October, 1989). Although stride length and frequency increase with pace, the length of increase should also be comfortable and natural for each individual (Fig. 16-A and 16-B). Care should be taken to prevent overstriding, which not only causes a braking

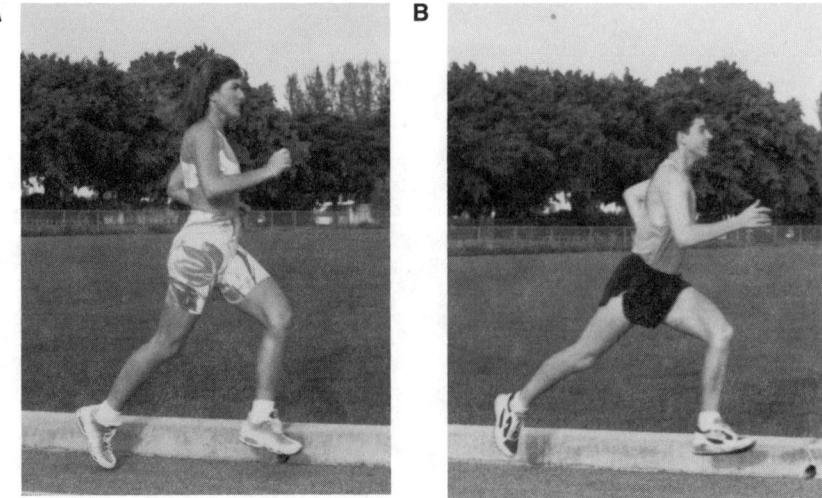

Figure 3-16. A. In jogging, use a shorter stride and less arm action. **B.** In running, the stride is increased and arm action is stronger.

action and inefficiency, but a susceptibility to injury. To prevent overstriding, concentrate on the feeling of running with knees rather than the feet. An overstrider contacts the ground with the leg fully extended and the ankle in front of the kneesee Fig. 3-17B). Proper stride length is characterized by a slightly bent knee as the foot contacts the ground and a heel strike directly under the knee. Stride angle should be 90° for the recreational runner (65° in front and 25° in the rear) and 100° for the competitive runner (70° in the front and 30° in the rear). (See Figure 13-7A above.) Also, watch for excessive knee lift or kick up (Figs. 3-16 and 3-17).

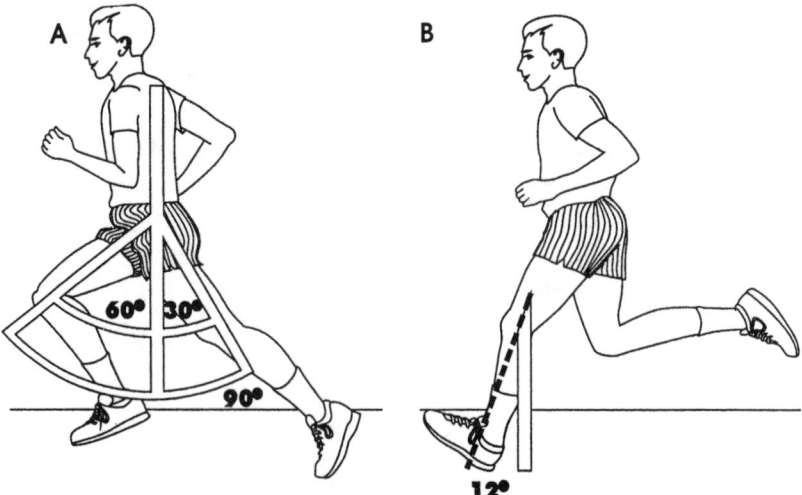

Figure 3-17. A. Example of a 90°stride angle. **B.** Overstriding.

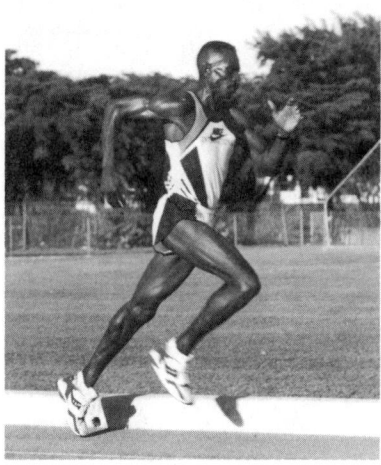

Figure 3-18. Pushing action and knee lift.

As the foot plants under the knee, the heel strikes first and the weight shifts on the outer edge to the ball of the foot. If the heel is kept on the ground longer by allowing the knee to bend forward, the calf muscle will stretch further and will result in greater stride length and power. The final push-away is off the toes with the big toe imparting the most force. Pulling action takes place as the leg leaves the ground and prepares to reach forward. Hip flexion causes the leg to swing forward. The pushing action, which is diagonally backwards, begins at contact and increases as the body moves forward. The knee and ankle lift to assist with the push (Fig. 3-17). Push-off must be forward, not upward, to eliminate bouncing.

Practice Suggestions

The suggestions listed in the fitness walking section may be used for jogging or running. Videotapes on jogging or running and mechanics of jogging or running should be substituted for walking references. Use Lab 3.3, "Jogging/Running Mechanical Analysis."

Another practice concern may be to improve running economy, which leads to improving times in races. Improving economy will enable the walker/runner to move with less effort than previously required. Running economy tends to be a better predictor of racing success than VO_2 max which will be discussed later. Chapter 5 will discuss strength training and running economy. Jack Daniels in *Running Research News* (July/August, 1988) suggests the following practice to improve running economy:

Repetition training — Complete a number of 400 meter runs at a rapid but not maximal velocity (less than 5K race pace). Do not exceed 5% of weekly mileage in total distance involving 400 meter runs. The rest period between runs should be 4 or 5 times the amount of time for the 400 meter run. The objective is to be well rested in order to practice good running form during the entire 400 meters. Eight is the maximum of these workouts that should be attempted during a six-weeks period. Then, the next type of economy training should be employed.

Downhill running — Run down a slight downhill grade, approximately 2%, to train the legs to run faster without a dramatic increase in effort. Run downhill for a minute or less at a faster speed than normal training runs, but not maximum speed. Rest totally before each run and do not exceed 5% of the weekly mileage during the downhill workout. After 8 downhill sessions in six weeks, downhill running should be replaced by the next type of economy training.

Uphill running — Find a steady, but not steep, grade of 200 uphill yards. Steadily run, not sprint, uphill for 30-45 seconds. Rest for two and a half minutes between each run. This will improve the power of the buttocks muscles. Uphill runs should not exceed 10% of the total weekly mileage.

Bounding drills — Use easy bounding by exaggerating strides while running until fatigue sets in. After resting repeat the bounding. Include several of these during easy workout runs.

Owen Anderson in *Running Research News* (March/April 1992) commented that even a three percent increase in running economy can improve a three hour marathon time by 6 minutes and a 40 minute 10K by 60-90 seconds. He suggests bouncing up hills by not leaning forward and by using a vertical springing action up onto the toes which improves the elasticity of the muscles, tendons and ligaments. Swedish researchers and Arthur Lydiard have advocated this type of hill workout. Bouncing hill workouts and speed economy workouts (repetitions) should alternate in one's training schedule. It is important to incorporate these types of economy workouts 2-4 times per month over a long period of time in order to affect economy.

Breathing Techniques

Joggers/runners should breathe naturally and rhythmically through the mouth and nose. Americans typically breathe more rapidly and shallower than the rest of the world. In order to breathe deeper and less often, it is suggested to use the diaphragm more extensively and the lungs more passively, particularly while jogging, running, or racewalking. This will help to prevent a "side stitch" or pain in the side. Keeping the diaphragm and chest muscles in shape can help keep the VO_2 max high even though the lungs lose elasticity as one ages.

Aerobic activity can help strengthen breathing muscles. However, supplementary exercises can be beneficial to provide additional strengthening and reduce workout fatigue.

Diaphragm breathing may be practiced by lying down with books on the abdominal area. The objective is to move the books up and down through abdominal breathing. Also, to strengthen the diaphragm, lie down on a bench and hold a weight behind the head. Take a deep breath using the diaphragm, then slowly and forcibly exhale. Repeat up to 15 times. (See Figs. 3-18 and 3-19.)

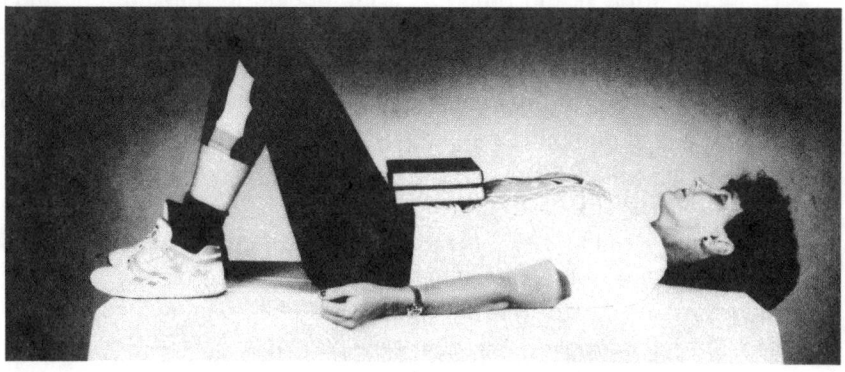

Figure 3-18. Diaphragm breathing practiced by using books on abdominal area.

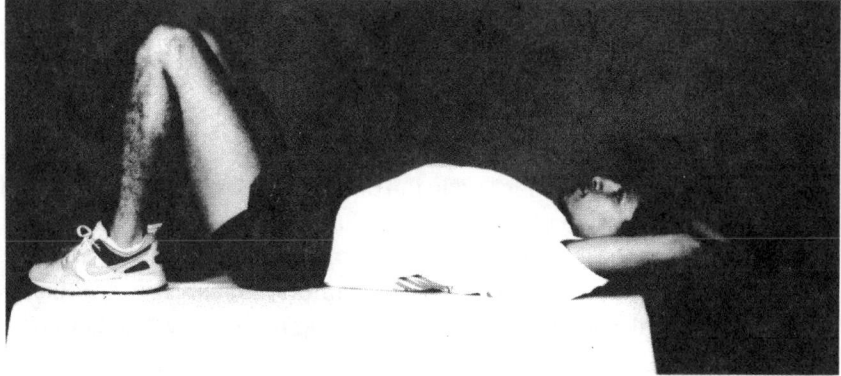

Figure 3-19. Strengthening the diaphragm by using weights.

Working against resistance can help your lungs. Pucker the lips to vary the opening of the mouth. Breathe through the mouth, making an opening progressively smaller until the size is a quarter of an inch or less. Breathe in and out to a ratio of 1:2 or 1:3. Pranayama, yoga exercises, can also help with breathing control.

Additional exercises include breathing in and out forcefully replicating a steam engine. A second method is to speed up and breathe as fast as possible, then slow down until the breath is held for a count of four and exhale to an 8+ count. Another exercise is to sit on the edge of a chair or bench. Use the 4/8 count as in the previous exercise. Inhale quickly, concentrating on minimal effort, rock forward, then hold for a 4 count. While exhaling to a count of 8, contract the buttocks. These exercises should help develop breathing with a short, rapid inhalation and a long exhalation.

Progression From Jogging to Running

To increase pace and progress from jogging to running, one must increase stride length slightly, move feet quicker by spending less time supporting the body and by flexing and lifting the knees more as the leg swings forward, use a stronger push-off using a more forceful heel lift, flex trunk slightly, and pump the arms quicker, higher, and more vigorously.

Use of Hand Weights

Jogging or running with weights held in the hands is controversial. If the purpose of the weights is solely to elevate oxygen uptake and heart rate, then carrying one to three pound weights while jogging or running will accomplish that purpose. It should be noted that carrying one pound weights does not significantly increase oxygen uptake or heart rate. If a person wants to become a faster runner, then carrying weights is not recommended. Use of weights decreases the speed of the workout rather than allowing practice at a quicker pace to improve speed.

PHYSIOLOGY

Aerobic/Anaerobic

Walking, jogging, and running are classified as aerobic activities. **Aerobic** means "with oxygen" or "in the presence of oxygen." To walk, jog, or run aerobically while training or racing, an individual must use oxygen efficiently at a pace for which he or she is trained. These aerobic activities will improve the functioning of the respiratory system; an aerobically trained individual will be capable of ventilating more air with less effort.

Aerobic capacity is inherited. However, through aerobic activities such as walking, jogging, and running, the potential of this capacity can be reached by each individual. **Maximum oxygen uptake (VO_2 max)** is the maximum amount of oxygen that the body can consume. It is a good predictor of endurance potential, but not the only factor. The VO_2 max of elite runners and racewalkers may vary even though times at certain distances are similar. Two contributing factors to VO_2 max are (1) the heart's ability to pump blood (cardiac output) and (2) the muscle's ability to use oxygen and produce energy. A normally active male will have 44-47 milliliters of oxygen per kilogram of body weight per minute with females having slightly less. A typical adult will have 20-30 ml/kg x min. Top female runners will have over 65 ml/kg x min and top male runners will have over 70 ml/kg x min. To estimate VO_2 max use either formula below (if both results are different, take the average of both):

VO_2 max = 133.61   (13.89 x minutes for 1 mile run)

VO_2 max = 120.8 — (1.54 x minutes for 10K/6.2 mile run)

Untrained individuals who begin a walking, jogging, or running program can increase their current VO_2 max by 15-20% as they become trained. Once a person is trained, after 6 months to two years of regular, progressive aerobic workouts, his/her potential is reached and little improvement in VO_2 max can be achieved.

If a person walks, jogs, or runs at a pace and/or distance exceeding that for which he/she has trained, the exercise will become **anaerobic** ("without oxygen"). The body will not have enough oxygen to service the demand; oxygen debt will occur when this **anaerobic threshold** is reached. At this time, waste in the form of lactic acid builds in the muscles and produces fatigue. After the VO_2 max potential has been reached, further training can improve the percentage of the VO_2 max at which a person can exercise aerobically before the anaerobic threshold is reached. Elite runners are capable of exercising to 85-90% of their VO_2 max before reaching their anaerobic threshold.

In summary, even though VO_2 max is hereditary, the potential can be reached through a planned aerobic exercise program. Further training can improve the intensity or percentage of VO_2 max at which one can exercise before reaching his/her anaerobic threshold.

Cardiorespiratory Response

Undoubtedly the most publicized benefit of participation in walking, jogging, running, and other aerobic activities is the improvement in the cardiorespiratory system which protects against heart disease. Aerobic activities, and particularly walking, have been used by cardiac patients to rehabilitate from heart attacks and heart surgery. Millions of other individuals have started aerobic exercise programs to decrease the risk of being afflicted with cardiovascular disease, to reduce the risk of heart attacks, to decrease the severity of a heart attack, and to increase the chance of surviving a heart attack.

The cardiorespiratory system distributes oxygenated blood throughout the cells of the body and regulates the body temperature. A complete circuit takes approximately one minute with an output of 5 liters of blood. Greater output occurs during maximum exertion with the untrained individual output averaging 16 liters/minute and the trained individual output increasing up to 40 liters/minute.

Numerous cardiorespiratory benefits are realized by individuals who participate in a regular program of walking, jogging, or running. They will develop a stronger and often larger heart. A stronger heart is characterized by thicker walls, larger ventricular muscles which improve ventricular functioning, and increased diastolic or filling volume. This results in a slower heart rate. The resting heart rate will decrease 10-20 beats per minute or more. Upon examination, the impact of this is tremendous. Just a slight decrease of 10 beats per minute will result in 600 less beats an hour, 14,400 less beats per day, 100,800 less beats per week and 5,241,600 less beats in a year. Those statistics alone dramatically indicate the valuable energy-saving benefit for the heart. Not only will the resting heart rate decrease, but the heart rate during a similar exercise workload will decrease. Also, a trained individual's heart rate will return to normal more quickly following exercise.

Further benefits of aerobic exercise to the heart include an increased blood volume and stroke volume, which means more blood is pumped with each beat of the heart. The heart's pumping chamber is able to fill more completely and the increased strength of the ventricular muscle causes more blood to be pumped with each beat. Blood vessel improvements include increased capillary size, number of open capillaries, peripheral circulation, and coronary circulation, plus decreased blood pressure for some individuals. Aerobic exercise also contributes to an increase in the number of high density lipoproteins (HDL or "good cholesterol") and to an increase in the body's ability to extract oxygen from the blood.

Aerobic exercise can contribute to lowering of blood pressure. This contribution often is coupled with the reduction of body fat, a common result of aerobic exercise. **Blood pressure** is the pressure of the blood against the walls of the blood vessels. Since most pressure is higher in the arteries than veins, the blood pressure reading involves arterial pressure. The upper reading is obtained during the strongest pressure or systolic phase when the heart contracts. The lower reading is obtained during lowest pressure which occurs during the relaxation or diastolic phase. A normal reading for males is 120/80 and for females, 110/70. An acceptable range is **(120 + or - 20) / (80 + or - 10)**. A reading above 140/90 indicates hypertension. This causes undue stress on the blood vessels and the heart, often leading to a heart attack or stroke. If diagnosed with high blood pressure, an individual should exercise cautiously.

Finally, walking, jogging, and running improve bone density and reduce the risk of osteoporosis, help to relieve stress, increase the efficiency of the immune system, and prevent certain forms of cancer. The cancer preventing benefit was cited in a study conducted by Steve Blair at the Institute for Aerobic Research in Dallas, Texas, and published during the fall of 1989 in *Journal of the American Medical Association.* Further research is needed to determine why aerobic exercise prevents cancer. Information on body fat reduction and stress management benefits of aerobic exercise will be found in later chapters in this book.

Ultimately, regular exercise not only improves the quality of one's life, but can extend life. Dr. Larry Gibbons, medical director of the Cooper Institute for Aerobic Research, projects that **a person extends his or her life by two hours for every hour of exercise.**

In conclusion, the heart of an aerobically trained person is more efficient and circulates more oxygen to the muscles. An improved cardio-vascular system which supplies more oxygen to the muscles will improve energy output. This should improve an individual's performance capabilities both physically and mentally.

Muscular Response

Mitochondria are the powerhouses located in the muscles that produce energy to drive the muscle cells. Oxidative enzymes in the mitochondria break down food, changing the food energy to **adenosine triphosphate (ATP)**. ATP, as well as oxygen, is used by the body to perform muscular contractions. Aerobic activities such as walking, jogging, and running contribute to the development of larger quantities of mitochondria and to the improvement in the size of mitochondria produced by the body. ATP produced by the mitochondria provides more sustaining energy than stored ATP, which lasts 3-5 seconds, and ATP produced from muscle glycogen, which lasts 20-30 seconds. Walking, jogging, and running produce an increase in oxygen and an increase of mitochondria, resulting in an energy increase.

Research indicates that both aerobic and anaerobic training contribute to the increase in mitochondria. However, anaerobic training is necessary to increase enzymes needed for anaerobic energy production. Therefore, runners and racewalkers who wish to improve their racing speed must include anaerobic speed training in their workout regimen. These programs will be discussed in the next chapter.

The type of muscle fibers which a person possesses will affect performance in endurance-type activities such as walking, jogging, and running. Individuals possess slow and fast twitch fibers to varying degrees. **Fast twitch fibers** burn sugar and provide more speed, but burn out and fatigue more quickly. Sprinters possess a high percentage of these fibers. **Slow twitch fibers** burn fat and provide more sustaining energy for endurance activities, but do not provide the energy for a finishing kick needed in a race. Slow twitch fibers contain more mitochondria and oxidative enzymes. Trained slow twitch fibers will have a greater endurance capacity than trained fast twitch fibers. However, fast twitch fibers can be trained to burn fat and act similar to slow twitch fibers. Therefore, an individual possessing a greater number of fast twitch fibers can participate in endurance activities such as walking, jogging, or running, but will not be an elite distance runner or racewalker.

PSYCHOLOGY

It is important to understand the motivation needed to walk, jog, or run and the psychological benefits derived from these activities. Motivation is often needed to begin and continue a walking, jogging, or running program and motivation is involved in race participation and achievement. Often individuals select and/or continue a program because of the psychological benefits derived.

Motivation

Two of the more difficult aspects of a walking, jogging, or running program are getting started and then continuing the program. People develop excuses and often procrastinate on beginning an aerobic exercise program even though they are aware of the positive benefits. Unfortunately, it often takes an extreme situation such as a heart attack, heart surgery, or cardiac arrest to motivate an individual or family and friends to begin to exercise aerobically. Thousands of people begin an aerobic exercise program each year, but the majority usually quit within the first six months.

Motivating factors to begin an exercise program vary with each individual. Common reasons to start a walking, jogging, or running program are: concern for good heath and fitness, prevention of heart disease, participation in a fad, improvement of physical appearance, participation in a social activity, weight loss or control, stress reduction, recapturing of youth, and preparation for or improvement in a strenuous sport activity. There are numerous suggestions to assist an individual to continue with a walking, jogging, or running program. Some or all of the following tips may be used, depending upon individual preference:

1. **Gain knowledge on the subject.** Numerous books, films, videos, and magazines are available which provide valuable information on walking, jogging or running. The well-informed exerciser tends to continue.

2. **Develop a schedule.** It is important to make walking, jogging, or running a top priority on the list of daily activities. Make it a part of the daily schedule and attempt to exercise at the same time daily.

3. **Set goals.** Make sure the goals are realistic and within range of accomplishing. Follow suggestions in Chapter Four for goal suggestions. Review the goals every day to etch them in the mind.

4. **Don't overdo it.** Stick to the goals. Overexertion can cause soreness and fatigue which can discourage a beginner and cause him/her to discontinue the exercise program.

5. **Record progress.** Keep a log or diary. Write down achievements (time or distance), feelings, and description of the environment. Pulse rate and body weight may also be recorded.

6. **Strive for success.** Set out to meet the goal for each workout. Reward yourself for accomplishing a major exercise goal.

7. **Seek support from family and friends.** Support from significant others to continue a walking, jogging, or running program is a major factor in prevention of quitting.

8. **Use music.** Walking, jogging, or running while listening to music enhances the workout and helps the time pass quickly. Upbeat music can help to liven the pace and stimulate the workout. Music may be used in a safe environment, but is not recommended for use on busy streets.

9. **Make it social.** Seek companionship of a partner or group for walking, jogging, or running workouts. Group efforts add fun to the workout and provide additional stimulation and support. Joining a walking/jogging/running club is a way to meet people for socialization as well as exercise.

10. **Make a list of advantages and disadvantages.** Writing out a list of the advantages of a walking, jogging, or running program and a list of disadvantages from not following an aerobic exercise program

can be helpful. Post and review this list regularly to reinforce the decision to work out regularly.

11. **Reduce barriers.** To reduce roadblocks which prevent continuing an exercise program, use any techniques that will be helpful. These may include setting out the exercise outfit the night before, reviewing and committing to the exercise schedule and goals every morning, and placing cue cards in strategic places at home or at work to motivate working out.

12. **Enter a running or walking event.** The incentive of working toward a goal of preparing for and participating in such an event helps motivate a person to continue workouts.

The key to beginning and continuing a training program for fitness through walking, jogging, or running as well as training and racing at an advanced level is to tap your inner power and use positive mind control. The mind can ensure that the body achieves the goals set forth. By using the mind positively to project accomplishment in the areas of exercise and fitness, a walker, jogger, or runner can reap the benefits of the self-fulfilling prophecy. Willpower and relaxation techniques can help control jitters before races and stimulate better performances. Although a sprinter needs to be at a high level of anxiety, distance runners or walkers need to be more relaxed to prevent muscles from tightening and inhibiting performance. Meditation, relaxation techniques, and visualization of accomplishment can help promote relaxation and positively channel the jitters. Using the power of the mind can not only help a person pull through a tough event, but can enable a person to soar physically beyond the seeming limits of the body. Numerous accounts have been written about extraordinary physical performances under great adversity. One must block out negativity and allow the mind and body to work as partners to experience greater achievements in training as well as competition. Planning is suggested along with mind/body coordination. This prevents a person new to exercise from overdoing it by exercising too long or too strenuously and being too sore to work out in succeeding days. It will also prevent a top level athlete from peaking too early or burning out. Moderation in motivation is also suggested. Too little motivation may cause dropout and too much motivation may cause burnout.

During a race, runners and racewalkers must develop mental coping strategies to maximize their potential. Once pre-race jitters are under control and the race gets underway, efforts must be made to keep a relaxed state of mind. As the race progresses, the competitor feels bored, tired and/or hot, the legs feel like lead, and/or the muscles may feel sore. At that point, often the competitor wants to slow down or quit. It is then that mental coping strategies must be employed. These strategies may be used not only during races, but also while participating in training workouts.

The three most common types of coping methods cited by *Running Research News* (March/April, 1985) are association, dissociation, and positive self-talk. When using **association**, the competitor concentrates on body sensations, monitors respiration, temperature, muscle fatigue, etc., and attempts to keep relaxed and loose while adjusting pace and stride. To employ **dissociation** techniques, body sensations are blocked out and the competitor focuses his/her mind on pleasant thoughts or subjects unrelated to the race. A competitor employing **positive self-talk** repeats positive phrases such as "I can do it," "I move easily and swiftly," "I have unlimited energy," etc. Elite racers typically use association, while the average racer tends to use dissociation. However, psychologists indicate that both association and dissociation may need to be employed at different times during a race. Total dissociation may be dangerous since an injury may be ignored and result in serious physical problems. Association helps to monitor one's pace and to remember to drink fluids and relax muscles in the latter part of a workout or race. Association contributes to the ability to exercise or race at a faster pace. However, one must practice using association in order to improve the technique and to continue associating for long periods of time. Another suggestion for improving the association technique is to keep a training log and include information on your thoughts during a workout or race.

In 1984 Jeff Galloway suggested other coping techniques to use during training or racing—ignoring, distraction, projection, and relaxation. To **ignore**, one must let negative thoughts pass through the mind and get back to positive thinking. **Distraction** is similar to dissociation by thinking of things other than the race. The competitor may observe the houses, cars or businesses along the route or concentrate on power line poles or runners ahead. **Projection** involves focusing on the goal and visualizing achievement of the goal or the end of the race or training run. Finally, to achieve **relaxation** it is important to concentrate on relaxing and allowing the body movements to flow easily.

Benefits

As early as the ancient Greeks, assertions were made that a strong, fit body contributed to a sound mind. Numerous recent studies reveal positive psychological benefits from aerobic exercise.

A relaxed feeling and a sense of well-being are typical after a walking, jogging, or running workout. Research indicates that a reduction of tension occurs to a greater extent after a more strenuous workout. Walking, jogging, and running have been cited as antidotes to anxiety, minor depression and other mental difficulties. This may be a result of an increase in brain emission of alpha waves during the workout. Studies also support the tranquilizing effect of aerobic activity; aerobic exercise may be as effective as an average dose of valium in producing relaxation.

Walking, jogging, and running improve the ability to cope and adapt to stress and result in greater stability and calmness within the participant. Stress has less negative impact on individuals who walk, jog or run regularly. Therefore, they have fewer health problems related to stress. As a result of aerobic exercise, powers of concentration increase. Walkers, joggers, and runners have a greater quality of concentration and can concentrate for longer periods of time. Creativity, problem-solving, and mental alertness are also improved. Psychological rejuvenation and improved personality traits have been observed particularly in older and female walkers, joggers, and runners. This may be attributed to reports that regular aerobic workouts help build positive self-esteem, develop self-discipline, and result in a feeling of accomplishment. In addition, improved sleeping and prevention of insomnia are cited benefits.

Walkers, joggers, and runners often allude to the "high" or euphoric state achieved during their workout. This high is characterized by mental clarity and a feeling of well-being. Due to this euphoric state, many claim they are addicted to walking, jogging, or running. The cause of the "high" feeling has often been attributed to **endorphins** released in the body's central nervous system; however, research has failed to support this notion.

TRAINING PRINCIPLES: FITT

Aerobic activity is the key to providing the physiological and psychological benefits discussed earlier in this chapter. For over twenty years the guiding principle of aerobic exercise has been the **FIT exercise prescription guidelines** recommended by the American College of Sports Medicine (ACSM). FIT prescribed a minimum of 3 days per week of vigorous activity at 60-90% of one's predicted maximum heart rate to be performed in 20-60 minute continuous sessions. FIT formula has been used for cardiac rehabilitation, as a training plan for athletes and individuals whose occupation required a high level of fitness. Some individuals who wanted a quick fix of fitness followed the minimum of 3 days for 20 minutes. However, many individuals were turned off to exercising vigorously and continuously.

Research conducted during the past 20+ years prompted **lifetime activity recommendations** in 1995 by the Centers for Disease Control and Prevention (CDC), the ACSM, and the President's Council for Physical Fitness and Sports. Russell Pate, former president of ACSM, summarizes the **lifetime activity recommendation:** "Every U.S. adult should accumulate 30 minutes or more of moderate-intensity physical activity on most, preferably all, days of the week." The following segments in this book will compare both recommendations for adults using FITT—frequency, intensity, time and type. Recommendations for children and adolescents/young adults (11-21 years of age) will then be summarized. The reader may then choose the plan most suitable for his or her goals.

Frequency

Frequency refers to how many days per week that a person exercises or is physically active. **FIT exercise prescription guidelines** recommend a minimum of 3 days. The **lifetime activity recommendations** suggest most, preferably 7, days per week. Beginning exercisers following either plan should consider starting with 3 non-consecutive days and then progress to more days. Vigorous exercisers should consider rest or moderate activity one or two days per week in addition to five or six days of vigorous activity to enable the body to recuperate and avoid injury.

Intensity

Intensity involves the amount of exertion during the activity. **FIT exercise prescription guidelines** recommend a person exercise at 60-90% of his/her predicted maximum heart rate. Initially, 40-50% should be used by very low fit individuals. Others may start at 60-70% and then move into a 70-85% zone. Each individual must calculate his/her target heart zone and maintain the heart rate in that zone throughout the workout. To achieve that goal, the heart rate must be monitored periodically during the workout, and adjustments made in intensity.

Intensity is measured in METS. One MET is equivalent to the quantity of calories expended while at rest. Two METS require twice as much energy, three METS require three times as much energy, etc. The **lifetime activity recommendations** advocate moderate activity of 4-6 MET energy expenditure, such as brisk walking, but does not discourage vigorous activity of 7 METS or higher, such as jogging or running.

Monitoring Heart Rate

Those who choose to monitor their heart rate must find their pulse at the carotid or radial artery. Locate the **carotid artery** by placing the fingers on the "Adam's apple" and sliding them lightly toward the notch area at the side of the neck, or start at the outside corner of the eye and slide the fingers down the face to the neck. A radial pulse check is often recom-

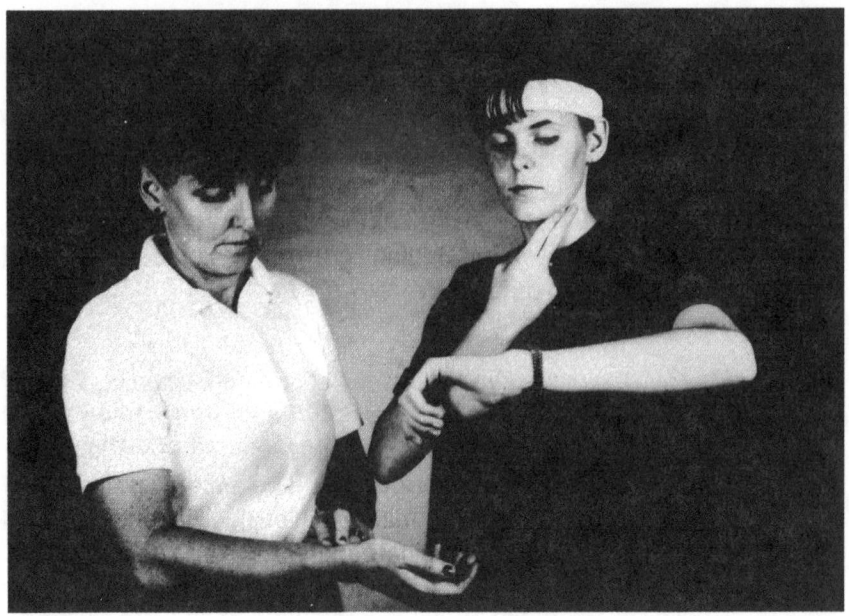

Figure 3-20. Monitoring heart rate at radial pulse (left) and carotid pulse (right).

mended, particularly for older adults and walkers and for those who press too hard at the carotid artery or have irregular beats. The **radial pulse** may be taken by placing the fingers at the wrist of the opposite hand (palm up) below the base of the thumb. Once the pulse is located, count the number of beats for six seconds and add a zero to obtain the minute pulse rate. It may also be counted for 10 seconds multiplying by 6, or 15 seconds multiplying by 4. For many, the simplicity of adding the zero onto the 6-second count is easier. This short break to monitor the heart rate will not cause the pulse to slow down long enough to drop below the minimum level of the target heart zone. A more accurate measurement is provided by using a heart rate monitor. Wearing a heart monitor eliminates the necessity of pausing during exercise to locate and count one's pulse. More sophisticated heart monitors can provide a recall of exercise heart rates throughout the exercise period and computer printouts of the heart rates. Training with a heart monitor will be discussed in Chapter 4.

Determining Target Heart Zone

For a quick determination of the **target heart zone**, the chart below will serve that purpose. However, a more personalized computation of the target heart zone may be achieved by using a specific formula. First, determine the **resting heart rate (RHR)**. The resting heart rate should be taken as described previously; however, it should be counted for the entire minute. The resting heart rate (RHR) should be determined after a person has been sleeping or napping and has awakened naturally without an alarm. Count without moving from the reclined position. Once the resting heart rate has been determined, the formula that follows may be used. Find the **maximum heart rate (MHR)** by subtracting age from 220 (older adults may use 200).

It has been suggested that women may subtract from 226. For individuals over 45 who are non-smokers with a resting heart rate over 70 beats per minute, a more accurate equation is suggested for finding the maximum heart rate. Men should subtract (.8 x age) from 214. Women should subtract (.7 x age) from 209. Current runners can determine a more accurate maximum heart rate by first warming up with a 20-minute run. Then do two very hard 800 meter runs on a measured track and jog for one minute between each. The heart rate taken immediately after the second 800 should be the maximum heart rate.

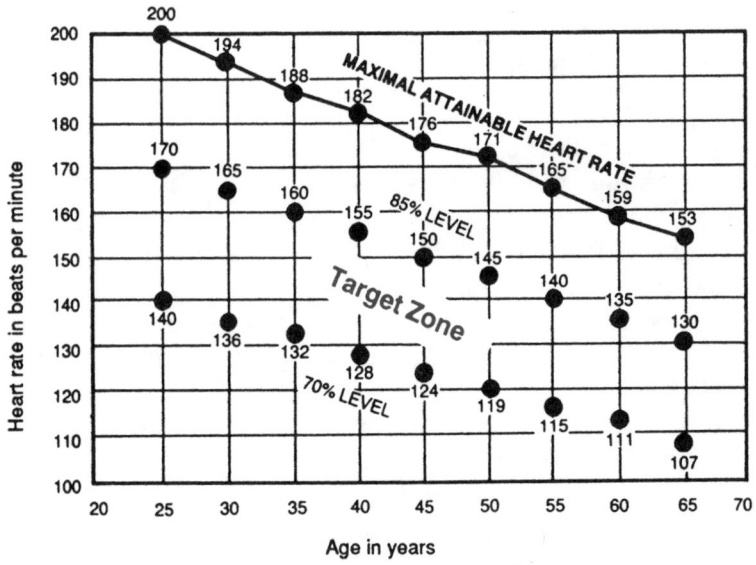

Figure 3-22. Heart Rate Chart

This figure shows that as we grow older, the highest heart rate which can be reached during all-out effort falls. These numerical values are "average" values for age. Note that one-third of the population may differ from these values. It is quite possible that a normal 50-year-old man may have a maximum heart rate of 195 or that a 30-year-old man might have a maximum of only 168. The same limitations apply to the 70% and 85% of maximum lines. (From L. Zohgman, M.D., *Beyond Diet: Exercise Your Way to Fitness and Heart Health,* CPC International, Englewood Cliffs, NJ.)

One should never exercise above his/her maximum heart rate to avoid injury or undue stress to the heart. Older individuals, recently sedentary individuals, and cardiac rehabilitation patients should reduce the percentage to a level recommended by their physician. Patients taking beta blockers should realize that their pulse reading is lower and they should use a lower percentage to determine their target heart zone. As an individual progresses in his/her exercise program, the resting heart rate should be checked and the formula recomputed. Also, those exercising at a lower percentage level may increase the percentage based upon their physician's advice. To compute one's target heart rate, refer to lab 3.4.

Time

Time involves the number of minutes of activity each day. The **FIT exercise prescription guidelines** recommend 20-60 minute sessions of continuous exercise within the target zone described above exclusive of warm-up and cool-down.

The **lifetime activity recommendations** suggest 30 or more minutes accumulate in numerous sessions throughout the day. At this time a minimum of 5 minutes per session is recommended. A person may also choose one session of 30 or more continuous minutes.

Type

Type indicates activities that contribute to aerobic fitness. The **FIT exercise prescription guidelines** recommend activities that elevate the heart rate into the chosen target heart zone and can be performed for a continuous 20-60 minute time period. The commonly selected activities include brisk walking, jogging, running, brisk cycling, cross country skiing, lap swimming, water jogging, aqua fitness exercising, aerobic dancing, step aerobics, rowing and inline skating. Numerous computerized and non-computerized machines have been manufactured to simulate many of these activities, such as stationary bicycles, rowing machines, treadmills, stair climbers, and cross country skiing machines.

The **lifetime activity recommendations** emphasize moderate activities. Moderate activities include brisk walking, racquet sports, mowing the lawn with a power mower, housework, cycling, moderate swimming, golf (walking), walking up stairs, and skating. Vigorous activities may also be selected, such as very brisk walking, walking uphill, jogging, running, brisk cycling, active sports, aerobic dance, speed skating, and mowing the lawn with a hand mower.

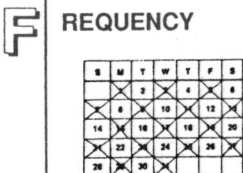

F REQUENCY

I NTENSITY

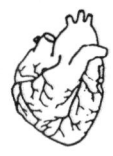

T IME

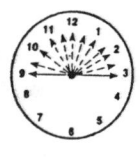

T YPE

	Exercise Prescription Guidelines ACSM	Lifetime Activity Recommendations CDC/ACSM/PCPFS	
		Moderate	Vigorous
FREQUENCY	**Minimum 3 days/week**	**Most Days** Preferably All Days	**Most Days** (Additional Days Moderate)
INTENSITY	**60-90% Max Heart Rate** (Initially 40-50% for very low fit individuals	**4-6 METS**	**7+ METS**
TIME	**20-60 continuous minutes**	**30+ cumulative minutes** (Minimum 5 min. per session)	**30+ cumulative minutes** (Minimum 5 min. per session)
TYPE	**Activities that elevate heart rate and can be continuous for 20+ min.:** brisk walking, jogging, running, cycling, skating, lap swimming, rowing, cross country skiing, step aerobics	**Moderate Activities:** brisk walking, racquet sports, moderate swimming, cycling, skating, mowing lawn (power), housework	**Vigorous Activities:** very brisk walking, jogging and running, lap swimmng, fast cycling, skating, mowing lawn (hand), aerobic dance, active sports

Children and Adolescent/Young Adult FITT

Activity recommendations for children under the age of 11 suggest A MINIMUM OF 30 MINUTES, preferable 60 cumulative minutes, of moderate activity most, preferably all, days of the week. Skill/movement learning can be included in the 60 minutes. According to Salis, Patrick and Long in 1994, activity **recommendations for adolescents and young adults ages 11-21** indicate they "should be physically active daily, or nearly every day, as part of play, games, sports, work, transportation, recreation, physical education, or planned exercise, in the context of family, school, and community activities." Whenever possible, adolescents and young adults should be involved at least 3 times a week in moderate to vigorous activity for a minimum of 20 continuous minutes.

The Overload Principle and Progression

In order to improve aerobically, the **overload principle** must be applied to increase the demands made on the body. The body is an adaptive mechanism. If the same level of intensity is maintained, the body will adapt and improvement will cease. Therefore, a **progression** plan must be established which involves **overloading** by increasing the degree of difficulty of each workout or workout week. For walking, jogging, or running, distance or length of time of the workout may be increased in order to achieve this overload. It is recommended that the increase not exceed 10% a week. For an example, if a person walked, jogged, or ran 9 miles the previous week, he/she may add .9 miles to the next week's workout. This may be achieved by adding .9 miles to one day or splitting the .9 miles and adding .3 miles to each of 3 days. Once a person reaches a point when his/her schedule will only permit a certain amount of time for working out, overload intensity may be achieved by increasing the pace. For additional overload, the number of workout days per week may be increased.

Walking is less intense than jogging, running, or racewalking. In order to elevate the heart rate into the target heart zone by means of walking, pace and intensity of the arm swing must be increased. Once the body has adapted, walking with weights, hill walking, or stair walking may be used to achieve overload and to move the exercise heart rate into the target heart zone. Another option would be to progress from walking to jogging then running, or from walking to racewalking, in order to achieve overload and to exercise within the training zone.

In summary, it is important to strive for progression. In order to progress when the body adapts to a walking, jogging, or running workout, a person must overload by increasing the frequency, intensity, or duration of his/her workouts.

Retrogression

Throughout a walking, jogging, or running program, plateaus occur. When a plateau is reached, improvement is curtailed. It is difficult to maintain the current workout level and a performance decrease often results. **Retrogression** may be a message from the body that it is attempting to adjust to the overload. Once the adjustment is complete, performance levels increase and improvement is evident.

CONCLUSION

Once a person becomes aerobically fit through a regular progressive walking, jogging, or running program, or other activity program, the program must be continued in order to maintain that fitness. Fitness is not similar to skill and/or knowledge which are learned and retained. If a fitness program is abandoned, the person will decline to his/her previously unfit state. Aerobic fitness will decline significantly after ten to twelve weeks of inactivity. It will take three to five months to totally lose the aerobic fitness achieved. Those who achieved a higher fitness level will take longer to decline than those who did not achieve a high level of fitness. Therefore, to retain aerobic fitness, participation in a walking, jogging, or running program or other activity programs must be a lifetime commitment.

CHAPTER SUMMARY

Walking, jogging, and running have good posture as a basis for proper mechanics. Good form and efficient mechanics enhance performance. Walking, jogging, and running are popular aerobic activities that provide numerous psychological and physiological (particularly cardiovascular) benefits. Motivation is often needed to begin and continue a walking, jogging, or running program. In order to become aerobically "FITT," an individual has choices. The first choice is to follow the lifetime activity recommendations. To achieve this, "don't measure it, just do it" by accumulating thirty minutes or more of moderate intensity or vigorous activity most days per week. The second choice is to achieve a high fitness level. To achieve that level, one must exercise continuously within one of the training zones that elevates the heart rate over 60-90% of maximum 3 or more days per week. To retain aerobic fitness, the walking, jogging, running, or other exercise plan must continue throughout life.

CHAPTER FOUR

Training Programs

DETERMINING THE STARTING LEVEL

Value and Purpose of Testing

Testing is important to determine an individual's current level of aerobic fitness. Once that level is determined, the appropriate walking, jogging, or running programs can be followed. As suggested in Chapter Two, before testing and beginning a walking, jogging, or running program a medical examination is important. This examination is essential for individuals who have not been engaging in sports activities on a regular basis or who are over the age of 45. Because of the more sedentary lifestyle and poor dietary habits characteristic of the youth of today, inactive, fast food-eating individuals are showing signs of heart disease before the age of 21 and, in some cases, as early as 2-3 years of age. Based upon the results of the physical examination, the physician can provide advice about plans to begin an aerobic exercise program.

TESTS

Test A. RISKO

The RISKO test (reprinted by permission of the American Heart Association) is a quick check to determine a person's risk for developing heart disease. Results of the RISKO test may serve as a warning and an indicator of the necessity to consult a physician. This test should be taken before any of the following tests are administered. See Lab 4.1 in Appendix D.

After medical approval to begin a walking, jogging, or running program has been obtained, at least one or more of the following tests should be taken. These tests can help to determine the current aerobic condition of an individual and can serve as a guide to selecting or developing a walking, jogging, or running program.

If a person wishes to participate in a walking program exclusively, then the Rockport Walking Test should be used as an assessment tool. This test is an excellent means by which to determine an individual's aerobic level. If a person wishes to begin a walking program and progress to jogging, to begin a jogging program which may or may not progress to running, or to continue a jogging or running program, he/she should select the 1.5 mile test or the 1 mile test. These tests involve jogging, running, or the combination of jogging and walking for the prescribed distance or time. Finally, to assess the aerobic fitness level for either walkers, joggers, or runners, if a measured surface is not available for test administration or for a group test with a mix of walkers, joggers, and runners, the 3 minute bench (12" box) step test may be used. This test is popular for use with a group with mixed exercise goals. The one drawback is the accuracy and honesty of the pulse counting involved in the testing. Therefore, the other tests mentioned above are preferred over the 3 minute bench step test.

Test B. Rockport Walking Test

To prepare for the test, stretch for 5-10 minutes and practice taking a pulse reading, preferably using the carotid artery at the side of the neck or the radial artery at the wrist (refer to Chapter Three). Wear comfortable shoes, preferably walking shoes, and loose-fitting, preferably workout, clothing.

To take the test, find a measured mile and walk a mile as fast as possible, attempting to keep a steady pace. Time the mile and check the pulse immediately after completing the mile. Since the heart rate begins to slow down after stopping, count for 15 seconds only and multiply by 4 to get the minute pulse rate.

Use the charts on the next two pages to determine the fitness level indicated by the walking test. Age and sex will determine the chart to use. Find the point where the time and pulse rate results meet to obtain the fitness rating.

Rockport Walking Test

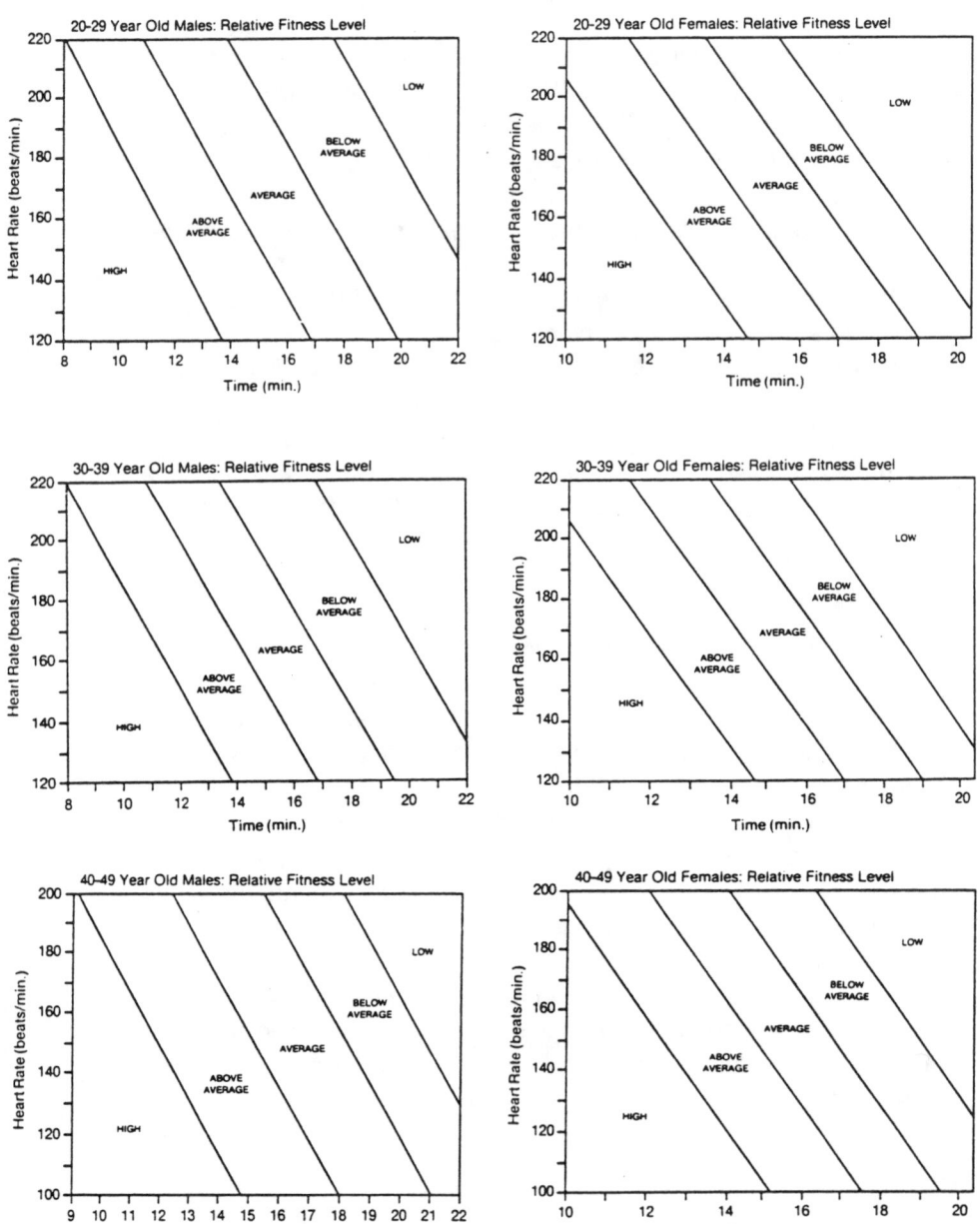

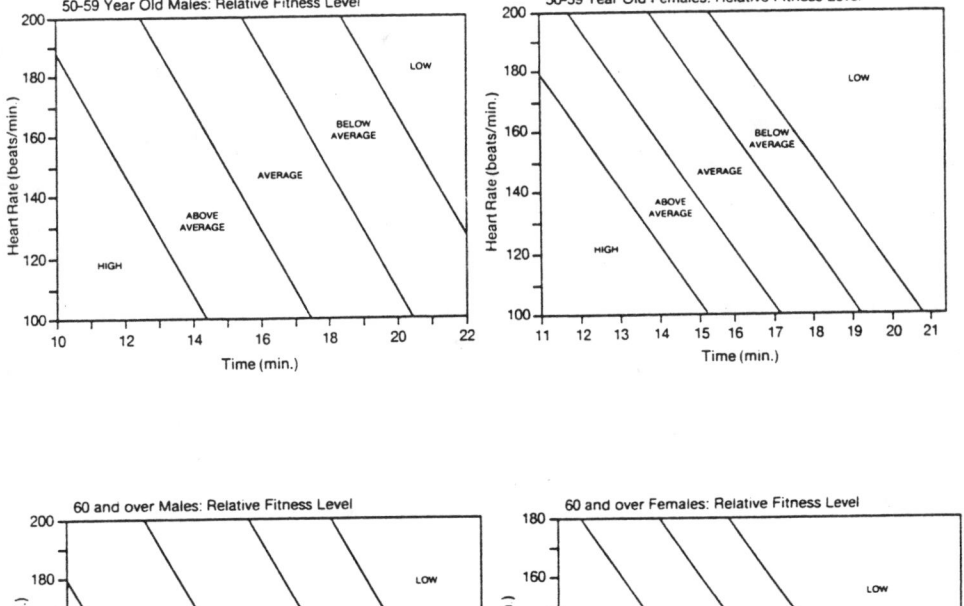

Exercise Level:

Low = Introductory Level   Above Ave = Intermediate
Below Ave = Beginner   High = High Intermediate to Advanced
Ave = Advanced Beginner

Use the charts beginning on the next page to determine the exercise program level indicated by the walking test. Age and sex will determine the chart to use. Find the point where the time and pulse rate results meet to obtain the program level. (Exercise levels have been added by authors.)

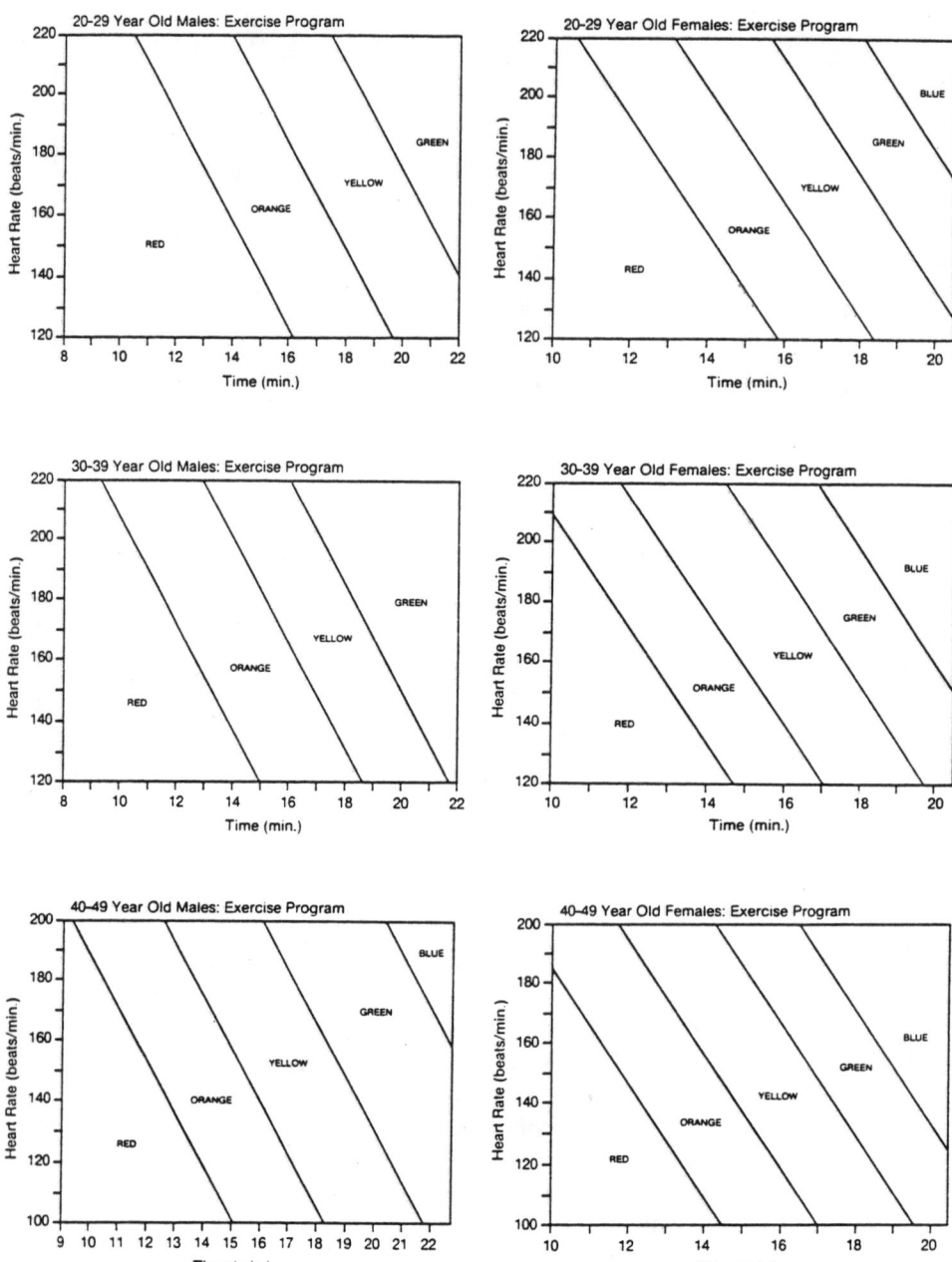

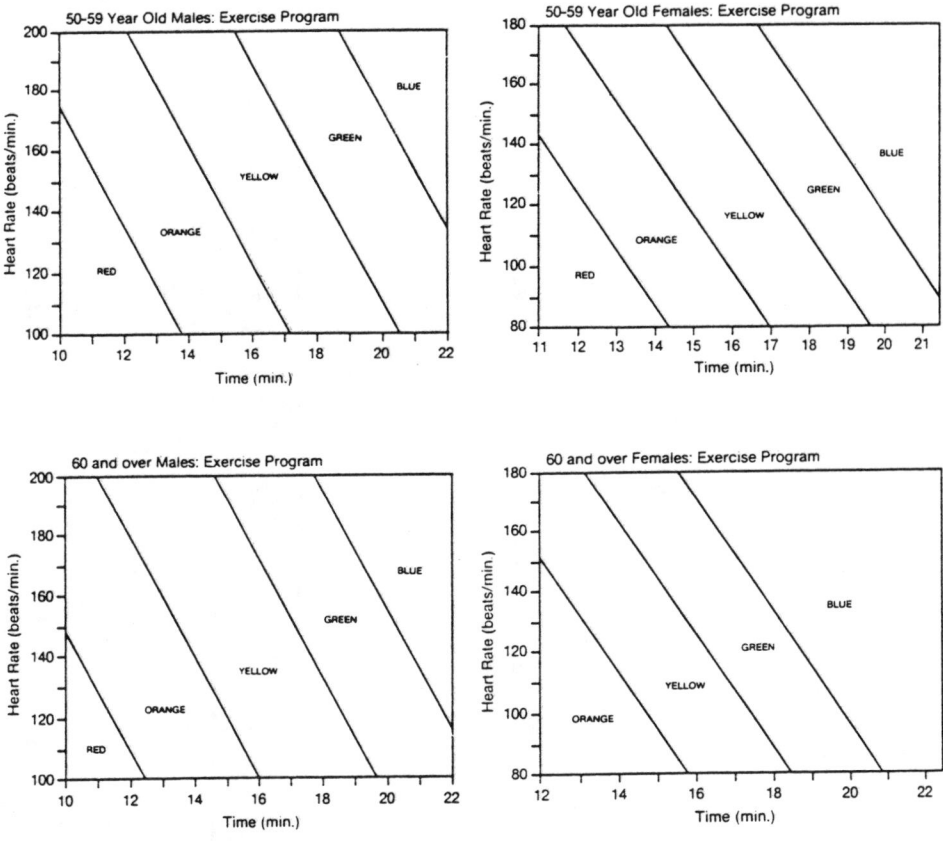

Test C. 1.5 Mile Test

Warm up with 5-10 minutes of stretching exercises before starting the test. Those already participating in a jogging or running program may wish to run, jog, or fast walk for 5-10 minutes after stretching and prior to taking the test. One should wear loose-fitting clothing or workout clothing designed for the weather of the day and wear workout shoes, preferably running shoes.

The objective of the test is to walk/jog, jog/run, or run a distance of 1.5 miles as fast as possible, attempting to use a steady pace. Time the 1.5 miles with a stopwatch or running watch. The watch should be started at the beginning of the test and stopped or time read upon completion of the distance. Use the charts on the next page to determine fitness level and suggested exercise program level according to sex, age, and time for the 1.5 mile test.

1.5 MILE RUN

MALES (BY AGE)

FITNESS CATEGORY	13-19	20-29	30-39	40-49	50-59	60+	EXERCISE LEVEL
Superior	<8:37	<9:45	<10:00	<10:30	<11:00	<11:15	Advanced
Excellent	8:37 - 9:40	9:45 - 10:45	10:00 - 11:00	10:30 - 11:30	11:00 - 12:30	11:15 - 13:59	High Intermediate
Good	9:41 - 10:48	10:46 - 12:00	11:01 - 12:30	11:31 - 13:00	12:31 - 14:30	14:00 - 16:15	Intermediate
Fair	10:49 - 12:10	12:01 - 14:00	12:31 - 14:45	13:01 - 15:35	14:31 - 17:00	16:16 - 19:00	Advanced Beginner
Poor	12:11 - 15:30	14:01 - 16:00	14:46 - 16:30	15:36 - 17:30	17:01 - 19:00	19:01 - 20:00	Beginner
Very Poor	>15:31	>16:10	>16:31	>17:31	>19:01	>20:01	Introductory

FEMALES (BY AGE)

FITNESS CATEGORY	13-19	20-29	30-39	40-49	50-59	60+	EXERCISE LEVEL
Superior	<11:50	<12:30	<13:00	<13:45	<14:30	<16:30	Advanced
Excellent	11:50 - 12:29	12:30 - 13:30	13:00 - 14:30	13:45 - 15:55	14:30 - 16:30	16:30 - 17:30	High Intermediate
Good	12:30 - 14:30	13:31 - 15:54	14:31 - 16:30	15:56 - 17:30	16:31 - 19:00	17:31 - 19:30	Intermediate
Fair	14:31 - 16:54	15:55 - 18:30	16:31 - 19:00	17:31 - 19:30	19:01 - 20:00	19:31 - 20:30	Advanced Beginner
Poor	16:55 - 18:30	18:31 - 19:00	19:01 - 19:30	19:31 - 20:00	20:01 - 20:30	20:31 - 21:00	Beginner
Very Poor	>18:31	>19:01	>19:31	>20:01	>20:31	>21:01	Introductory

1.5 Mile Run from *The Aerobics Program for Total Well Being* by Kenneth H. Cooper, M.D., M.P.H., copyright 1982 by Kenneth H. Cooper. Used by permission of Bantam Books, a division of Bantam, Doubleday, Dell Publishing Group, Inc. (Exercise levels have been added by authors.)

Test D. 1 Mile Run Test

Instructions for taking this test are identical to the 1.5 mile test except the distance is reduced to 1 mile. This test is often used when a marked 1.5 mile cannot be found. It is also used when a group of people that include a mixture of walkers, joggers, and runners will test together. Walkers will follow the Rockport Walking instructions and the joggers and runners will walk/jog, jog, jog/run, or run for time and use the chart below to determine fitness level and suggested exercise program level.

1 MILE RUN TEST

Grade	Sex	Age 13 - 19	20 - 29	30 - 39	40 - 49	50 - 59	60+	Exercise Level
A+	Women	7:00	7:30	8:00	8:30	9:00	9:30	Advanced
	Men	6:00	6:30	7:00	7:30	8:00	8:30	
A	Women	7:30	8:00	8:30	9:00	9:30	10:00	High Intermediate
	Men	6:30	7:00	7:30	8:00	8:30	9:00	
B	Women	8:30	9:00	9:30	10:00	10:30	11:00	Intermediate
	Men	7:30	8:00	8:30	9:00	9:30	10:00	
C	Women	9:30	10:00	10:30	11:00	11:30	12:00	Advanced Beginner
	Men	8:30	9:00	9:30	10:00	10:30	11:00	
D	Women	11:00	11:30	12:00	12:30	13:00	13:30	Beginner
	Men	10:00	10:30	11:00	11:30	12:00	12:30	
F	Women	11:01+	11:31+	12:01+	12:31+	13:01+	13:31+	Introductory
	Men	10:01+	10:31+	11:01+	11:31+	12:01+	12:31+	

Reprinted with permission of *Runner's World*. (Exercise levels have been added by authors.)

Test E. One-Half Mile Test

Walk a flat, measured half-mile (twice around a quarter-mile track) as briskly as possible. Determine your fitness level by using the chart below. (This scale was developed by noted cardiologist, James M. Rippe.)

	Age	20-29	30-39	40-49	50-59	60+	Exercise Level
Women	High	< 5:37	< 5.55	< 6.17	< 6:40	< 7:07	Adv./H. Intermediate
	Above Ave.	5:37 - 6:27	5:55 - 7:00	6:17 - 7:21	6:40 - 7:53	7:07 - 8:31	Intermediate
	Average	6:28 - 7:31	7:01 - 8:05	7:22 - 8:45	7P:54 - 9:16	8:32 - 10:29	Advanced Beginner
	Below Ave.	7:32 - 8:59	8:06 - 10:09	8:46 - 10:29	9:17 - 11:12	10:30 - 12:04	Beginner
	Low	> 8:32	> 10:10	> 10:30	> 11:13	> 12:05	Introductory
Men	High	< 5:14	< 5:37	< 5:55	< 6:09	< 6:24	Adv./H. Intermediate
	Above Ave.	5:14 - 6:12	5:37 - 6:27	5:55 - 7:00	6:09 - 7:21	6:24 - 7:31	Intermediate
	Average	6:13 - 7:21	6:28 - 7:31	7:01 - 8:18	7:22 - 8:45	7:32 - 9:00	Advanced Beginner
	Below Ave.	7:22 - 8:31	7:32 - 8:45	8:19 - 9:49	8:46 - 10:09	9:01 - 10:49	Beginner
	Low	> 8:32	> 8:46	> 9:50	> 10:10	> 10:50	Introductory

Reprinted with permission of *Merrell Footwear*.

Test F. 3 Minute Bench Step Test

Walkers, joggers, and runners may all participate in this test. The equipment needed includes a 12" high bench, a metronome, and a stopwatch or watch with a second hand. This test may be difficult to self-administer and a helper to administer the test is suggested. Comfortable, loose activity clothing and athletic shoes are recommended attire for participation. It is suggested that participants rest a minimum of 10 minutes prior to taking the test.

The test involves stepping up on a 12" bench first with one foot then the other to stand with both feet on the bench and legs straight momentarily. Next is to step down with one foot then the other. Twenty-four of these two steps up and two steps down sequences should take place each minute. In order to achieve this, a metronome (an instrument which marks time with a choice of settings) may be used and set to 96 beats per minute. The test administrator can assist by saying, "up, up, down, down," with each sequence. The stepping sequences should continue for 3 minutes. After 3 minutes the participant should sit down immediately, find his/her pulse and 5 seconds after completion of the stepping, begin a 1 minute pulse count. Immediately after the pulse check, the participants should get up and walk. For a more accurate pulse check when only one person is testing, it is suggested that the test administrator use a stethoscope for the pulse count.

Participants in this test should be cautioned that if they feel dizzy or lightheaded they should discontinue the test and walk slowly until their heart rate is below 100 beats per minute (bpm). Also, if the rate of stepping cannot be maintained, the participant should discontinue the test. Stopping the test is important, since slowing down would decrease the intensity of the test and, therefore, not reflect a proper fitness rating. If the test is discontinued for either reason, the participant receives a very poor rating.

Using the 1 minute pulse count, scrutinize the chart which follows to determine the fitness rating and suggested exercise program level.

3 MINUTE BENCH STEP TEST			
Fitness Rating	Male	Female	**Exercise Level**
EXCELLENT	<71	<97	High Intermediate — Advanced
GOOD	71 - 102	97 - 127	Intermediate
FAIR	103 - 117	128 - 142	Advanced Beginner
POOR	118 - 147	143 - 171	Beginner
VERY POOR	148+	172+	Introductory

WALKING, JOGGING, AND RUNNING PROGRAMS

Determining Programs Based Upon Fitness Rating

The level for fitness programs in walking, jogging, or running should be selected or designed based upon the results of the test used. Rockport walking programs are color-coded by degree of difficulty. Check the Rockport Walking Test result charts which are coded according to suggested walking programs to determine the appropriate program to follow. Once the 20 week program has been completed, Rockport suggests retesting with the mile walk test to determine the next program to follow. Older women, age 60+, should be aware that fast, hard walking may be risky according to a 1990 University of Florida study by Dr. Michael Pollock. The authors advise older women to consult with their physician before engaging in a fitness walking program. Other test results suggest starting exercise levels for jogging and running programs. Individuals should refer to the information provided next, based upon their exercise level, to determine if they will develop their own program or follow one of the suggested programs. Use Lab 4.2, "Monthly Walking/Jogging/Running Schedule/Goals" to plan your workout routine for each month. Retesting upon completion of a program will determine which program level should be followed next.

Walking, jogging, running programs are organized as follows:

Introductory/ Beginner Level	*Adv. Beginner/ Intermediate Level*	*High Intermediate/ Advanced Level*
Walking: Rockport Blue Rockport Green American Heart Association Beginner Sample Introductory **Walking/Jogging:** Sample Introductory Sample Beginner	**Walking:** Rockport Yellow Rockport Orange **Jogging:** Sample Advanced Beginner Sample Intermediate	**Walking:** Rockport Red **Running:** Ullyot Intermediate Sample High Intermediate

Introductory to Beginner Level

Most experts agree that fitness walking, jogging, or running programs should alternate hard and easy days. If working out only three days, each workout day should be followed by a day off to represent the easy day. In beginning walking, jogging, or walking and jogging programs, perform that exercise for a period of time rather than mileage. In planning to overload while developing an exercise program, weekly workout time or distance should not be increased by more than 10% per week. A greater increase is not recommended due to the risk of injury. To determine pace for walking or jogging, strive to achieve a steady and comfortable speed and be able to carry on a conversation with a companion. Dr. Kenneth H. Cooper, noted aerobics expert, suggests that beginning programs range from 15-30 minutes in length and that instead of a fast or long workout on the weekend, a person should enjoy a vigorous activity which is either aerobic or stop and go, such as racquetball, tennis, basketball or soccer.

Walking Programs

Walking Program A.   *Rockport Blue Program*

Week	Warm-up	Mileage	Pace (mph)	Heart Rate (% Max)	Cool-down	Frequency (times/wk.)
1	5-7 mins. before-walk stretches	1.0	3.0	60	5-7 mins. after-walk stretches	5
2	5-7 mins.	1.0	3.0	60	5-7 mins.	5
3	5-7 mins.	1.25	3.0	60	5-7 mins.	5
4	5-7 mins.	1.25	3.0	60	5-7 mins.	5
5	5-7 mins.	1.5	3.0	60	5-7 mins.	5
6	5-7 mins.	1.5	3.5	60-70	5-7 mins.	5
7	5-7 mins.	1.75	3.5	60-70	5-7 mins.	5
8	5-7 mins.	1.75	3.5	60-70	5-7 mins.	5
9	5-7 mins.	2.0	3.5	60-70	5-7 mins.	5
10	5-7 mins.	2.0	3.75	60-70	5-7 mins.	5
11	5-7 mins.	2.0	3.75	70	5-7 mins.	5
12	5-7 mins.	2.25	3.75	70	5-7 mins.	5
13	5-7 mins.	2.25	3.75	70	5-7 mins.	5
14	5-7 mins.	2.5	3.75	70	5-7 mins.	5
15	5-7 mins.	2.5	4.0	70	5-7 mins.	5
16	5-7 mins.	2.5	4.0	70	5-7 mins.	5
17	5-7 mins.	2.75	4.0	70-80	5-7 mins.	5
18	5-7 mins.	2.75	4.0	70-80	5-7 mins.	5
19	5-7 mins.	3.0	4.0	70-80	5-7 mins.	5
20	5-7 mins.	3.0	4.0	70-80	5-7 mins.	5

Walking Program B. *Rockport Green Program*

Week	Warm-up	Mileage	Pace (mph)	Heart Rate (% Max)	Cool-down	Frequency (times/wk.)
1	5-7 mins. before-walk stretches	1.5	3.0	60-70	5-7 mins. after-walk stretches	5
2	5-7 mins.	1.5	3.0	60-70	5-7 mins.	5
3	5-7 mins.	1.75	3.0	60-70	5-7 mins.	5
4	5-7 mins.	1.75	3.0	60-70	5-7 mins.	5
5	5-7 mins.	2.0	3.0	60-70	5-7 mins.	5
6	5-7 mins.	2.0	3.5	60-70	5-7 mins.	5
7	5-7 mins.	2.0	3.5	70	5-7 mins.	5
8	5-7 mins.	2.25	3.5	70	5-7 mins.	5
9	5-7 mins.	2.25	3.5	70	5-7 mins.	5
10	5-7 mins.	2.5	3.75	70	5-7 mins.	5
11	5-7 mins.	2.5	3.75	70	5-7 mins.	5
12	5-7 mins.	2.55	3.75	70	5-7 mins.	5
13	5-7 mins.	2.75	3.75	70	5-7 mins.	5
14	5-7 mins.	2.75	3.75	70-80	5-7 mins.	5
15	5-7 mins.	3.0	4.0	70-80	5-7 mins.	5
16	5-7 mins.	3.0	4.0	70-80	5-7 mins.	5
17	5-7 mins.	3.25	4.0	70-80	5-7 mins.	5
18	5-7 mins.	3.25	4.0	70-80	5-7 mins.	5
19	5-7 mins.	3.5	4.0	70-80	5-7 mins.	5
20	5-7 mins.	3.5	4.0	70-80	5-7 mins.	5

Walking Program C. *American Heart Association Program*

In this program, the American Heart Association recommends walking a minimum of 3 times per week and using a target heart zone based upon a 60 to 75% range. To determine this target heart zone, use the formula discussed in the FITT section of Chapter Three.

Week	Target Zone Exercising	Total Time in Minutes
		(warm-up + target zone exercising + cool down)
1	Walk briskly 5 min.	15 min.
2	Walk briskly 7 min.	17 min.
3	Walk briskly 9 min.	19 min.
4	Walk briskly 11 min.	21 min.
5	Walk briskly 13 min.	23 min.
6	Walk briskly 15 min.	25 min.
7	Walk briskly 18 min.	28 min.
8	Walk briskly 20 min.	30 min.
9	Walk briskly 23 min.	33 min.
10	Walk briskly 26 min.	36 min.
11	Walk briskly 28 min.	38 min.
12	Walk briskly 30 min.	40 min.

13 on: Check your pulse periodically to see if you are exercising within your target zone. As you get more in shape, try exercising within the upper range of your target heart zone. Remember that your goal is to continue getting the benefits you seek while enjoying your activity.

Beginning Walking Program table. Reproduced with permission. *Walking for a Healthy Heart,* 1984. Copyright American Heart Association.

Walking Program D. *Sample Introductory Program*
Daily Plan for 3-6 Weekly Workouts

EW = Easy Walk; BW = Brisk Walk

Week	Daily Workout (min.)	Total (min)
1	EW 20	20
2	EW 9 BW 1 EW 9 BW 1	20
3	EW 8 BW 2 EW 8 BW 2	20
4	EW 7 BW 3 EW 7 BW 3	20
5	EW 6 BW 4 EW 6 BW 4	20
6	EW 5 BW 5 EW 5 BW 5	20
7	EW 4 BW 6 EW 4 BW 6	20
8	EW 3 BW 7 EW 3 BW 7	20

Walking Program E. *Sample Beginner Program*

Daily Plan for 3-6 Weekly Workouts

EW = Easy Walk; BW = Brisk Walk

Week	Daily Workout (min.)	Total (min)
1	EW 2 BW 8 EW 2 BW 8	20
2	EW 1 BW 9 EW 1 BW 9	20
3	BW 10 EW 1 BW 9	20
4	BW 20	20
5	BW 22	22
6	BW 24	24
7	BW 26	26
8	BW 28	28
9	BW 30	30

Walking Program F. *Cooper Aerobic Exercise System*

Dr. Kenneth Cooper has developed a number of exercise programs for walking, walking/running, running, cycling and other activities. By participating in a program, aerobic points are accumulated to reach a weekly goal total. Programs have been devised based upon age and, more recently, based upon the results of a 12 minute test. A ranking is given based upon the distance covered by walking, jogging, and/or running during the time period. Programs are selected based upon the ranking achieved. Books authored by Dr. Cooper contain rankings and programs, and may be found in most libraries and bookstores. (See Appendix A, References.)

Walking Program G. *Reebok Walking Program*

Reebok has adopted walking and walking/running programs from *PALS — Personalized Aerobics Lifestyle System* developed by the Institute for Aerobic Research in Dallas, which was founded by Dr. Cooper. Information on this program may be obtained by writing the Cooper Institute for Aerobics Research at 12330 Preston Road, Dallas, Texas 75230.

Walking-Jogging Programs

Joan Ullyot, author of *Women's Running,* suggests that women begin with 10 minutes on Mondays, Wednesdays, Thursdays, 20 minutes on Saturday; and rest on Tuesday, Friday, and Sunday. Women in better shape and men should try for a mile of slow jogging. When tired, one should substitute walking and, after a while, try jogging again. Strive to increase jogging time until developing the capability of jogging the entire mile. Then continue to increase jogging distance until capable of jogging two miles.

Frank Rosato, author of *Jogging for Health and Fitness,* suggests walking for several weeks, followed by alternate walking and jogging for several weeks and, finally, slow jogging for the entire workout.

Bill Dellinger, author of *The Running Experience,* suggests working out six days a week using a step counting system. This involves alternating walking and jogging for a certain number of counts for 20 minutes on alternate days and walking only for 20 minutes on the other days. Each count represents 10 foot plants by the right foot. Beginning level would start with 10 counts of jogging alternating with 20 counts of walking. Jogging counts are gradually increased and then walking counts decreased until jogging for the entire 20 minutes is achieved. If more than 3 days are desired for aerobic exercise, he suggests brisk walking on alternate days for 20 minutes.

Jeff Galloway, author of *Galloway's Book on Running,* suggests starting by walking 30 minutes 3 or more times per week until it feels easy. Then increase the pace to brisk walking for the 30 minutes, attempting to push the heart rate into the training zone. Once this can be accomplished regularly, 3-4 short jogs of 100 or more yards can be inserted. Wait to insert the jogs until a good walking pace has been established. Amount and frequency of the jogs should then be increased until the entire 30 minutes is jogging. Some people are not interested in going beyond this level and choose to continue 30 minute jogging workouts with occasional walking breaks.

Dr. Kenneth Cooper has a number of programs involving jogging or running at different levels as discussed previously in the walking program section. Basically, Cooper advocates 15-30 minutes of walking, jogging, running, or other aerobic activities a minimum of three times per week. The pace does not have to be extremely fast or the distance long. On weekends instead of a long run, Cooper suggests participating in a vigorous aerobic type sport or stop and go activity such as racquetball, tennis, basketball or soccer.

Sample programs suggested by the authors follow:

Walking/Jogging Program A. *Sample Introductory Program*

Daily Plan for 3-6 Weekly Workouts		
(EW = Easy walk; BW = Brisk walk; J = Jog)		
Week	**Daily Workout (Minutes)**	**Total Minutes**
1	EW 5 - BW 5 - EW 5 - BW 5	20
2	EW 3 - BW 7 - EW 3 - BW 7	20
3	EW 1 - BW 9 - EW 1 - BW 9	20
4	BW 20	20
5	BW 8 - J 2 - BW 8 - J 2	20
6	BW 7 - J 3 - BW 7 - J 3	20
7	BW 6 - J 4 - BW 6 - J 4	20
8	BW 5 - J 5 - BW 5 - J 5	20

Walking/Jogging Program B. *Sample Beginner Program*

Daily Plan for 3-6 Weekly Workouts		
(BW = Brisk walk; J = Jog)		
Week	**Daily Workout (Minutes)**	**Total Minutes**
1	BW 5 - J 5 - BW 5 - J 5	20
2	BW 4 - J 6 - BW 4 - J 6	20
3	BW 3 - J 7 - BW 3 - J 7	20
4	BW 2 - J 8 - BW 2 - J 8	20
5	BW 1 - J 9 - BW 1 - J 9	20
6	J 10 - BW 1 - J 9	20
7	J 20	20
8	J 20 (pick up pace and cover more distance)	20

Advanced Beginner to Intermediate Level

As a person progresses out of the beginner level of a walking or jogging program he/she should plan to alternate hard and easy days or plan a day of rest after each workout day, and should increase weekly time or distance by not more than 10%. However, the jogging program usually changes from a time based to a mileage based program once a person can jog for the entire 20 to 30 minute workout time. To determine the mileage covered during the exercise time, the 20 to 30 minute jog should be performed on a marked trail or track. This distance is then used as a base for establishing a fitness program based upon mileage. To progress in the program, distance is regularly increased according to desired goals. These goals may be limited by time constraints of a personal daily schedule. Often at this stage, the number of workout days are increased in the program before or after the distance has been increased, not to exceed 6 days total.

Walking Programs

Using the Rockport walking program, once a particular level program has been completed, the walker can more on to another level program after retesting to determine the proper level or may follow a maintenance program.

Walking Program G. *Rockport Yellow Program*

Week	Warm-up	Mileage	Pace (mph)	Heart Rate (% Max)	Cool-down	Frequency (times/wk.)
1	5-7 mins. before-walk stretches	2.0	3.0	70	5-7 mins. after-walk stretches	5
2	5-7 mins.	2.25	3.0	70	5-7 mins.	5
3	5-7 mins.	2.5	3.0	70	5-7 mins.	5
4	5-7 mins.	2.5	3.0	70	5-7 mins.	5
5	5-7 mins.	2.75	3.0	70	5-7 mins.	5
6	5-7 mins.	2.75	3.5	70	5-7 mins.	5
7	5-7 mins.	2.75	3.5	70	5-7 mins.	5
8	5-7 mins.	2.75	3.5	70	5-7 mins.	5
9	5-7 mins.	3.0	3.5	70	5-7 mins.	5
10	5-7 mins.	3.0	3.5	70	5-7 mins.	5
11	5-7 mins.	3.0	4.0	70-80	5-7 mins.	5
12	5-7 mins.	3.0	4.0	70-80	5-7 mins.	5
13	5-7 mins.	3.25	4.0	70-80	5-7 mins.	5
14	5-7 mins.	3.25	4.0	70-80	5-7 mins.	5
15	5-7 mins.	3.5	4.0	70-80	5-7 mins.	5
16	5-7 mins.	3.5	4.5	70-80	5-7 mins.	5
17	5-7 mins.	3.5	4.5	70-80	5-7 mins.	5
18	5-7 mins.	4.0	4.5	70-80	5-7 mins.	5
19	5-7 mins.	4.0	4.5	70-80	5-7 mins.	5
20	5-7 mins.	4.0	4.5	70-80	5-7 mins.	5

Yellow Maintenance Program

Warm-up: 5-7 minutes before walk stretches
Aerobic Workout: mileage: 4.0 - pace: 4.5 mph
Heart Rate: 70-80% of maximum
Cool-down: 5-7 minutes after walk stretches
Frequency: 3-5 times per week
Weekly Mileage: 12-20 miles

Walking Program H. *Rockport Orange Program*

Week	Warm-up	Mileage	Pace (mph)	Incline/ Weight	Heart Rate (% Max)	Cool-down	Frequency (times/wk.)
1	5-7 mins. before-walk stretches	2.5	3.5		70	5-7 mins. after-walk stretches	5
2	5-7 mins.	2.75	3.5		70	5-7 mins.	5
3	5-7 mins.	3.0	3.5		70	5-7 mins.	5
4	5-7 mins.	3.0	3.5		70	5-7 mins.	5
5	5-7 mins.	3.25	3.5		70	5-7 mins.	5
6	5-7 mins.	3.5	4.0		70	5-7 mins.	5
7	5-7 mins.	3.5	4.0		70	5-7 mins.	5
8	5-7 mins.	3.75	4.0		70	5-7 mins.	5
9	5-7 mins.	4.0	4.0		70	5-7 mins.	5
10	5-7 mins.	4.0	4.0		70	5-7 mins.	5
11	5-7 mins.	4.0	4.0		70-80	5-7 mins.	5
12	5-7 mins.	4.0	4.0		70-80	5-7 mins.	5
13	5-7 mins.	4.0	4.0		70-80	5-7 mins.	5
14	5-7 mins.	4.0	4.0		70-80	5-7 mins.	5
15	5-7 mins.	4.0	4.0	+	70-80	5-7 mins.	5
16	5-7 mins.	4.0	4.0	+	70-80	5-7 mins.	5
17	5-7 mins.	4.0	4.0	+	70-80	5-7 mins.	5
18	5-7 mins.	4.0	4.0	+	70-80	5-7 mins.	5
19	5-7 mins.	4.0	4.0	+	70-80	5-7 mins.	5
20	5-7 mins.	4.0	4.0	+	70-80	5-7 mins.	5

Orange/Red Maintenance Program

Warm-up: 5-7 minutes before walk stretches

Aerobic Workout: mileage: 4.0; pace: 4.5 mph; weight/incline: add weights to upper body or add hill walking as needed to keep heart rate in target zone (70-80% of predicted maximum).

Heart Rate: 70-80% of maximum

Cool-down: 5-7 minutes after walk stretches

Frequency: 3-5 times per week

Weekly Mileage: 12-20 miles

Jogging Programs

Galloway suggests that time of the jogging program should increase from 30 to 40 minutes. Then increase one of the weekly sessions to 60 minutes.

In Dellinger's program described earlier, jogging is increased and walking is decreased during the count system days. Also, the 20 minute walking days begin to interject jogging. After 10 weeks the program should build to 20 minutes of jogging only each day. At that point a distance schedule is employed, striving to build hard and easy days to achieve a 20 mile week. Speed intervals may be interjected on the low distance (easy) days.

Jogging Program A. *Sample Advanced Beginner Jogging Program*

3 Day Workout Plan — Rest 1 Day Between Each Workout
4-5 Day Workout Plan — Eliminate 1 or 2 Rest Days and Repeat Day 2 or 3 at the End of the Week

Week	Daily Workout (Minutes)			
	Day 1	Day 2	Day 3	Day 4
1	20	20	20	
2	22	22	22	
3	24	24	24	
4	26	26	27	
5	28	28	27	
6	30	30	30	
7	30	30	30	10
8	30	30	30	20

Jogging Program B. *Sample Intermediate Jogging Program*

4 Day Workout Plan — Rest After Day 2 and Before and After Day 4
5 Day Workout Plan — Repeat Day 1 After Day 4

Week	Daily Workout (Mileage)			
	Day 1	Day 2	Day 3	Day 4
1	3	3	3	3
2	3	3	3	4
3	3	3	3	5
4	3	3	6	
5	3	4	3	6
6	3	5	3	6
7	3	5	3	7
8	3	6	3	8

High Intermediate to Advanced Level

If fitness is the only goal, program distance may stabilize and an increase in pace is used as the means to push the heart rate into the target heart zone or achieve overload. This increase in pace will progress a jogger to a runner and could progress a walker into using a racewalking technique.

Walking Programs

Walking Program I. *Rockport Walking Red Program*

Week	Warm-up	Mileage	Pace (mph)	Incline/ Weight	Heart Rate (% Max)	Cool- down	Frequency (times/wk.)
1	5-7 mins. before-walk stretches	3.0	3.5		70	5-7 mins. after-walk stretches	5
2	5-7 mins.	3.25	3.5		70	5-7 mins.	5
3	5-7 mins.	3.5	3.5		70	5-7 mins.	5
4	5-7 mins.	3.5	4.5		70-80	5-7 mins.	5
5	5-7 mins.	3.75	4.5		70-80	5-7 mins.	5
6	5-7 mins.	4.0	4.5		70-80	5-7 mins.	5
7	5-7 mins.	4.0	4.5	+	70-80	5-7 mins.	3
8	5-7 mins.	4.0	4.5	+	70-80	5-7 mins.	3
9	5-7 mins.	4.0	4.5	+	70-80	5-7 mins.	3
10	5-7 mins.	4.0	4.5	+	70-80	5-7 mins.	3
11	5-7 mins.	4.0	4.5	+	70-80	5-7 mins.	3
12	5-7 mins.	4.0	4.5	+	70-80	5-7 mins.	3
13	5-7 mins.	4.0	4.5	+	70-80	5-7 mins.	3
14	5-7 mins.	4.0	4.5	+	70-80	5-7 mins.	3
15	5-7 mins.	4.0	4.5	+	70-80	5-7 mins.	3
16	5-7 mins.	4.0	4.5	+	70-80	5-7 mins.	3
17	5-7 mins.	4.0	4.5	+	70-80	5-7 mins.	3
18	5-7 mins.	4.0	4.5	+	70-80	5-7 mins.	3
19	5-7 mins.	4.0	4.5	+	70-80	5-7 mins.	3
20	5-7 mins.	4.0	4.5	+	70-80	5-7 mins.	3

Orange/Red Maintenance Program

Warm-up: 5-7 minutes before walk stretches
Aerobic Workout: mileage: 4.0; pace: 4.5 mph; weight/incline: add weights to upper body or add hill walking as needed to keep heart rate in target zone (70-80% of predicted maximum).
Heart Rate: 70-80% of maximum
Cool-down: 5-7 minutes after walk stretches
Frequency: 3-5 times per week
Weekly Mileage: 12-20 miles

Previous programs used to advance a person from walking to jogging or beginning jogging can be employed by substituting jogging for walking and running for jogging in each program if 20 or 30 minutes is the goal workout time frame. Another suggested progression begins with 5 minutes of jogging, alternating with 1 minute of running (not sprinting or speed work), and continues by decreasing the jogging time by one minute and increasing the running time by one minute until the entire session is involved with running. Remember, this running involves a gradual increase of pace — not a sprint or speed work. A person changing from walking to a race-walking technique for fitness workouts may use the same increase plan for jogging to running by substituting walking for jogging and racewalking for running. If a person wishes to become a runner/racer or a racewalking/racer, then a competitive training program (to be discussed later in the chapter) must be followed.

Running Programs

Running Program A. *Joan Ullyot Intermediate Programs*

Sun	Mon	Tues	Wed	Thurs	Fri	Sat	Total
8	2	5	7	3	0	5	30 miles
12	3	5	10	5	0	5	40 miles

Running Program B. *Sample High Intermediate Program*

Week	Day 1	Day 2	Day 3	Day 4	Day 5
		Daily Mileage			
1		3 hills	6	3	8
2	2	3 hills	6	3	9
3	3	4 hills	6	4	9
4	4	4 hills	7	4	10
5	5	4 hills	8	4	11
6	5	4 hills	8	4	12
7	6	4 speed	8	4	12
8	6	4 speed	8	4	12

RUNNING AND RACEWALKING PROGRAMS FOR RACE COMPETITORS

Introduction to Running Programs

Many programs have been written in magazines and books about preparing for race competition and how to run faster at different race distances. The most common length of distance races are 5 (K) Kilometer (3.1 miles), 10 (K) Kilometer (6.2 miles), half marathon (13.1 miles), and the marathon (26.2 miles), although 5 miles and 15 (K) Kilometer (9.3 miles) are distances gaining in popularity.

Programs will vary depending on the race distance for which a person is training and the author. However, several similar underlying suggestions exist. First, alternate hard and easy days of training. Easy means working out at a comfortable pace and distance or taking the day off. Another alternative is to cross train using opposite muscles even if it is a hard workout. Never follow a long workout with a speed workout or vice versa. Do not increase by more than 10% weekly. On days when long, slow distance is involved, run 1 1/2 to 2 minutes slower than race pace. Include speed work or hill work, but not for more than 10% of the weekly mileage and only after a strong mileage base has been built. To train for longer distance races, mileage must be gradually increased and longer runs must be longer. The long training run should be longer than race distance. However, marathoners generally do not run 26 miles regularly. Running 26 miles or more once or twice before the marathon and scheduling long distance runs on alternate weeks is suggested. To build up mileage, competitors will often participate in two workouts a day.

Several competitive training programs will be discussed for possible adoption by the reader. For training suggestions to prepare for specific distance races, reference should be made to running magazines and running books.

Running Programs

Jeff Galloway's Training Pyramid

This training program takes four to six months to accomplish. Each phase of the program must be completed before moving on to the next phase. It can be used by a runner or racewalker attempting to peak for a particular race or striving to improve performance and fitness. The following pyramid diagram summarizes this training plan.

Base training for several months is extremely important to build a solid foundation. It is often difficult for racers to accept that long, steady

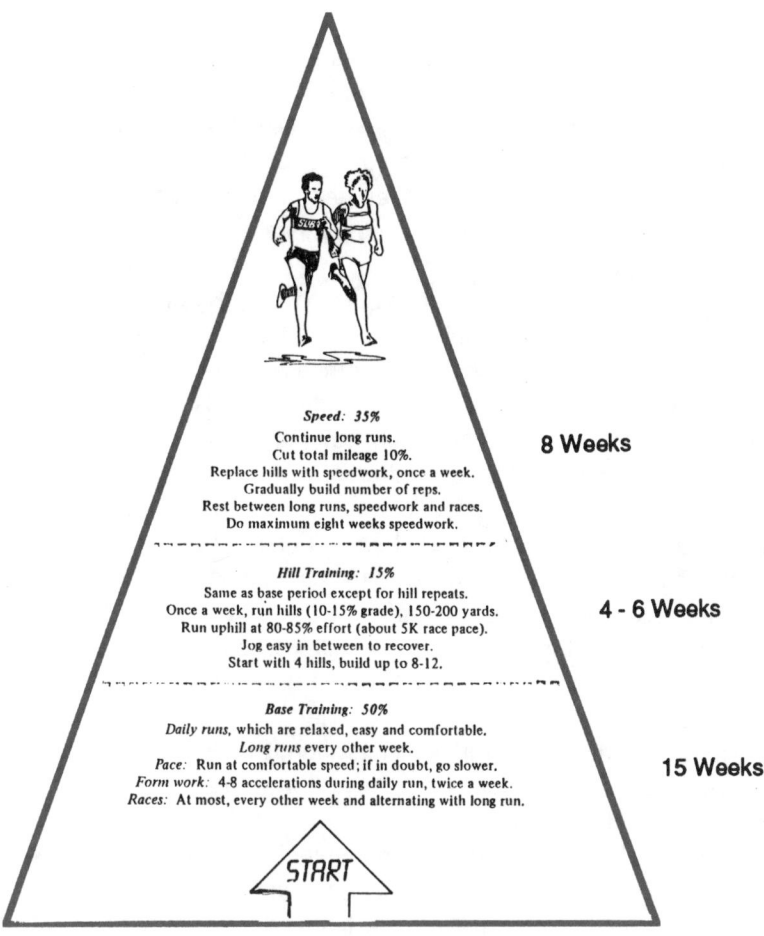

Speed: 35%
Continue long runs.
Cut total mileage 10%.
Replace hills with speedwork, once a week.
Gradually build number of reps.
Rest between long runs, speedwork and races.
Do maximum eight weeks speedwork.

8 Weeks

Hill Training: 15%
Same as base period except for hill repeats.
Once a week, run hills (10-15% grade), 150-200 yards.
Run uphill at 80-85% effort (about 5K race pace).
Jog easy in between to recover.
Start with 4 hills, build up to 8-12.

4 - 6 Weeks

Base Training: 50%
Daily runs, which are relaxed, easy and comfortable.
Long runs every other week.
Pace: Run at comfortable speed; if in doubt, go slower.
Form work: 4-8 accelerations during daily run, twice a week.
Races: At most, every other week and alternating with long run.

15 Weeks

START

Excerpted from *Galloway's Book on Running,* © 1983 by Jeff Galloway. $8.95 Shelter Publications, Inc., P.O. Box 279, Bolinas, CA 94924. Distributed in bookstores by Random House. Reprinted by permission.

workouts will help improve speed. During this time period the distance of normal daily runs can be maintained. These daily workout sessions should be at a comfortable, relaxed pace with form work accelerations inserted during two of the days. These accelerations should begin after a minimum 10 minutes of steady running. Strive to accelerate to one mile race pace for 100-200 yards while employing good form as described in Chapter Three. Start with 4 accelerations and increase to 8 per session. It is important to recover between each acceleration by continuing with the comfortable, relaxed pace.

Long workouts are the key to base training. After determining the longest workout of the past three weeks, start with that distance and schedule a long workout weekly increasing the distance by 1 mile per week to 12 miles. At that point, long workouts should be scheduled every two weeks with an increase of two miles each session to allow the body to recover between sessions. The biggest mistake in distance training is to schedule long distance workouts every week which builds up a residual tiredness. Suggested long distance buildup for 10K racers is 16 miles and for marathoners 20 miles at this phase of training. Races should be limited at this time to alternate weeks from distance workouts and preferably once a month. A full race effort should not be attempted. A race pace of halfway between normal race pace and daily training pace is suggested.

Hill training should be added next to the training schedule for 4-6 weeks to build strength needed for speed work. Improvement in strength will be realized in the quadriceps, hamstrings, and calf muscles. Working out on hills should be inserted in the existing training program once a week, preferably midweek, if distance training is on the weekends. This allows for recovery between long workouts and hill workouts. Choose a moderate grade hill of approximately 10-15% which rises 1 foot in 15 and no more than 1 foot in 10, and is 150-200 yards in length. The uphill workout should be at an 85% maximum effort, which is slightly faster than 10K race pace. The downhill should be a slow recovery effort with additional recovery distance on the flat, if needed, before the next uphill effort. A starting level of four hills should be increased by one a week to 8-12 hills. While working out on hills, keep posture erect. Don't be tempted to lean forward uphill or backward downhill. Shorten stride and keep relaxed breathing going uphill; lengthen stride only slightly and let gravity do the work going downhill.

Speed training should begin only after base training and hill training have been completed, and should continue for only 8 weeks. This is important to prevent injury. It will replace hill training in the workout schedule and allow the long workout to continue on alternate weeks. The purpose of this training is to pace faster and improve racing times. Beginners and those without a time improvement goal should not include speed work in their program. After 8 weeks, speed work should be discontinued and a new pyramid cycle begun.

The primary **speed work** benefit is to teach the body to work out anaerobically. Generally, participants in speed work have reduced times in all race distances. Various coaches and exercise physiologists have developed plans for speed work. Most running coaches caution that no more than 5-10% of weekly training should be speed work. Speed work should be incorporated slowly and the intensity and duration should increase gradually over time in order to prevent injury. Refer to magazines and books for suggestions. The common types of speed training are Fartleks, or speed play, and different types of intervals.

Fartleks involve faster than race pace accelerations interspersed with endurance pacing. They should be started only after 10 or more minutes of easy pacing. The accelerations are of varying distances by the choice of the individual and can be playful in nature. Other variations are hill Fartleks or timed segments. Hill Fartleks involve a starting pace of one minute slower than 10K race pace followed by a series of faster than race pace accelerations up and over hills with recovery easy pacing. Timed segments involve faster than race pace accelerations that are timed for one, two, three or more minutes followed by recovery easy pacing. The number of accelerations in any type of Fartlek is up to individual preference.

Intervals involve speed repetitions at a specific distance such as 440 yards, 880 yards, or mile. Common distance for 10K training is 440 yards or 400 meters. However, the distance can increase or decrease according to the race distance goal. Repetitions should be faster than race pace but not all-out, and be followed by slow pacing recoveries of equal distance, or less if recovery time is less. 440 yards should be run 5-7 seconds faster than goal pace; 880 yards, 10 seconds faster; and one miler, 15-20 seconds faster. Goal pace is determined by the pace which will lead to achieving goal time for a desired race distance. In the first session repetitions should be few, but increase each week striving to reach 20. It is important to warm up sufficiently before starting the repetitions. Galloway suggests walking 5-10 minutes, slow pacing 10-20 minutes, and then a stretching session. Next perform 5-10 accelerations of 100-200 yards and slow pace down for 3-5 minutes. Afterward, take time to finish with a slow pace for 10 minutes followed by 15-20 minutes of gradually slower walking. Plan to workout easily for two days following speed training to provide rest and recuperation.

Racers who follow Galloway's pyramid can expect to improve 20-40 seconds if current 10K time is 32-35 minutes, or as much as 3-5 minutes if 10K time is above 50 minutes. Faster marathoners may improve 2-5 minutes and 4:30 marathoners may improve up to 30 minutes.

A sample 10K training schedule which follows the Galloway Training Pyramid is shown next. Goal times for hill and speed work depends on current race pace of the individual. As race pace potential increases the distance scheduled, on days other than speed and hill work days, should increase.

PROGRAM
10K GOAL: 45 MIN.

BASE TRAINING builds endurance.

Week Number	Mon	Tue (Form)	Wed	Thur (Form)	Fri	Sat	Sun (Longer runs)
1–14.	0–2 mi.	5–6	0–2	5–6	0–2	0	Starting with longest run in last 2 weeks, increase 1 mile per week up to 12.

HILL TRAINING develops leg strength

Week Number	Mon	Tue (Form)	Wed	Thur (Form)	Fri	Sat	Sun
15	0–2 mi.	5 (Hills)	0–4	5–6	0–2	0	12
16 easy	0–2	6 (Hills)	0–2	5–6	0–2	0	6
17	0–2	7–8 (Hills)	0–4	5–6	0–2	0	12
18	0–2	8–10 (Hills)	0–4	5–6	0–2	0	6
19	0–2	5–6 (Hills)	0–4	4–6	0–2	0	13
20 easy	0–2	4 (Hills)	0–2	4–6	0–2	0	6
21	0–2	5–6 (Hills)	0–4	4–6	0–2	0	14
22	0–2	5–6 (Hills)	0–4	6–7	0–2	0	6–7

SPEEDWORK trains you to run faster

Week Number	Mon	Tue (Form)	Wed	Thur (Form)	Fri	Sat	Sun
23	0–2 mi.	8×440 @1:42	0–4	4–6	0–2	0	15
24 easy	0–2	10×440 @1:42	0–2	4–6	0	5k	6–8
25	0–2	12×440 @1:42	0–4	5–7	0–2	0	15
26	0–2	14×440 @1:42	0–4	6–7	0	10k race	6–8
27	0–2	16×440 @1:42	0–4	5	0–2	0	15
28 easy	0–2	18×440 @1:42	0–2	4–6	0–2	0	6–8
29	0–2	20×440 @1:42	0–4	5–6	0	5k race	15
30	0–2	6–8×440 @1:40	0–4	4–6	0	10k dry run	6–8
31	0–2	7×440 @1:40	0–2	4–6	0	5k race	12–14
32	0–2	7×440 @1:40	0–2	4–6	0	10k goal race	

Excerpted from *Galloway's Book on Running* © 1983 by Jeff Galloway. $8.95 Shelter Publications, Inc., P.O. Box 279, Bolinas, CA 94924. Distributed in bookstores by Random House. Reprinted by permission.

Lydiard's Training Program

World famous coach Arthur Lydiard, from New Zealand, is a strong proponent of hill training combined with anaerobic work. After building a high mileage base, he advocates including a tortuous hill and anaerobic workout in the training program. Each hill workout involves 4 cycles. Each cycle involves running hard up a 1/2 mile hill, jogging 4-5 minutes (approximately 1/2 mile) at the top for recovery, then running a fast but relaxed downhill pace. At the bottom, resume jogging for a short distance for recovery, then begin a series of sprints 3 x 220 yard or 6 x 50 yards. Each sprint should be followed by an equal distance of jogging recovery. It takes a strong runner to complete 4 cycles with few runners making it past two. Lydiard's hill training also includes springing drills in order to develop ankle power and flexion. He recommends bouncing up less steep hills on one's toes. Be cautious when trying these drills, since they can result in injury. The outstanding runners from Kenya conduct most of their training on hilly terrain rather than special hill workouts. This produces powerful quadriceps and improves running economy. Hill training has not been commonly used by racewalkers.

Benson's Training Program

Roy Benson is a long-time runner, coach, and exercise physiologist. He advocates three components of training to improve performance in running or walking. These components are endurance, stamina, and speed work. **Endurance training** is aerobic and performed at a level 70% of maximum or approximately 1 1/2 - 2 1/2 minutes per mile slower than 10K race pace. This is important to increase the distance that can be covered before fatigue sets in. Once endurance has been built, at least one run per week should be increased to 2-3 miles longer than race distance.

Stamina training will help the competitor maintain race pace through-out a race. This type of training improves the circulatory system by increasing the number of capillaries throughout the muscles, resulting in an increase of energy. Stamina work is performed at 85% of maximum which involves a workout hard enough to reach anaerobic threshold or slightly into oxygen debt. This pace would be 20-25% slower than 10K race pace and must be maintained for one-half to two-thirds of the goal race distance. Stamina workouts should be preceded and followed by easy days of endurance training.

The third component, **speed work**, is performed 15-20% faster than 10K race pace or 90-95% of max. This type of training develops an individual's maximum oxygen uptake. The suggested distance is 440 yards. Start with 8-10 440s and increase to 10-12 involving a recuperation jog of equal distance between each effort. A suggested training program is shown below:

Sun	Mon	Tues	Wed	Thurs	Fri	Sat
10-12 miles endurance	2-4 miles endurance	Speed	2-4 miles endurance fast down	Hills easy up	2-4 miles endurance or race	2-4 mi. stamina
A day of rest may be substituted for Friday or Thursday if such an intense schedule is not desirable.						

Costill's Program

David Costill is one of the foremost researchers in exercise physiology. As a result of his research, he advocates using three types of interval training: aerobic, aerobic-anaerobic, and anaerobic.

Aerobic intervals involve faster paced workouts (5-6 seconds per minute slower than 10K race pace) with short rest periods (10-15 seconds) in between to receive the same benefits as a long easy paced workout. Twenty repetitions of a 400 meter distance is the suggested goal.

Aerobic-anaerobic interval training is designed to develop the leg muscles to race fast. These intervals involve race-pace speed workouts with medium rest periods of 60-90 seconds following each interval. Ten repetitions of a 400 meter distance is the suggested goal.

Finally, **anaerobic intervals** performed faster than race pace are suggested to improve leg strength and improve ability to remove lactate from the muscles. These are similar to intervals discussed previously in the chapter. Ten repetitions of a 200 meter distance with two minutes rest in between is the suggested goal.

Daniels' Program

Jack Daniels is a former Olympic medal winner in the modern pentathlon event and is currently coaching at the State University of New York at Cortland. Through years of coaching and research he has devised a threshold-pace training system which is individualized according to a person's fitness level. This training does not exceed 90% of the maximum pulse rate and the pace pushes a person just short of the level at which lactic acid build-up in the blood accelerates. Therefore, a person will improve his/her pace and recuperation will be quicker. The chart on the opposite page indicates the threshold pace based upon current 5K or 10K times. This pace can be changed every three weeks as 5K or 10K times improve. The chart may be used as a guide or the pace can be increased by 4 seconds per mile every 3 weeks.

THRESHOLD-PACE CHART

Fitness Level		Threshold Pace Per		
5-K	10-K	880	1320	Mile
27:00	56:03	4:41	7:02	9:22
25:12	52:17	4:23	6:35	8:46
24:08	50:03	4:13	6:04	8:26
23:09	48:01	4:03	6:04	8:06
22:15	46:09	3:53	5:50	7:47
21:25	44:25	3:45	5:38	7:30
20:39	42:50	3:37	5:26	7:15
19:57	41:21	3:30	5:15	7:00
19:17	39:59	3:24	5:06	6:48
18:40	38:42	3:18	4:57	6:36
18:05	37:31	3:12	4:48	6:24
17:33	36:24	3:07	4:40	6:13
17:03	35:22	3:01	4:32	6:03
16:34	34:23	2:56	4:25	5:53
16:07	33:28	2:52	4:18	5:44
15:42	32:35	2:48	4:12	5:36
15:18	31:46	2:44	4:06	5:28
14:55	31:00	2:40	4:00	5:20
14:33	30:16	2:37	3:55	5:14
14:13	29:34	2:33	3:50	5:07
13:54	28:55	2:30	3:45	5:00
13:35	28:17	2:27	3:40	4:53
13:18	27:41	2:24	3:36	4:48
13:01	27:07	2:21	3:32	4:42

"Cruise Control" by Jack Daniels from *Runner's World*, June, 1990, Volume 25, Number 6, pp. 80 and 82. Reprinted with permission of *Runner's World*.

Several alternatives are available for determining threshold pace. One is to work out 10-15 seconds slower than 10K race pace. Another is to use a heart rate monitor set to work out at 85-92% of maximum heart rate provided an accurate maximum heart rate has been determined. The latest suggestion by Daniels is to use breathing rate to establish threshold pace. For most people, a breathing rate of 2-2 (2 steps while breathing in and 2 steps while breathing out), 2-3, or 3-2 indicates threshold pace. To determine one's threshold breathing rate, do a workout at 10-15 seconds lower than 10K pace and monitor the breathing pattern.

Three types of **lactate threshold-pace workouts** are tempo runs, cruise intervals and cruise repetitions. **Tempo runs** involve 20 minutes at threshold pace during a workout. It is suggested that tempo running should be preceded by a warm-up run of one to two miles and a warm-down run of two miles. Since the threshold pace is individualized, a person should run alone and not be tempted to increase pace. The only variance to the threshold pace would be the adjustment necessary for hills, wind, and heat.

Cruise intervals involve threshold-pace running in segments with 30-60 second recovery jogs. These intervals should be preceded by a one to two mile warm-up and followed by a warm-down run. The distance should not exceed 8% of the weekly mileage and cruise intervals are generally performed once a week. The example on the next page can serve as a guide.

A **cruise repetition** workout is similar to a cruise interval workout, but involves a full recovery after each run of 880 yards, 1320 yards, or 1 mile. Three or four repetitions are sufficient and may be performed early the week preceding a race to provide quality training without undue stress.

For **intense workouts to improve speed,** Daniels advocates three types of workouts. These workouts can be alternated each time the training schedule indicates an intensity session, or a portion of each can be combined in one workout. Another possibility would be for a person to concentrate on one type of workout for several weeks, then switch to another type which may help a competitor peak for longer periods of time. The first type is **intervals** for 2-3 minutes at 5K race pace with equal recovery time between each set. The second type is **repetitions** which involves working out with 20-400 meter repetitions at a pace of 5 seconds faster per 400 meters than 5K race. Long recoveries should follow each repetition. The third workout is a **lactate threshold "tempo" workout** discussed previously.

Cruisin' For a PR (Personal Record)

A successful cruise-interval workout must meet *your* pace needs only. Below you'll find workouts for three runners of very different abilities and training levels.

As different as these runners are, all three will find that they'll feel better if they do four to five strides (not sprints) of 100 to 220 yards after the last cruise interval. Strides should be run just a little faster than cruise-interval pace, with complete recovery between them. — J.D.

Runner A

Current 10-K time: 46:00

Current training: 20 miles/week

Cruise-interval pace (from chart): 7:45/mile

Workout: Warm up, then run 3 x 880 in 3:52, with 30- to 60-second recovery jogs. Warm down.

Runner B

Current 10-K time: 40:00

Current training: 40 miles/week

Cruise interval pace (from chart): 6:48/mile

Workout: Warm up, then run 4 x 1320 yards in 5:06, with 60-second recovery jogs. Warm down.

Runner C

Current 10-K time: 34:00

Current training: 60 miles/week

Cruise-interval pace (from chart): 5:50/mile

Workout: Warm up, then run 5 x 1 mile in 5:50, with 60-second recovery jogs. Warm down.

"Cruise Control" by Jack Daniels from *Runner's World,* June 1990, Volume 25, Number 6, pp. 80 and 82. Reprinted with permission of *Runner's World.*

Heart Rate Monitor Training

Training with heart rate monitors is the latest trend. Styles of heart rate monitors are now more compact and comfortable to wear both training and racing. They are used by fitness walkers and joggers, as well as competitors. These monitors provide accurate monitoring of one's pulse and can be set for the desirable training or racing heart rate range. If one's heart rate deviates either higher or lower than the desired range, the monitor will provide a signal. In addition, higher tech models provide a recall and even a computer printout of heart rates at various times or mile markers during training or races.

The training zones suggested are a specific percentage of one's maximum heart rate and exercise programs often contain workouts in a variety of zones. The basic training zones are as follows:

Fitness

Moderate Zone:	50-60%
Weight Management (fat burning) Zone:	60-70%
Aerobic Zone:	70-80%

Competitive

Anaerobic Threshold Zone:	80-90%
Red (speedwork) Zone:	90-100%

Several books have been written which act as a guide to training with a heart rate monitor to achieve personal goals. *The Heart Rate Monitor Book* by Sally Edwards is a comprehensive guide. Roy Benson's *Precision Running with Your Polar Electronic Heart Rate Monitor* provides guidance in the use of a heart rate monitor to follow his training program for competitors which was described earlier. *Target Your Fitness and Weight Management Goals* by James M. Rippe focuses on designing a fitness or weight control program assisted by a heart rate monitor. Refer to these books for assistance in developing a personal program using a heart rate monitor.

Miscellaneous Training Ideas

1. To boost VO_2 Max, do a 10-15 minute jog, then pick up the pace to 87% of the maximum heart rate. After settling in to that pace, accelerate to 90-95% for 2 minutes or more. When fatigue sets in, back down to 87% until comfortable, then accelerate again to 90-95% for two minutes. Continue alternating speeds for at least 15 minutes. With each workout of this type, increase the total time until the workout lasts for 30 minutes.

2. In addition to running or racewalking, training on an exercise cycle has proven to increase VO_2 Max and improve race times. Cycling workouts for up to 50 minutes at 80% of maximal heart rate provides moderate race improvement. However, workout intensities of 80-85% or 90-95% provide as much as 15% increase in VO_2 Max. Cycling intervals at 95-100% for 30-60 seconds (while standing up), for five minutes (while seated), for

a combination of three 150 seconds and six 75 second intervals with alternating rest periods of the same time as the workout, have resulted in dramatic race time improvements.

3. Hill workouts have been described in this chapter and in Chapter 3. Research indicates that working out on hills helps leg muscles resist soreness and helps to prevent a loss in fitness when training must be reduced. In order to race faster on hills, training on hills is important. Generally, for 10K races or shorter, less steep hills of 100-200 yards with no more than 20% grade are suggested. Hills on a golf course or softer surface are ideal. After warming up, start with 4 uphill repeats at 10K pace with a downhill jog recovery and increase weekly toward 8-12 repeats. For longer distance racers, such as marathoners, longer hills of up to a mile are preferred. After warm-up, run one uphill repeat at marathon pace with downhill jog recovery and increase weekly toward 4 repeats. Concentrate on form when running uphill by focusing on knee lift, arm swing, and breathing.

Downhill running can help to quicken pace by working on leg turnover and stride length. Be cautious with overstriding which can cause shin splints. After warm-up, run five to ten 100-400 meter downhill repeats, thinking of quick leg action rather than a sprint. Recover by jogging uphill.

Another variation of hill training is to combine uphill and downhill work. Concentrate on form uphill and quickness downhill building to a series of 5-10 series repeats. Always warm up and stretch before all uphill, downhill, or combination workouts and follow the workout with a cool-down jog and stretch.

4. 15K races provide better preparation for 10K races than running 10-12 mile training runs.

5. Run as often as possible on soft surfaces such as grass or trails to reduce pounding and the risk of injury.

Long Distance Racing

Often after a series of 10K races has been conquered, runners are intrigued by the challenge of participating in a half-marathon and ultimately a marathon. The key to preparing for a longer distance race is to increase the distance of the long training run to race mileage or beyond. For many years coaches and runners advocated high weekly mileage training including a weekly long distance run. Often a breakdown of the body and injuries were the result. The beginning marathoner often trains by increasing his/her weekly mileage and including a long run of not more than 15-20 miles. This often results in "hitting the wall" or struggling during the last 10K of the marathon generally due to insufficient training and/or a complete depletion of muscle glycogen.

More recently Galloway, Tom Osler, author of the *Serious Runner's Handbook,* plus Joe Henderson and other *Runner's World* editors advocate a more sensible approach which works and results in fewer injuries. A runner can continue his/her current training program and increase the long run gradually by increments of 1-2 miles every 14 days. Long run increase goals for a half-marathon would be 13-14 miles and for a marathon would be 26-28 miles. This long training run should be scheduled for alternate weeks, not weekly. Once the long run reaches 18 miles, an increase every third week for the long run should be considered. A runner may want to decrease the weekly mileage while increasing the long run to provide for recovery. A marathon training program can begin with a current training schedule of as little as 5 days of 30 minutes per day and a long run of an hour. Strength training should also be included.

A beginning half-marathoner and marathoner should concentrate on the training program and a goal of finishing. Hill work is not necessary unless the target race is on a hilly course. Speed work is not essential; occasional pickups during training runs are sufficient. Racing in occasional shorter races while training is not essential but can help with lactate threshold training. It is desirable to be rested before attempting the long training run. To help the capability of participating in a long distance training run and increasing the mileage more rapidly, Osler suggests walking for 5 minutes every half hour. Galloway suggests running the long run very slowly (2 minuts slower than you could run on that day) and taking walk breaks of 1-2 minutes every 2-8 minutes. The pace of the long run should be slow, 1.5 to 2 minutes slower than 10K race pace. The distance of the long run should be continuous, not split into a morning and evening run, in order for the body to adjust to the stress of the desired race distance.

For an experienced half-marathoner or marathoner who has established a good training base and wishes to decrease his/her race time, several weeks of hill work may precede increasing the long run to over 12 miles. If the race course is hilly, occasional hill workouts should be continued. For half-marathoners the long run goal should be 16+ miles. Marathoners should build up to long runs of 20+ miles and include at least one 26 mile training run. To reduce fatigue and injury possibilities, no more than 6 runs of 20+ is suggested.

Weekly speed work is important for marathon training, preferably mile repeats or intersperse a series of 20 second accelerations at 5K race pace in the middle of longer workouts. Another speed workout called "Yasso 800s" by Amby Burfoot has been successful at helping marathoners reach goal times. After determining a realistic marathon goal, start running a series of four 800 meter runs in minute/second equivalents of marathon goal time two months before the marathon. For example, if the marathon goal is 4 hours, run the 800 meters in 4 minutes. If the marathon goal is 3 hours and 30 minutes, run the 800 meters in 3 minutes and 30 seconds. Jog for an equivalent time between each 800 and increase by one 800 each week until reaching the goal of 10 fourteen to seventeen days before the marathon. Amby polled 100 marathoners and found that these equivalent 800s correlated to marathon times.

Lactate threshold workouts are essential in order to improve marathon times. Some runners use 5K and 10K races for threshold training. Owen Anderson, editor of *Running Research News,* reports that research indicates the last two months before the marathon one to two times per week is ideal for building lactate threshold running speed (LTRS). Marathoners should use a mixture of the following workouts:

(a) Run two 10-minute repeats at current 10K pace and jog easy for 4-6 minutes between. This pace is faster than LTRS.

(b) Do steady 25-minute runs at a pace 12 seconds per mile slower than current 10K pace. This pace approximates LTRS.

(c) Do 6 mile runs at a pace about 24 seconds per mile slower than current 10K pace. This pace is slightly lower than LTRS.

(d) Run 8-10 miles at a pace about 35 seconds per mile slower than current 10K pace. This pace is approximately marathon pace.

Good nutrition while training for a marathon is essential. A diet of 65% carbohydrates for an energy boost and 15% protein to assist with repair is suggested. Be certain to eat and hydrate before and during long workouts. It is also important to replenish glycogen stores within 15 minutes after a long run by consuming a high carbohydrate drink or fruit juice.

Rest and recovery days are important during marathon training in order to allow healing of microscopic damage to muscles and connective tissues as a result of increased mileage and vigorous training. Forty-eight hours of rest can provide recovery and reduce the risk of overtraining injuries. Galloway suggests completing goal training mileage in fewer days by running more miles on workout days. Consider chilling out for 10 minutes after a long run by soaking legs in cold water, using ice massage, ice packs, or hosing legs with cold water to help constrict blood vessels and muscle tissues and assist with recuperation. Extra sleep can also be helpful to the marathoner in training. Sleep should not be sacrificed for extra mileage.

Whether a novice or experienced marathoner, it is important to taper prior to the big race by running the last 20+ mile run no less than three weeks prior to the race and decreasing other training runs. It is important to keep the same intensity while cutting back on mileage. Cut back by 75% three weeks away. Cut back to 50% two weeks away with the maximum run no more than 12 miles. During the last week cut back to 30%, eliminate hard training and run on soft surfaces. In the last three days, run two days and rest one while stretching frequently. *Running Research News* suggests a stair step tapering plan for a month prior to the marathon, reducing by 80%, 60%, 45%, and 30%.

If the race course is hilly the occasional hill workout must be program and speed work or a race may be inserted during the off week from the long run. Whether a novice or experienced marathoner, it is important to taper prior to the big race by running the last long run no less than two weeks prior to the race and decreasing other training runs. The last 26+ mile run should be no closer than 21 days prior to a marathon. Take at least one or two days off prior to the event. After the race, walk at least 10 minutes and in the days following remember to rest 1 day for each mile of the race. Rest may involve walking and jogging the distance of a normal workout, waiting 10 or more days to run 12-14 miles and 21 days for a 20+ run, and not participating in a strenuous speed workout or race.

The authors suggest race preparation in the last one to two weeks before the marathon:

1. Set your biological clock by going to bed and awakening at times planned for marathon day.
2. Begin training runs at the starting time of the marathon.
3. Eat and drink in the evening, before, and during workouts as you would the night prior to and the morning of the marathon.
4. Drink the same electrolyte fluid that will be supplied at the marathon to test the reaction of your stomach.
5. Load up on carbohydrates, preferably liquid, for 6-7 days prior to the marathon to help glycogen reserves and hydration.
6. Plan race pace times and write them on a small card to carry with you. Consider using Greg Myers Pace Goal for four segments of the marathon. Multiply each number by your projected finish time in seconds in order to determine pace per mile: 9-12 miles (3.756); 12-18 miles (3.8086); 18-23 miles (3.8725); and 23-26 miles (3.950).

During the marathon, Galloway suggests taking walking breaks every mile starting with the first mile; advanced runners may want to fast shuffle instead of walking. These breaks will keep the muscles resilient. At 18-20 miles experienced marathoners should be able to eliminate the breaks, pick up the pace and run in with negative splits.

After the race, walk at least 10 minutes and in the days following remember to rest one day for each mile of the race. Rest may involve walking and jogging the distance of a normal workout, waiting 10 or more days to run 12-14 miles and 21 days for a 20+ run, and not participating in a strenuous speed workout or race. In order to recuperate adequately and reduce the risk of injury, Bill Rodgers and Priscilla Welch suggest that marathoners under age 40 eliminate hard training or racing one day for each mile and that marathoners age 40 or over eliminate hard training or racing one day for each kilometer.

Sample Half-Marathon/Marathon Training Programs

(Note: Half-marathoners can follow these programs, but would not increase mileage beyond 16 for long run.)

Marathon Goal: 4 Hours

BASE TRAINING builds endurance.

Week Number	Mon	Tue (Form)	Wed	Thur (Form)	Fri	Sat	Sun (Longer runs)
1–15	0–2 mi.	4	0–2	4	1–2	0	Starting with longest run in last 2 weeks, increase 1 mile per week up to 12.

HILL TRAINING develops leg strength

Week Number	Mon	Tue	Wed	Thur (Form)	Fri	Sat	Sun
16	0–2 mi.	4–5	0–2	4–5	1–2	0	4 (Hills)
17	0–2	4–5	0–2	4–5	1–2	0	14
18	0	3	0	4	1	0	6 (Hills)

SPEEDWORK trains you to run faster

Week Number	Mon	Tue (Form)	Wed	Thur (Form)	Fri	Sat	Sun
19	1–2 mi.	2–3	1–3	4–5	1–2	0	16
20 easy	0	2–3	0–2	3–6	1–2	0	2×1 mile @8½ min.
21	1–3	4–5	0–2	4–5	1–2	0	18
22	0–2	2–3	1–3	4–6	1–2	0	4×1 @8½
23	1–3	4–5	0–2	4–5	1–2	0	20
24 easy	0	2–3	0–2	3–6	1–2	0	6×1 @8½
25	1–3	3–6	1–3	4–6	1–3	0	22
26	1–3	3–6	1–3	4–6	1–3	0	10k race in 50–54 min.
27	1–3	4–6	1–3	4–6	1–3	0	24
28 easy	0	2–3	0–2	3–6	1–2	0	10k race in 48–52 min.
29	1–3	4–6	1–3	4–6	1–3	0	26
30	1–3	4–6	1–3	4–6	1–3	0	10k race in 46–50 min.
31	0–2	2–3	0–2	3–6	1–2	0	12 easy
32	0	2–3	0	3–6	1–2	0	Marathon!

Excerpted from *Galloway's Book on Running* © 1983 by Jeff Galloway. $8.95 Shelter Publications, Inc., P.O. Box 279, Bolinas, CA 94924. Distributed in bookstores by Random House. Reprinted by permission.

Program

Marathon Goal: To finish

Week Number	Mon	Tue (Form)	Wed	Thur (Form)	Fri	Sat	Sun
1	0–2 m.	2	0–2	2	0–2	0	2
2	0–2	2	0–2	2	0–2	0	3
3	0–2	2	0–2	3	0–2	0	4
4 easy	0	3	0	2	0	0	4
5	3	0–2	4	0–2	3	0	5
6	0–2	3	0–2	4	0–2	0	6
7	4	0–2	3	0–2	4	0	7
8 easy	0	4	0	3	0	0	8
9	4	0–2	3	0–2	4	0	9
10	0–2	4	0–2	4	0–2	0	10
11	4	0–2	4	0–2	4	0	11
12 easy	0	4	0	4	0	0	6
13	4	0–2	4	0–2	4	0	12
14	0–2	4	0–2	4	0–2	0	6
15	4	0–2	4	0–2	4	0	14
16 easy	0	4	0	4	0	0	7
17	4	0–2	4	0–2	4	0	16
18	0–2	4	0–2	4	0–2	0	8
19	4	0–2	4	0–2	4	0	18
20 easy	0	4	0	4	0	0	9
21	4	0–2	4	0–2	4	0	20
22	0–2	4	0–2	4	0–2	0	10
23	4	0–2	4	0–2	4	0	22
24 easy	0	4	0	4	0	0	11
25	4	0–2	4	0–2	4	0	24
26	0–2	4	0–2	4	2	0	12
27	4	0–2	4	0–2	2	0	26
28 easy	0	4	0	4	0	0	13
29	4	0–2	4	0–2	4	0	12 easy or 5k race
30	0	4	0	2	1	0	Marathon!

This program is not designed for speed, but for finishing a marathon comfortably and with reduced injury risk. Hence there will be no hills or speedwork in your training program. Thousands of runners have followed this program and successfully completed marathons. As you can see, it's quite a bit different from other marathon training schedules; the unique features are the low daily mileage and the long run every other week.

Shown here is a 30 week program. This assumes that your current long run is 2 miles. If your long run is longer than this, start with the week that has your current long run in it.

Excerpted from *Galloway's Book on Running* © 1983 by Jeff Galloway. $8.95 Shelter Publications, Inc., P.O. Box 279, Bolinas, CA 94924. Distributed in bookstores by Random House. Reprinted by permission.

Prediction Time Chart for Half-Marathon and Marathon

10-K Time	1/2 Marathon Time	Predicted Marathon
30 min. *	1:07	2:20
31 min.	1:09	2:25
32 min.	1:11	2:29
33 min.	1:14	2:34
34 min.	1:16	2:38
35 min.	1:18	2:43
36 min.	1:20	2:48
37 min.	1:23	2:53
38 min.	1:25	2:57
39 min.	1:27	3:02
40 min.	1:29	3:07
41 min.	1:31	3:11
42 min.	1:34	3:16
43 min.	1:36	3:20
44 min.	1:38	3:25
45 min.	1:40	3:30
46 min.	1:43	3:34
47 min.	1:45	3:39
48 min.	1:47	3:43
49 min.	1:49	3:48
50 min.	1:51	3:53
51 min.	1:54	3:57
52 min.	1:56	4:02

* all times rounded to nearest minute

"Predicting your time chart," *Training Smart,* p. 38. Reprinted by permission.

Racewalking Programs

According to racewalking expert Henry Laskau, racewalking training is similar to training for running. Racewalkers training for longer races must include longer training walks. Speed work is important to improve racewalking times, but hill work is not suggested. Downhill racewalking may be included as a type of speed work to train the legs to move faster.

General Information for Program Development

Research indicates that intervals can also increase the ventilation (lactate) threshold. This threshold is the rate of oxygen consumption above which lactic acid begins a dramatic increase, which in essence will postpone the onset of fatigue. Some researchers claim speed work will increase VO2 max while others claim long workouts will cause the increase. Incorporation of both in a program appears to be the solution.

Many programs involve working out at a certain percentage of max which refers to VO_2 max. Computing VO_2 was outlined in Chapter Three. To determine pace for the workout, first multiply the desired percentage by the VO_2 max. Then add 5.24 to the result and divide that result into 329 to arrive at the workout pace.

$$\frac{329}{(\% \times VO_2 max) + 5.24} = \text{Workout Pace}$$

A variety of paces are suggested for speed workouts. The programs discussed previously have recommended including several types of speed workouts with different goals paced in an individual's training schedule. Many writers support 90% max for speed training segments over one minute and max speed for segments less than one minute. Recommendations for the number of weeks to include speed workouts in one's training schedule vary from 7 to 14 weeks. Although more improvement is seen in the first 7 weeks, those who participate in speed workouts for more weeks show greater overall improvement. Some writers suggest more intense workouts for 10K distance or less should be limited to 8 weeks, while less strenuous marathon speed work may continue through 12-14 weeks. Number of days per week for speed work is controversial. Two speed work days have resulted in the same benefit as 4 days. However, most runners, with the exception of elite racers, select 1 day a week for speed work. Fewer days and sessions per week are most often selected because the risk of injury increases as weeks of speed work increase and amount of sessions per week increase. Selection of interval length varies. However, longer, slower intervals stress the aerobic capacities more, which leads to generating less lactic acid during workouts and races. Many racers complete a variety of distances during their speed work to be certain to gain a variety of benefits. Often with interval training, racers will begin training at a slower pace with more repetitions, then increase the pace and decrease the repetitions. The decision for building an interval plan and making personal adjustments is up to each individual. Consultation with a coach is recommended by the authors.

Besides the classic intervals involving a number of repetitions at the same distance, a ladder plan may be used. In the early stages of speed work, the ladder could be 1 x 1 mile, 2 x 880 yds., 2 x 660 yds., 2 x 440 yds. and 2 x 220 yds. or shorter distances may be substituted. In later stages of speed work, a ladder could involve 5 x 110 yds., 4 x 220 yds., 3 x 440 yds., 4 x 220 yds., 5 x 110 yds. Adaptations for less intensity can be made by reducing distance or more commonly by reducing repetitions at the distances mentioned.

Tim Noakes, M.D., a noted physician, scientist, and runner from South Africa, has suggested in *The Lore of Running* the following **15 Laws of Training:**

1. Train frequently year-round (training year-round is better than planned layoffs and loss of conditioning that results.
2. Start gradually and train gently.
3. Train first for distance, only later for speed.
4. Don't set yourself a daily schedule (a weekly schedule is recommended to prevent individuals from training on a day when their body is not ready).
5. Alternate hard and easy training.
6. At first try to achieve as much as possible on a minimum of training.
7. Don't race when you are in training, and run time trials and races only infrequently.
8. Specialize (best racing results are achieved when an individual trains for a specific goal distance).
9. Incorporate base training and peaking (sharpening).
10. Don't overtrain.
11. Train with a coach.
12. Train the mind.
13. Rest before a big race.
14. Keep a detailed logbook. (Include how each workout feels, an effort rating of each workout, enjoyment rating of each workout, waking pulse rate, morning body weight, post-workout body weight, time one goes to be and number of hours of sleep, heart rate after each interval, and for women, their menstrual cycles.)
15. Understand the holism of training. (Realize that everything in one's life affects his/her training and try to achieve a balance. Don't let training become another stress.)

WALKING/JOGGING/RUNNING DURING PREGNANCY

Walking is considered the best activity during pregnancy. It does not involve the impact stress of jogging or running, but provides the needed activity to enhance or maintain the physical conditioning level of the expectant mother. Also, non-impacting cross training activities such as water walking/jogging or cycling may be selected. Medical reports indicate that mothers who are physically fit most often have an easier childbirth and recover more quickly afterward, but further research is needed to determine if the fetus benefits from the mother's exercise. Moderate exercise does not appear to have an adverse aspect on the fetus. Blood flow to a healthy placenta is adequate.

Most women who have been jogging or running regularly can continue to jog or run during pregnancy unless their physician specifies otherwise. There are valid reasons why certain women should not jog or run. However, if the physician does not suggest continuing a jogging or running program and does not provide a valid reason, seek another opinion. The authors recommend using an obstetrician who is sports oriented and knowledgeable of research on sports during pregnancy.

Suggestions for pregnant joggers and runners include not getting overheated or dehydrated (drink plenty of liquids), listening to one's body, and exercising at a comfortable pace for a specific length of time (not distance) while making adjustments. In addition, during pregnancy an individual's resting heart rate increases by 10-15 beats; therefore, it is important to avoid strenuous workouts or racing, always work out aerobically and exclude anaerobic sessions (slowing down may be necessary), and walk or rest if feeling stressed. In the last trimester the expectant mother may need to walk, stop, or rest if contractions occur. Dr. Cooper conservatively suggests walking as the only activity during this latter part of pregnancy. Some physicians recommend jogging or running in a swimming pool to decrease spinal stress. However, most women who began in good shape find they can continue jogging or running provided they let their body dictate each workout and make adjustments accordingly.

After childbirth rest is important. Walking only is suggested during the first two weeks. Jogging or running at a reduced pace can begin two weeks after giving birth if there are no complications and the physician gives approval. It is important to slow down and even rest if the body dictates.

General Guidelines and Recommendations
for Running During Pregnancy

1. Discuss your running goals during pregnancy with your physician.
2. Gradually reduce your mileage during the second and third trimesters. (Example: a woman averaging four miles a day might run three miles a day during the first trimester, drop to two miles in the second, and finally to to one and a half during the third.)
3. Avoid running when the temperature or humidity is high.
4. Try to run on flat, even running surfaces.
5. Allow the intensity of your exercise sessions to gradually decline. Pregnancy is a time to enjoy your workouts, but not be too competitive.
6. If running becomes uncomfortable during the second and third trimesters, try other forms of aerobic exercise, including swimming, running in water, bicycling, aerobic dance classes, etc.
7. Extend warm-up and cool-down periods.
8. Initially, body temperature should be taken immediately after exercise. Your rectal temperature should not exceed 101 degrees Fahrenheit (an oral temperature of 101 is too high). If body temperature exceeds 101, reduce your exercise intensity and duration, and move your exercise session to a cooler part of the day.
9. Use perceived exertion ratings versus fixed heart rates to monitor your exercise intensity. Run at a pace that is comfortable. A pounding heart rate, breathlessness, or dizziness are signs to reduce running pace.
10. Especially during the first trimester, eat a small snack before running to help avoid hypoglycemia.
11. Drink plenty of water before, during, and after running.
12. Do not overstretch or move in a way that is different from what is normally performed.
13. Stop exercising and immediately report to your doctor any unusual changes (vaginal bleeding, severe fatigue, joint pain, irregular heart beats, etc.)
14. Wear more supportive or protective running shoes.
15. Early on, be ready to modify your running or cross train if there are changes or complications in your pregnancy.

From *Running and FitNews,* July 1991 (Vol. 9, No. 7), published by the American Running and Fitness Association, 4405 East-West Highway, Suite 405, Bethesda, MD 20814. Used by permission.

PROGRAM EXECUTION

Individuals should follow the "Monthly Walking/Jogging/Running Schedule/Goals" (Lab 4.2) prepared earlier, to guide each daily workout. Each month, a new schedule should be planned according to the program selected, developed, or adapted. The "Weekly Walking/Jogging/Running Log" (Lab 4.3) should be used after each workout to record progress.

WHEELCHAIR WORKOUTS/RACING

Wheelchair aerobic workouts and racing have been popular with special populations. Special lightweight racing wheelchairs have been designed for this purpose. They vary according to weight, aerodynamics, and maneuverability.

Workout and racing mechanics vary and are based upon the capabilities of each individual. Numerous books and magazines are available to assist novices to racers with mechanics, conditioning, and training programs.

ADDITIONAL EXERCISE PROGRAM AND RACE PROCEDURES

Warm Up and Cool Down

It is important to warm up prior to an exercise workout or race and cool down afterwards. Warm-ups raise muscle temperature to help muscle contractions, enable more oxygen to be delivered to muscles (reducing oxygen deficit at the start of a race), increase speed of nerve impulses, prevent pulled muscles, and reduce stress to the heart. Cool downs help dissipate lactic acid more quickly and minimize stress on the heart caused by abrupt termination of exercise.

Warming up generally includes easy walking or jogging and stretching for a minimum of 5-10 minutes (refer to Chapter Five for suggested stretching exercises). The preferred method is to easy walk or jog for 2-10 minutes to gradually elevate the heart rate and to warm up the muscles, then stretch but not overstretch. For less strenuous workouts on "easy days," running coaches question the need for stretching. However, prior to hard workouts or races, the procedure of 10 minutes minimum of walking or jogging followed by stretching is emphasized. Further walking or jogging with accelerations should follow. General principles advocated in the research indicate 1) warm-up must be at least 5-10 minutes to enhance performance; 2) it must be moderate in intensity; 3) warm-up should involve the same activity to be performed (walking prior to brisk walking or racewalking and jogging or easy running prior to running); 4) to prevent loss of warm-up benefits, the strenuous workout or race should begin within one minute of the warm-up.

Cool-down generally involves slow jogging or walking 5-10 minutes followed by stretching. Some researchers indicate that more intense or longer workouts should involve a longer cool-down period. Others indicate cool-down walking or jogging can cease once the recovery heart rate of 100 bpm or less is achieved. More significantly, it has been found that slow jogging can continue to break down the glycogen in the legs thus causing further stress; therefore, a gradually slower walk until the heart rate lowers may be more beneficial.

Many people claim that dissipation of lactic acid through a cool-down procedure will help reduce muscle soreness. However, research does not support this claim and attributes most of the soreness to minor muscle fiber tears. Often this soreness is delayed until 8-12 hours after a long, hard workout and the soreness intensity peaks in 24-48 hours. New research suggests that including up to 30 minutes of downhill walking, jogging, or running or walking backward down hill in a workout program can reduce discomfort after a long race or workout once the muscles adjust to the downhill exercise.

Drinking and Eating

It is important to drink before, during, and after a workout or race. The suggested liquid is water for workouts or races less than one hour. The absorption of cool water is better than warm water since it absorbs some of the body's heat and exits the stomach sooner.

Research indicates that **electrolyte drinks** (containing water, sodium, potassium, calcium, magnesium, and chloride) provide no greater benefit than water except in long distance races or workouts of over an hour. However, sports drinks with 7% or less carbohydrates have a 30% faster absorption rate than water. (Caution: Drinks of 8% or more carbohydrates have slower absorption.) The type of electrolyte drink chosen is up to each individual. It is suggested that marathoners drink electrolyte solutions containing glucose (a sweet, syrupy simple carbohydrate) before and throughout the race to prevent blood volume depletion, hypothermia, and hypoglycemia involved in "**hitting the wall**." Although caffeine is

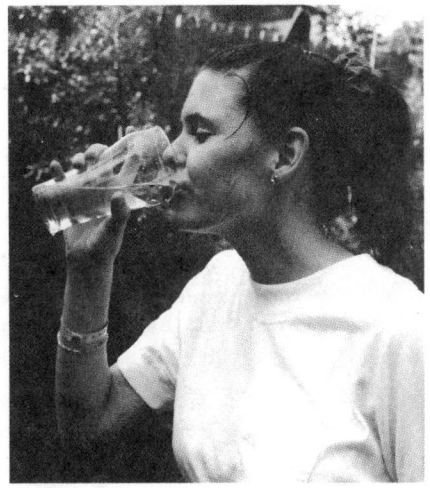

often consumed to increase blood fatty acids, it will not help conserve glycogen (stored carbohydrates) or increase blood fatty acids if the racer is carbohydrate loaded. **Carbohydrate loading** involves an elevated consumption of carbohydrates for 4 days prior to racing a half marathon distance and 6-7 days prior to a marathon. Caffeine helps with training intervals and short distance races, but does not help with marathons. Studies at the University of Guelph in Canada indicate that 2-3 cups of strong coffee ingested one hour before interval workouts can increase speed capacity and length of workout by 20%. 300 mg of caffeine or 2 cups of strong coffee one hour before a one-mile run can reduce time by 3-6 seconds. Taking 300 mg of caffeine in tablet form may also enhance 5K and 10K performances.

In warm weather, it is important to keep **hydrated** (body water at or slightly above natural level) by overloading on daily drinking. The body will then be more prepared to ward off **dehydration** (a condition where body water drops below normal level) and reduce amount of water needed during a race. Also, carbohydrate loading without prior **carbohydrate depletion** (depriving the body of carbohydrates for several days) can assist the body in storing water.

Drinking 6-8 glasses of fluids throughout the day can ensure hydration. Numerous exercise resources have indicated that dehydration can be avoided by drinking 16 to 32 ounces of fluid (water or beverages low in sugar and salt) 30 to 40 minutes prior to activity. Also, shortly before the start of a race or workout, 8 ounces of fluid should be consumed. The American College of Sports Medicine recommends drinking 10-12 ounces of water every 2 1/2 miles during a workout or race. This would mean 55 ounces or 7-cups consumption by fast racers and 28 ounces or less than 4 cups consumption by slower racers in an hour. Most racers would feel too bloated by following this suggestion and typically consume 16-20 ounces instead.

Recent research conducted by Nancy Rehrer, Ph.D., and colleagues at the University of Limburg in the Netherlands indicated endurance exercisers were more effectively hydrated when a "bolus" of water (20 ounces) was consumed just before a race or strenuous workout. During the race or workout 5 ounces of water is consumed every 20 minutes. This plan optimizes water absorption and enhances performance. However, exercisers may not be comfortable with the feeling of a full stomach as they exercise and it may take a number of workouts or races to adapt to that feeling. Tim Noakes, M. D., suggests an effective modification of 14 ounces of liquid at the start of an endurance workout/race followed by 3.5 ounces of fluid every 10 minutes during the workout/race. The American

Running and Fitness Association suggests drinking 4-8 ounces of liquid 15-30 minutes prior to exercise and 4-8 ounces of liquid every 15 minutes during exercise. Either of these three plans can optimize water absorption which is particularly needed during warm and humid weather conditions. Research has shown that the thirst mechanism cannot be relied upon as a gauge for fluid replacement. A general rule is to satisfy thirst and then drink more. If hydrated in advance and/or carbohydrate loaded prior to a long race, the racer should find that stored water will assist in preventing dehydration and reduce the necessity of extreme water consumption during races. **Overhydration** (a high body water level due to overcon-sumption of water or electrolyte drinks) during a race or workout can lead to nausea and gastrointestinal upset.

Water or an electrolyte drink should be consumed immediately after a race or workout. For each pound of weight loss, it is necessary to drink 2 cups (1 pint) of water. If the water isn't replaced the body stops producing sweat, body temperature increases sharply, and an imbalance in electro-lytes (water, sodium, potassium, magnesium, calcium and chloride) may occur. If the race or workout lasts over an hour, a high glucose drink should be consumed. The drink works more effectively than high carbohydrate food in replenishing glycogen stores. There are high glucose products on the market that can be used or the racer can make up his/her own drink by dissolving 17 tablespoons of sugar in a quart (.94 liters) of water. A general procedure to follow would be to drink half a quart of high glucose drink immediately following the long workout or race and another half quart two hours later. To be more precise, mix a solution of 20 tablespoons of sugar which equals 7.5 carbohydrate grams per ounce. Each individual uses his/her body weight and multiplies by .68. This will give the exact amount of high glucose liquid to be consumed. Divide that amount in half to follow the intake procedure suggested above.

Sodium and potassium (electrolytes) are necessary for the contraction of muscles, including the heart muscle. Salt (sodium chloride) is lost in substantial quantities during the initial stages of a walk, jog, run program. As the program is continued the body learns to conserve salt. Taking salt before and after a workout or race is not helpful nor desirable because of the interference with the absorption of water from the gastrointestinal tract. The normal daily intake of salt should not exceed 3 grams per day (1 teaspoon). The only time extra salt is needed is when very large quantities of water (four to six quarts within a twelve-hour period) are lost. Salt can be supplied to the body through a normal diet. The use of salt tablets is not recommended since more water than salt is lost during exercise. Potas-sium is lost as a person perspires. Individuals may become deficient in this electrolyte if they do not eat foods rich in potassium daily. Excellent sources of potassium are potatoes, dates, bananas, nuts, and citrus juices.

Light carbohydrate foods such as power bars, oranges, and bananas are commonly consumed as a pre-race meal. In early 1989, the American College of Sports Medicine cited new research that indicates better workout results if carbohydrates are consumed up to one hour prior to exercise. Previous research recommended that all eating should be completed 3 and preferably 4 hours prior to an endurance workout or race. Findings indicated that after eating carbohydrates, insulin levels elevated for 2-3 hours and individuals who exercised during that time would experience a drop in blood glucose levels and free fatty acids, the two sources of energy used by the muscles. Because of this information from past studies, most people are currently avoiding the eating plan suggested in the new research.

Another suggestion is to ingest a high carbohydrate drink three hours or less before a race and small amounts of high carbohydrate drink every 20 minutes during the race or workout. Cyclists have experienced improved performances using this method. However, walkers, joggers, and runners may want to try small quantities and gradually increase the amount of high carbohydrate solution, depending on the reaction of their stomach.

Fasting for 16 hours prior to an endurance workout or event is also common. Fasting stimulates fat cell breakdown enabling the muscle to use fats for energy and to save glycogen. Runners who fast break down more fats to provide energy, and racers who consume pre-race carbohydrates break down more glucose earlier in a race. However, research indicates that after 105 minutes blood glycogen levels tend to be the same for both groups. Therefore, neither practice appears better at delaying the onset of fatigue during a longer distance race or workout. However, the authors suggest consuming a pre-race/workout meal, since recent research indicates stronger or improved performances will result.

Remember Intensity

Remember that during the selected walking, jogging, or running program, not including warm-up and cool-down, it is important to exercise at an intensity level that will elevate and maintain the heart rate in the target heart zone. Monitor the pulse every 5 minutes during the exercise period to determine if the heart rate is in the target heart zone. If not, adjustments in intensity must be made.

Additional Pre-race, Race, and Post-race Procedures

Racers are advised to taper training a week or two prior to a big race with a longer tapering period prior to a longer race. This provides needed rest which increases energy stores, promotes healing and should lead to faster racing. Costill's research indicates 60% tapering leads to better performance. A day of total rest eliminating even minor activity is recommended prior to any race. Many racers have difficulty accepting that rest can be beneficial. Often it is claimed that "the edge" will be lost. However, it has been proven that even an extreme of 10 days rest does not cause a significant deterioration of fitness level.

Research at the University of Calgary indicates a significant increase in anaerobic capacity by following a training program of two weeks of hard workouts alternating with ten days of tapering. A study at McMaster University in Hamilton, Ontario, recommends a fast taper prior to competition. Mileage is reduced and replaced with fast 500 meter intervals. Joseph Houmard, Barry Scott and colleagues at East Carolina University suggest tapering by reducing to 15% of normal mileage and including 200 and 400 meter intervals for short races, 400 and 800 meter intervals for middle distance races, plus 80 and 1600 meters for marathoners. They have developed a seven-day fast taper for a 5K race which has been very effective. After warming up, 400 meter intervals are run at approximately 5K race pace with recovery periods of walking or resting until the heart rate drops to 100-110 beats per minute. The following schedule is used: Day 1, eight 400s; Day 2, five 400s; Day 3, four 400s; Day 4, three 400s; Day 5, two 400s and one 200; Day 6, two 400s; and Day 7, one 400. They contend that "intensity is the most critical factor during a tapering period." A 1994 study by David Jackson, Russ Pate and colleagues at the University of South Carolina verified the benefits of the East Carolina fast taper plan.

Don't go out too fast in the first mile of a race. A start that is too fast will result in a larger oxygen debt and deplete glycogen reserves which will slow the racer down for the rest of the race. Determine in advance the pace needed to achieve the race goal. Some racers write on their wrist the split time goals for each mile of the race. Monitor the splits to assist in keeping a steady goal pace. Examine the actual split times after the race to make adjustments in future races. A racer who is slow at the end requires a slower start adjustment and a racer who has a fast latter half of the race can pace faster during the race. However, negative splits can be effective

Adjusting Race Pace for Heat		
Estimated temperature at finish	*Slower than goal pace*	*8 min./mile pace becomes*
55-60°	01%	8:05
60-65°	03%	8:15
65-70°	05%	8:25
70-75°	07%	8:35
75-80°	12%	8:58
80-85°	20%	9:35
Above 85°	Forget it . . . Run for fun.	

Excerpted from *Galloway's Book on Running,* © 1983 by Jeff Galloway. $8.95. Shelter Publications, Inc. P.O. Box 279, Bolinas, CA 94924. Distributed in bookstores by Random House. Reprinted by permission.

and provide a psychological boost to the racer. To effectively drink water while maintaining race pace, squeeze one end of the cup and pour small amounts in the side of the mouth. Pace reduction will be necessary on warmer days as indicated by the chart above

To increase race times on hilly courses, run slower uphill to reduce lactate build-up. This allows for faster downhill running and reserve energy for the flats. To recover adequately after a race, wait one day for each mile (one kilometer for runners 40+) raced before engaging in a hard workout or another race. This will allow for better recuperation and prevent injury.

CHAPTER SUMMARY

Before starting a walking, jogging, or running program, an individual should participate in an aerobic exercise test to determine his/her starting exercise level. A physical exam prior to testing is important for sedentary individuals and those over the age of 45. Sample programs are provided for all levels from fitness walking to training for running races, or racewalking competition of various distances. Hill training and speed work are included to improve racing performance. After completion of a program, retesting is recommended to determine the next exercise level. The programs included in this chapter provide an opportunity to progress from walking to jogging to running or from walking to race walking. Warming up prior to walking, jogging, or running and cooling down afterwards should be standard procedure for each workout. Drinking is essential before, during, and after workouts or races. Eating should be completed 1-3 hours prior to the workout or race.

CHAPTER FIVE

Fitness Enhancing Programs

FLEXIBILITY
Principles

Flexibility, aerobic fitness and strength are the three components of fitness, and all three comprise the fitness triangle. A false belief is that strength training, particularly weight training, will restrict flexibility. However, if strength training is completed properly, through a full range of motion, flexibility will not be reduced. A well-rounded fitness program must include exercises for all three components of aerobics, flexibility and strength.

Flexibility can be defined as *a range of motion at a joint or a series of joints*. Flexibility is joint-specific since flexibility at one or more joints does not reflect flexibility at other joints. To achieve overall flexibility, specific stretching exercises must be performed at all joints. Several benefits from overall flexibility are: reduction of muscle soreness following exercise, prevention of injury when participating in strenuous activities, and greater freedom and ease of movement while performing everyday tasks.

Limitations on flexibility are bone structure, fat, connective tissue, muscles and tendons. All limitations except bone structure can be reduced and flexibility increased by following a planned program. Age, sex and inactivity affect flexibility. Women tend to be more flexible than men, particularly women with an early background of dance or gymnastics. As a person ages and/or becomes inactive, flexibility will decrease.

Increasing flexibility is a gradual process which may be achieved by regular performance of stretching exercises, preferably several times a day and 3-6 times per week. Several stretching techniques exist. **Static stretching** involves slow movement to achieve maximum range at a joint, then holding that stretching position from 10-60 seconds and repeating 3-5 times. A **ballistic stretch** involves moving the joint to the maximum range by means of bouncing or bobbing while stretching. Both of these types can be performed by the individual alone and are equally effective in achieving flexibility. However, ballistic stretching is no longer recommended due to the injury possibility while bouncing.

Another type of stretching is **proprioceptive neuromuscular facilitation (PNF)**. PNF has been used extensively by physical therapists and achieves the greatest increase in flexibility. However, since it requires a partner to assist, it may be inconvenient for many individuals. One effective type of PNF, slow-reversal-hold, begins with a partner moving a body part in the direction of the stretch to the point at which slight discomfort is felt by the exerciser. At that time the individual pushes against the partner for 10 seconds. The partner resists the push and prevents movement, which causes the push attempt to be an **isometric contraction** (muscle contraction without movement). After the 10 second contraction, both relax for 10 seconds. Next, the partner attempts to move the joint to increase the angle and establish a greater range of motion. At the greater joint angle position, the individual once again presses against the partner's resistance for 10 seconds and relaxes for 10 seconds. The sequence of increasing the angle, pressing, and relaxing is performing PNF. The partner must be knowledgeable since these types of stretching exercises are potentially dangerous if not performed properly.

A variation to PNF which involves isometric contraction, but does not require a partner, has demonstrated promising improvements in flexibility. This contract-relax technique involves a light stretch followed by a 7-8 second isometric contraction of the muscle previously stretched. Next, the muscle is relaxed for 2-5 seconds and than a 7-8 second maximal stretch of the muscle is attempted. The isometric contraction appears to enhance the ability of the muscle to achieve a maximum stretch. More research is needed before this method becomes widely accepted.

Rope assisted stretching is another variation for improvement of flexibility. While using a rope, an individual can often stretch through a greater range of motion than without and therefore increase flexibility. Using ropes of various colors can also add fun into a stretching routine and help ensure the continuance of a flexibility program.

To overload and improve flexibility through stretching exercises, the stretched position can be held longer. Also, as the flexibility program continues, attempts should be made to stretch further than the previous session, being careful not to overstretch.

The authors recommend static stretching, rope assisted or PNF to increase flexibility. Stretching exercises should be executed as part of the warm-up and cool-down procedure for walking, jogging, running and strength training. However, it may be more practical to use static stretching, with or without rope assistance, regularly for walking, jogging or running, and PNF as supplementary stretching whenever a knowledgeable partner is available to assist. Flexibility stretching exercises for all body areas should be performed 1-2 or more times per day, 3-6 times per week to achieve a greater increase in flexibility. As the static stretching flexibility program begins, the authors recommend holding for 10 seconds and repeating 3-5 times. After the 10 second stretch becomes comfortable, increasing to 15 seconds for 2-3 repetitions is recommended.

Suggestions for engaging in a safe, productive stretching program are:

1. Warm up muscles before starting by brisk walking, light jogging, or jogging in place for a minimum of 2 minutes. Another choice is to massage the quadriceps, hamstrings, groin, calves and feet and other body areas as a means of warm up prior to stretching.
2. Gradually assume the stretched position and try to go further with each repetition.
3. Avoid bouncing.
4. Don't overstretch. Always hold the stretch when feeling a tightness in the muscles.
5. Breathe normally or exhale while stretching. Never hold the breath.
6. Be careful if the joint is painful.

Stretching Exercises

Muscles which are being stretched are listed in parentheses and are shaded in the diagrams. For further location of muscles refer to the muscles of the body shown in the appendix.

Stretches for Walking, Jogging and Running

Group 1: These exercises are static stretches and are practical for warm-up since a comfortable surface to sit or lie on is not needed. After a brisk walk or easy jog, the individual can remain outside to perform these exercises.

1. Step one foot forward, bend knee at 90 degree angle, keeping knee above ankle. Extend opposite leg straight out behind; balance with hands on the ground and lift head up. *(Quadriceps, Adductor-longus, and Gracilis)*

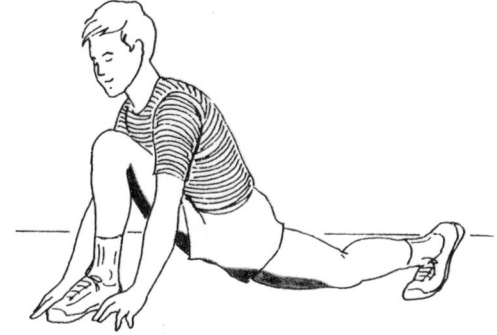

2.   Stand facing low bench or step. Place heel of one foot on bench or step and lean forward until a stretch is felt in the back of the thigh of the forward leg. Keep standing leg slightly bent. Repeat with opposite leg. *(Hamstrings and Back extensors)*

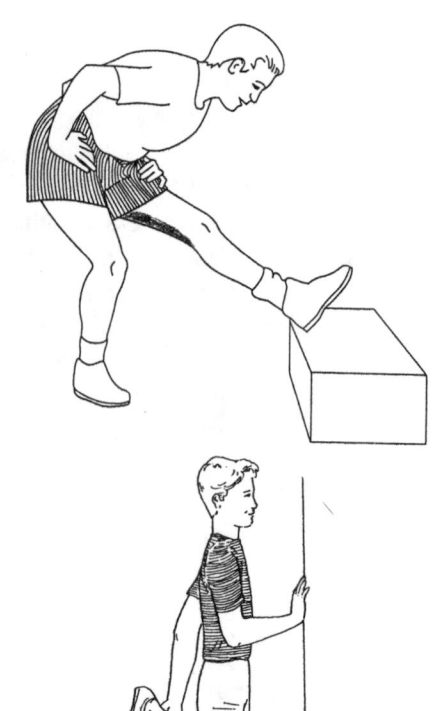

3.   Bend knee and lift heel to buttocks level. Use the opposite hand to hold the ankle and pull backward with opposite hand. With free hand, hold onto a stationary object for balance. *(Quadriceps)*

4.   Keep both feet flat on the ground and lean forward toward a wall with legs straight and arms bent. A variation is to position only one leg back *(Gastrocnemius and Achilles tendon)*

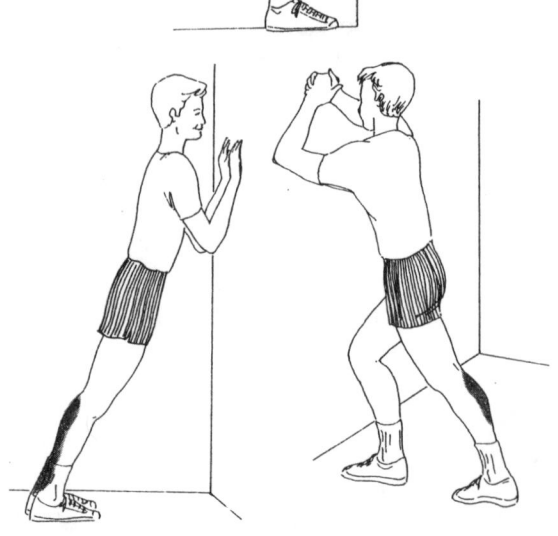

5. Keep both feet flat on the ground, bend knees, bend arms and lean forward toward a wall. A variation is to position only one leg back with the knee slightly bent. *(Soleus and Achilles tendon)*

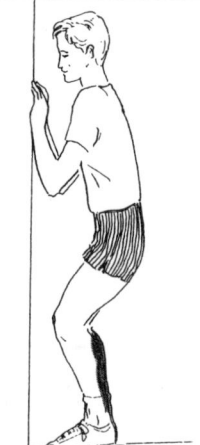

6. Reach arm over head and keep other arm down. Repeat with opposite arm. *(Deltoids, Latissimus dorsi and Obliques)*

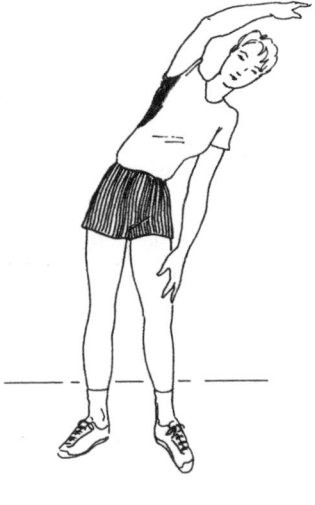

7. Hold hands behind the back, lean forward at waist with knees slightly bent, and lift arms as high as possible behind the body, keeping the head down. A variation is to hold a rope or towel with both hands, then lift the arms behind the body. *(Deltoids)*

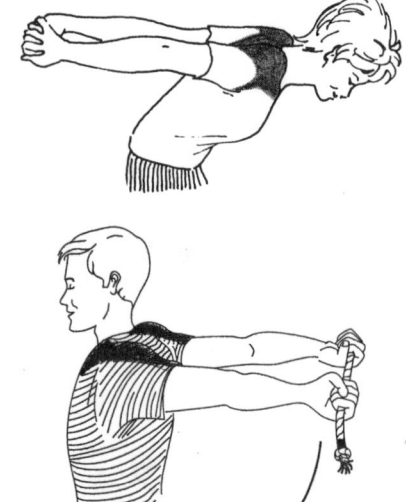

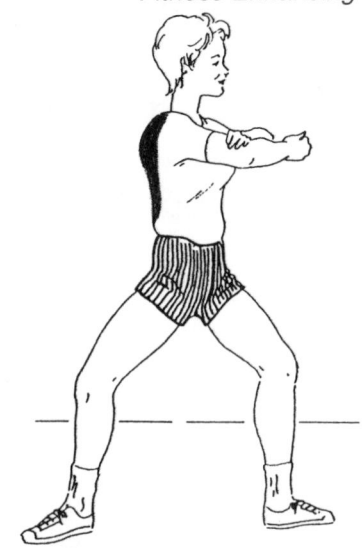

8. While standing, turn the trunk to the side while pulling the arms held at chest level. *(Obliques and Erector Spinae)*

Group 2: These exercises may be added to the list of exercises above and used for warm-up if a comfortable surface is available. However, they are excellent supplementary cool-down exercises once the walker, jogger or runner moves indoors for a shower or to continue the fitness workout. (Exercises 1-6 are static stretches; exercises 7-8 are rope assisted stretches; and exercises 9-15 are PNF stretches.)

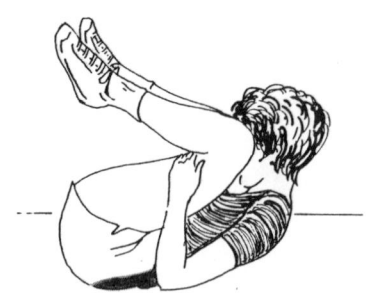

1. Lying on back, bend knees, hold hands behind knees and pull knees to chest. *(Lower back extensors)*

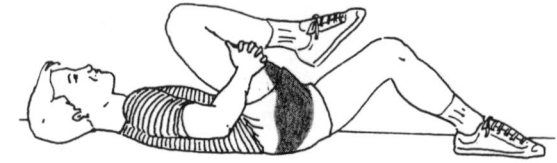

2. Repeat above, stretching one leg at a time. *(Hip extensors)*

3. Sit with legs spread. Reach with both hands toward the ankle and pull head to knee while keeping the leg straight. Then alternate legs. Variation is to sit with one knee bent with the bottom of the foot touching the extended leg. Bend and reach toward the straight leg. *(Hamstrings)*

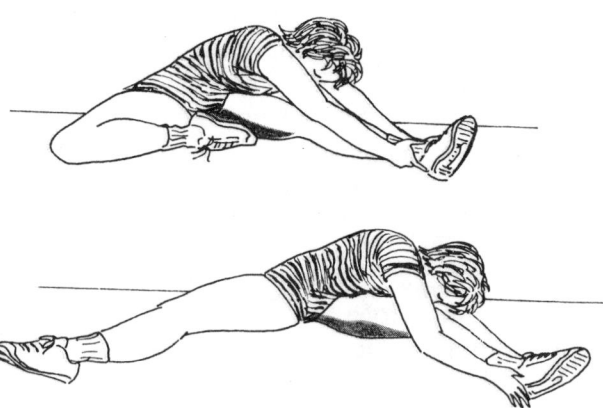

4. From a sitting position, place the bottom of both feet together, hold the ankles and press the knees to the floor using the elbows. *(Adductor-longus and Gracilis)*

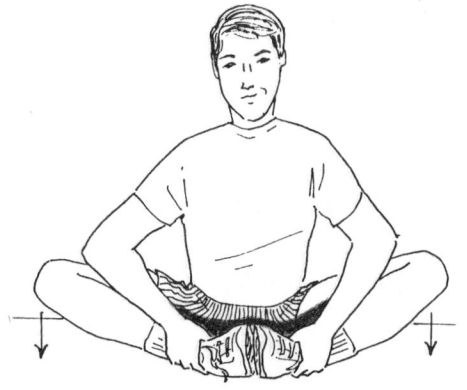

5. Sit on the floor and cross one leg over the other. Turn toward the crossed leg and reach arm over the knee of the crossed leg. Repeat to the other side. *(Obliques and Erector spinae)*

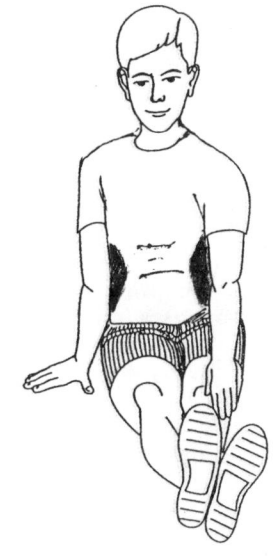

6. Lie on side. Bend higher leg and pull it back at the ankle using the higher arm. Lie on opposite side and repeat *(Quadriceps)*

7. Lying on back, with a towel or rope behind the ankle or sole of foot on one leg, lift the slightly bent leg upward, then toward the chest. Alternate legs. *(Hamstrings)*

8. Now allow the stretching leg to cross the straight leg in stages. Keep the knee bent and go all the way across. *(Hamstrings, Gluteus maximus, Obliques)*

9. A partner lifts the leg under the heel of a person in sitting position. With the opposite hand, the partner pushes the foot slowly forward toward the shin and follows the PNF sequence. Repeat with other leg. *(Calf and Achilles tendon)*

Additional Exercises for General Flexibility

Listed below are a few static exercises which can be used to supplement the flexibility exercises recommended for walking, jogging and running. Also, most of the static stretches below can be adapted to the PNF stretching method.

1. Spread legs in seated position, attempt to pull chest to the ground by pulling with hands on ankles. *(Hamstrings and Lower back extensors)*
2. From a seated position, place foot across opposite leg at thigh. Twist trunk to opposite side from crossed thigh. *(Obliques and Lower back)*
3. While standing, hold a towel behind the back with one hand holding at waist and the other above the shoulder. Pull towel downward with lower hand. *(Deltoids)*
4. Hold bent arm in front of the body and with opposite hand pull elbow toward opposite shoulder. *(Deltoids)*
5. From a standing position, bend forward from the waist toward a chair or table. Hold the chair and continue to press chest downward. *(Pectoralis major)*
6. Sit in a chair with legs spread. Lean forward between the legs and downward as far as possible. *(Back extensors)*
7. Lift arms above the head and lean back. *(Abdominals)*

Questionable/Risky Flexibility Exercises or Positions

Research has shown that a number of previously practiced flexibility exercises or positions, have caused damage to the body or overstretched ligaments thus reducing support and increasing risk of injury. The authors recommend that these potentially damaging exercises or **positions shown below** *should not* **be included in a flexibility program:**

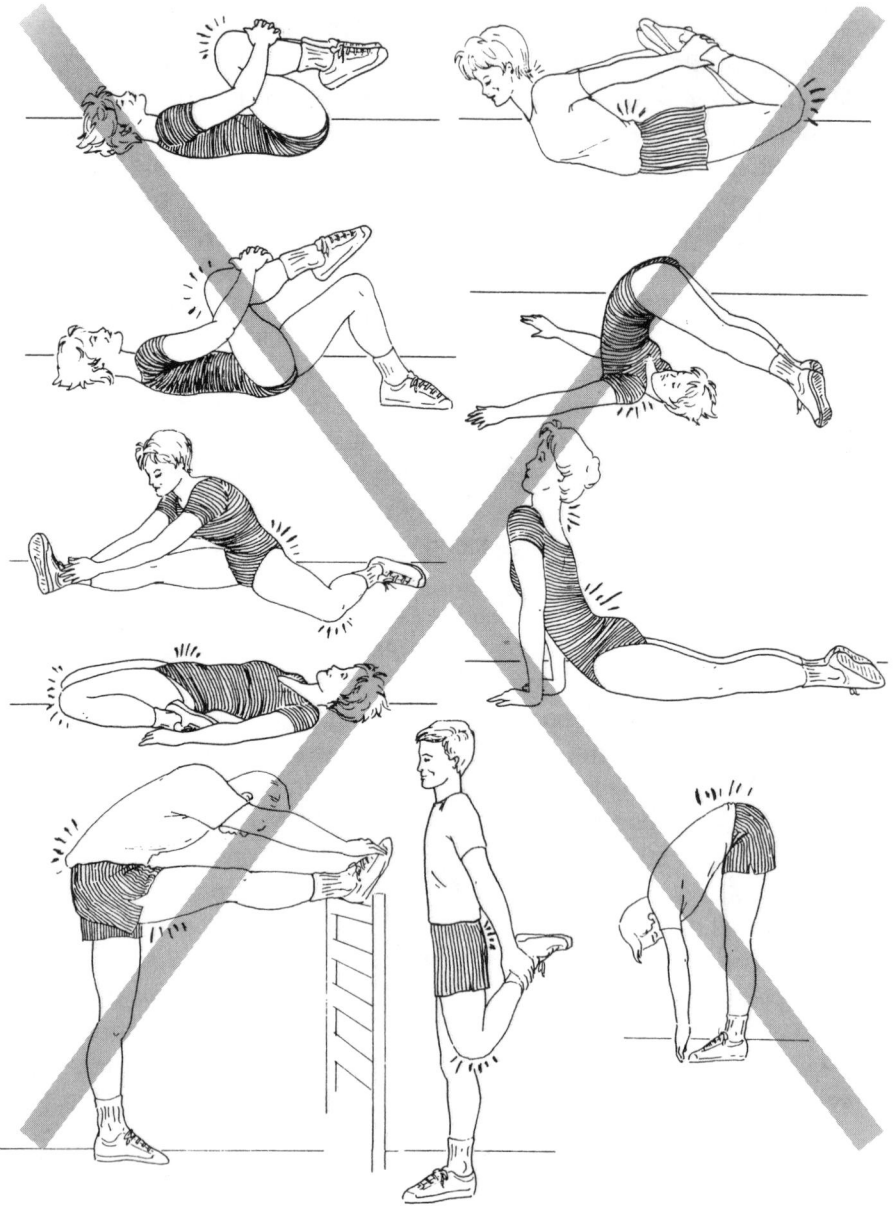

STRENGTH

Principles

Strength is the *amount of force that can be exerted by a muscle.* Improved strength helps to reduce fatigue, prevents muscle injuries and soreness, improves muscle tone and physical appearance, and improves performance in physical activities. Through strength training, muscle fibers enlarge and become stronger, connective tissue and tendons toughen, and neuromuscular efficiency increases. Research supports that strength training can improve running economy A runner who has never been involved in a strength training program while running can increase economy by 4-5 percent. This increase can result in a reduction of a minute or more for a 10K race. Racewalkers should realize similar improvement. Therefore, through strength training, walkers, joggers and runners will improve their fitness as well as their performance.

Runners have often questioned whether weight training for the legs will hamper their running. Research indicates that endurance training will inhibit strength training, but strength training will not have a negative effect on endurance training. Instead, velocity can be increased by both heavy weight training and light weight training with faster movements. This increase can help with sprinting and with a needed kick at the end of a race, but does not help endurance. Although more research is needed, some studies speculate that weight training can help to prevent strained or torn muscles during endurance training and can help to correct muscle imbalance by strengthening weak muscles. Weight training exercises for the upper body are important to provide the strength needed for pumping the arms. This pumping helps at the end of a long workout or race when the legs are tiring.

Often women are concerned that they will develop muscle bulk through strength training. The male hormone testosterone promotes bulking. Unless they inherited a larger than normal quantity of testosterone, females will become stronger without bulking. Typically, when women begin a strength program, a rapid increase of strength occurs, then they tend to plateau and the increase is less. Men, on the other hand, continue a steady increase as they follow a strength program.

Three types of strength training are isometric, isotonic and isokinetic. **Isometric** involves a maximum force with no movement. The muscle contracts and movement is prevented, thus the contraction is in a static position. The contraction is held 6-8 seconds and for up to 3 repetitions. Since sports activities are dynamic, strength building by this means is of limited value. Because of the static nature, isometrics do not contribute to muscular endurance. **Individuals with high blood pressure are cautioned not to use isometrics.** Finally, the motivation to exercise is diminished because isometric strength accomplishment is difficult to chart. Isometrics are more often used by weight lifters who are having difficulty at a certain point in the lift. They can position the muscle at that point and perform an isometric contraction.

Isotonic exercising is dynamic and involves muscular exertion through a full range of motion. **Calisthenics, weight training** with free weights, and weight training using variable resistance machines are types of isotonic exercises. Some strength programs utilize all three types of isotonic exercises. When utilizing weights, two types of contractions may be emphasized. One is concentric or positives where the length of muscle decreases and the circumference increases. This takes place as the weight is lifted. Eccentric or negatives occur when the weight is lowered slowly and the muscles elongate while still contracting. A good strength program should include both. Isotonic exercising is the most popular means of building strength. Therefore, most strength programs are comprised of isotonic exercises.

Isokinetic exercising involves near maximal contraction through the entire range of motion. This differs from isotonic, which typically begins with a need for near maximum effort followed by a diminished effort need as the lift is continued. Isokinetics are performed on machines with hydraulic, pneumatic or mechanical pressures causing resistance to be even throughout the movement. Movement is at the same speed regardless of the pressure exerted. Individuals of varying strength will perform the movement with a different exertion level but at the same speed. However, to obtain the maximum strength benefit, maximum force should be applied to each lift. If performed properly, this type of exercising can produce a greater increase in strength than the other two types. However, it is easy to cheat and not exert to the maximum, particularly on days when the exerciser feels lazy. Also, since amount of weight lifted is not recorded, improvement cannot be charted and motivation for this type of exercising decreases. Therefore, isokinetic exercising is less popular than isotonic exercising and is more commonly used for rehabilitation.

Since strength exercises using calisthenics, free weights, and variable resistance machines are more popular and equipment more readily available, the remaining discussion focuses on isotonic exercising for strength. For success in strength training, the overload principle must be applied. To overload, the muscle must be caused to work harder than normal in order for strength improvement to occur. For calisthenics such as sit-ups, push-ups, and pull-ups, overloading involves an attempt to increase the repetitions each time the exercise is performed. This will improve muscular endurance. For weight lifting the progressive resistance principle suggests a gradual overload by first increasing repetitions for lifting a particular weight each set. Once a muscle adapts to a particular weight, strength improvement does not occur and the amount of weight must be increased. This gradual increase of weight will also prevent injury. In order to determine the amount of weight to be lifted for each exercise when starting a program, start with lighter weights then try progressively heavier weights until a weight is selected that is a challenge to lift for 6 repetitions.

According to Dr. Michael Pollock of the University of Florida, a weight training prgram for health improvement should involve one set of 8-12 repetitions. The weight selected should cause the exerciser to struggle during the final repetitons. To overload, repetitions should increase to a maximum of 12 as exercise sessions continue. Once the weight can be lifted easily, the weight should be increased for the next workout.

Other variations exist and are used by individuals who are more experienced and have more advanced goals for weight lifting and body building. Also, if muscular endurance is desired as opposed to strength, a light weight may be lifted for 3 more repetitions. Weight training workouts should be conducted two to three times a week with a day of rest between. Calisthenics can be performed on successive days, but alternate days are preferred.

Following are suggested procedures to ensure a safe and productive weight training workout:

1. Warm up before starting and cool down following each workout (refer to warm-up/cool-down section in Chapter Four).
2. Wear loose comfortable clothing, supportive shoes and a weight belt if lifting heavy weights.
3. Follow proper techniques.
4. Learn the proper use of machines.
5. Use a spotter on designated lifts with free weights.
6. Don't show off and try to lift more than is safe.
7. Exhale as force is exerted and inhale during the relaxation phase.
8. Lift weight (positive) for 2 counts and lower weight (negative) for 4 counts.

9.   Select the correct weight.
10. Start each workout by exercising the larger muscles in the lower part of the body, then exercise the upper body.
11. Keep hands dry or use gloves, particularly with free weights.
12. Make sure plates are secure when using free weights.

Aerobic benefit can be obtained during a strength workout. This is popular using weight machines which are set up as a circuit. To keep the heart rate within the target heart zone, when one strength exercise is completed, a one minute aerobic exercise is performed before moving to the next strength exercise. This could be simply jogging in place, performing jumping jacks, or rope skipping. On the other hand, exercise bikes, rowing machines and other aerobic equipment may be strategically placed between the weight machines and can be used for the aerobic portion of the circuit.

Strength exercises are specific. Only the muscle group exercised will demonstrate an increase in strength. When planning a program to benefit a specific sport or activity or a general strength program, care must be taken to select exercises to accomplish the proposed strength goal. A general program should include at least one exercise for each major muscle group. To develop a personal strength plan and record progress use Lab 5.1, "Strength Workout Plan and Progress Chart."

Exercises

Specific for Walking, Jogging and Running

These exercises will help improve walking, jogging and running as well as contribute to overall strength fitness. Weight training exercises should be performed according to the principles discussed previously for weight training, and the strength exercises which do not involve weights should be performed according to the principles for the specific type of strength exercise. It is best to schedule these exercises after walking, jogging, or running, or on rest days. Muscles exercised are listed in parenthesis and are shaded in each figure that follows. To find the special location of each muscle, refer to the chart in Appendix B.

1. **Leg extension** *(Quadriceps).* From seated position on a chair or bench with lower leg at a 90 degree angle to the upper leg, extend lower leg and lower to the 90 degree bent position. After a number of repetitions, change legs and repeat. Weights may be added to the ankle. The same exercise may be performed on a leg extension machine which involves both legs extending simultaneously to lift the weight.

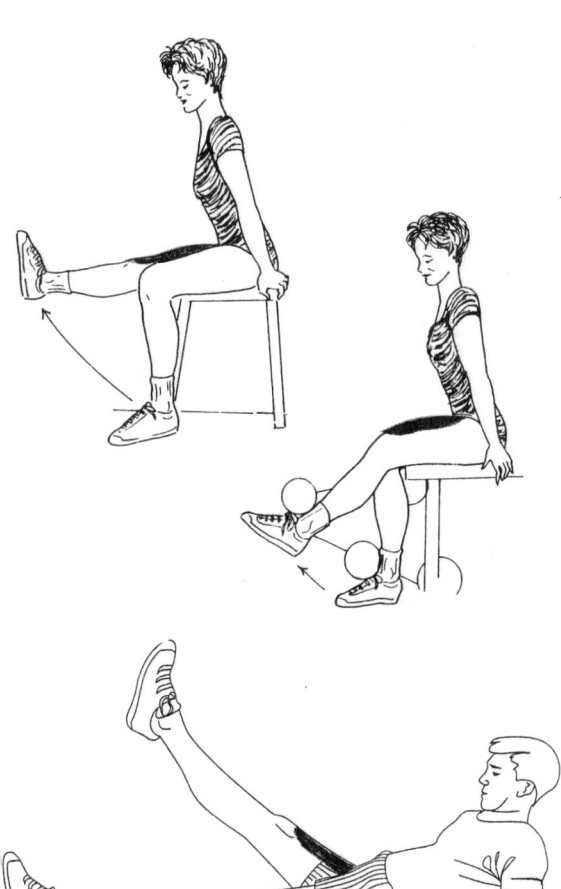

2. **Forward leg lift** *(Quadriceps and Hip flexors).* Sit on floor or mat and lean back supporting the upper body with the elbows. Lift one leg one foot off the floor repeatedly, keeping the leg straight. Repeat with other leg. Weights may be added to the ankle.

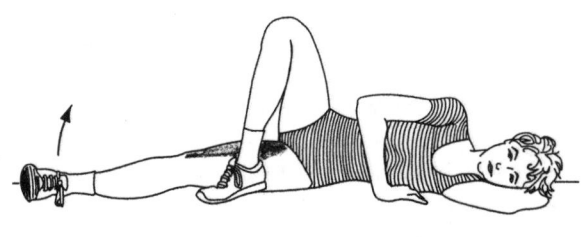

3. **Inside leg lift** *(Adductor longus and Gracilis).* Lie on the side, positioning the lower leg at a 90 degree angle to the body and placing the opposite foot on the floor in front of the lower leg. Lift the lower leg one foot off the floor keeping that leg straight. Change legs and repeat. Weights may be added to the ankle. These muscles can also be strengthened on an adductor machine.

4. **Outside leg lift** *(Tensor faciae latae and vastus lateralis)*. Lie on the side and lift the upper leg upward 1 - 1 1/2 feet. Repeat with opposite leg. Weights may be added to the ankle. These muscles can also be strengthened on an abductor machine.

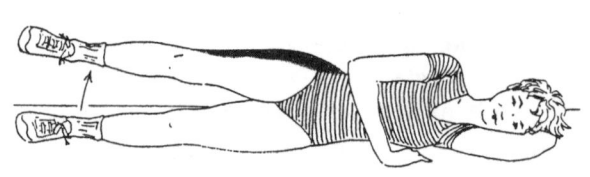

5. **Backward leg lift** *(Hamstrings and Gluteus maximus)*. Lie face down on floor or mat and lift one leg off the floor repeatedly, keeping the leg straight. Repeat with the other leg. Weights may be added to the ankle.

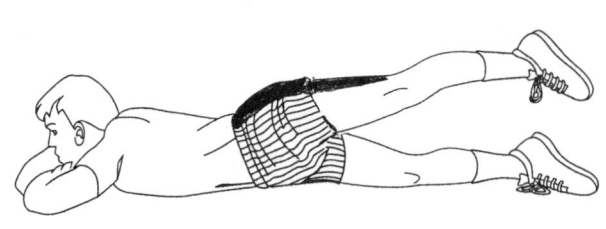

6. **Leg curls** *(Hamstrings)*. From a kneeling position with upper body bent forward and head resting on the hands, lift one leg to a position parallel to the floor. Alternately bend leg to a 90 degree angle and extend. Repeat with opposite leg. Ankle weights may be added. This exercise can also be performed on a leg curl machine.

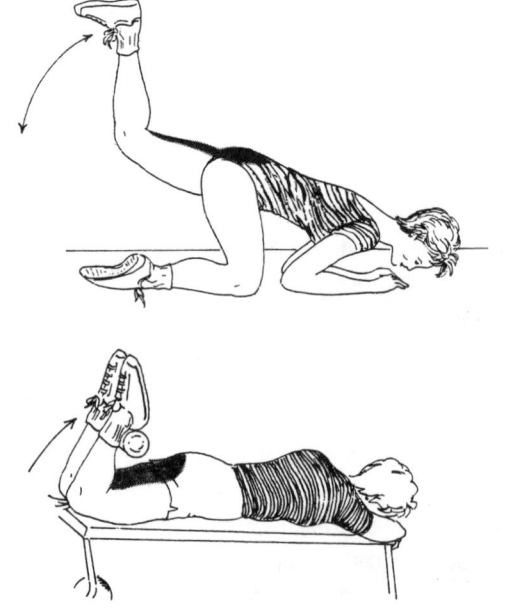

7. Buttocks Lift (*Gluteus maximus*). From kneeling position with body bent forward and head resting on the hands, keep knee bent and lift leg until thigh is parallel to the floor. Keep head in line with the body or down. From that position lift leg 3-4 inches using the buttocks. Ankle weights may be added.

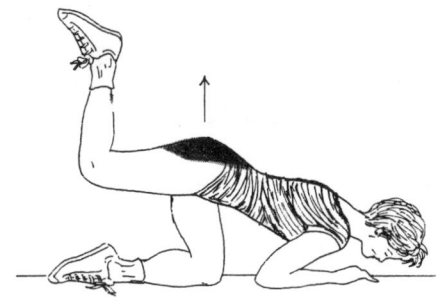

8. Hip Raises (*Gluteus maximus, Hip abductors*). Stand sideways on a step with one foot and the other foot positioned unsupported on the side of the step. Arm on the supported leg side holds onto the railing for balance. Keeping both legs straight, repeatedly lower the free leg several inches below the step level and raise it by moving the hip upward as high as possible. Change position on the step and repeat with the other hip.

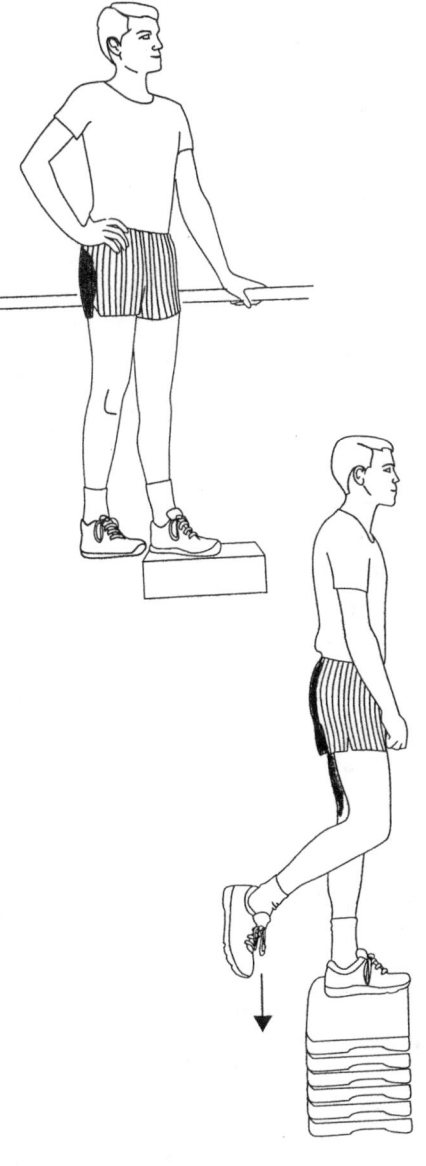

9. Bench Step-ups (*Gluteus maximus, Hamstrings, Quadriceps*). Use a bench that is approximately knee high. Start on top of bench. Step backward until heel of landing foot is on the floor. Push upward with landing foot and stand straight with bench leg. Repeat with the same leg until fatigue, then switch legs.

10. **Lunge** *(Quadriceps, Hamstrings, Gluteus maximus).* Step forward and bend knee to a 90 degree angle. Be certain that knee remains above the ankle. Opposite leg extends behind and head is looking forward. Repeat with opposite leg. A weight may be held across the shoulders.

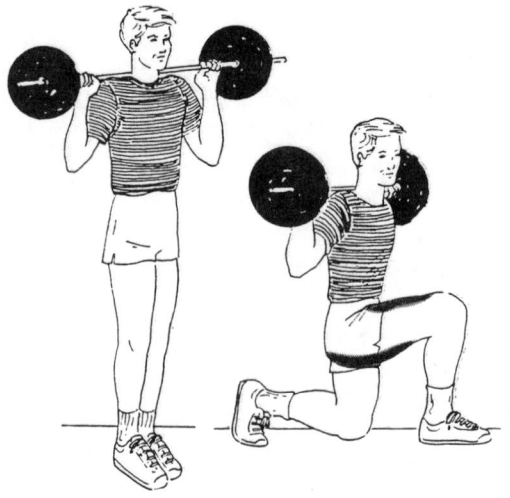

11. **Calf Raises** *(Gastrocnemius.* From a standing position, lift heels off the ground until standing on toes. Can be performed on the edge of a platform to allow heels to begin at a position lower than the toes. Repeat with toes in and then toes out. This may be performed while holding a weight or on a weight machine.

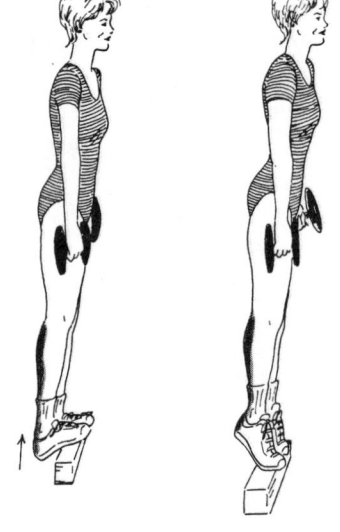

12. **Toe Presses** *(Calves).* Stand on a bench with one foot positioned with the heel off the bench. The other leg should be held in the air in bent position. For balance hold onto a wall or other support. Repeatedly lower heel and raise up onto the toes. Repeat with opposite foot.

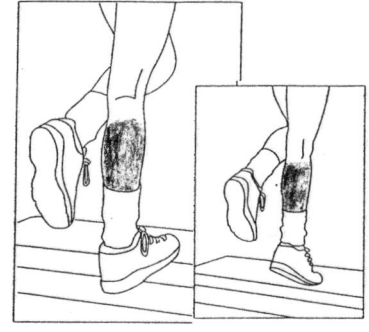

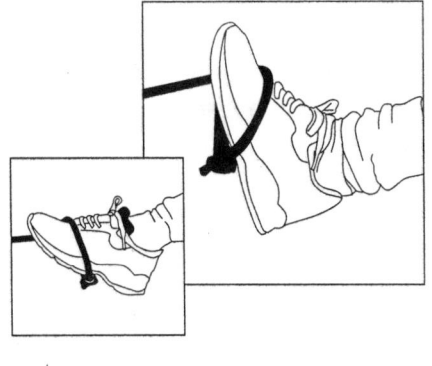

13. Resisted Ankle Pull *(Shins).* Place resistance band around foot. From a seated position, bend and extend foot. Can be performed with ankle weight attached to the foot. Repeat the exercise with the opposite foot.

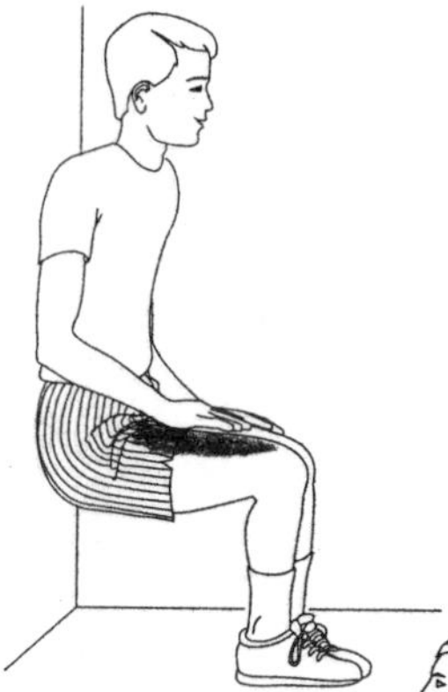

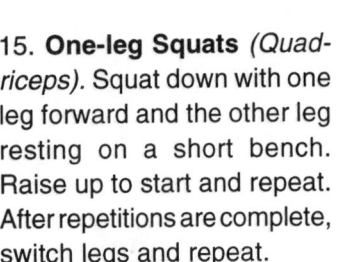

14. Wall Sits *(Quadriceps).* Sit on imaginary chair with the back against the wall. Legs should be bent at a 90 degree angle.

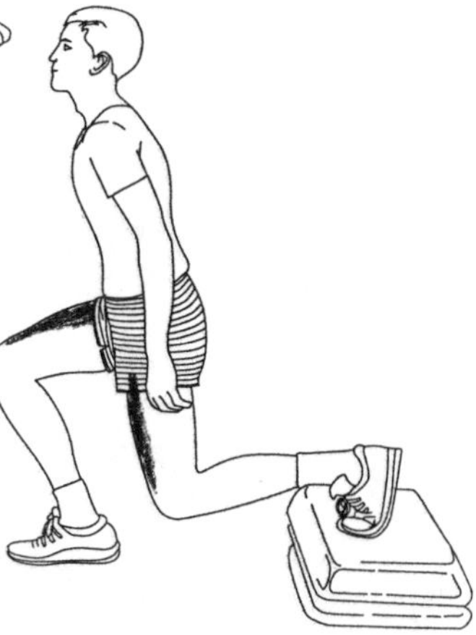

15. One-leg Squats *(Quadriceps).* Squat down with one leg forward and the other leg resting on a short bench. Raise up to start and repeat. After repetitions are complete, switch legs and repeat.

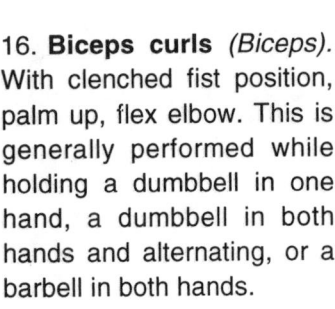

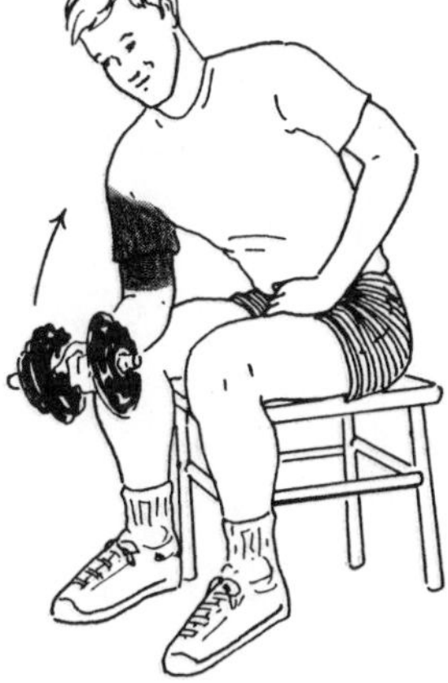

16. Biceps curls *(Biceps).* With clenched fist position, palm up, flex elbow. This is generally performed while holding a dumbbell in one hand, a dumbbell in both hands and alternating, or a barbell in both hands.

17. **Triceps Extension** *(Triceps).* From a standing position, bend over with arm flexed and fist clenched. Extend at the elbow until the arm is straight. Work one arm at a time. This is generally performed while holding a dumbbell.

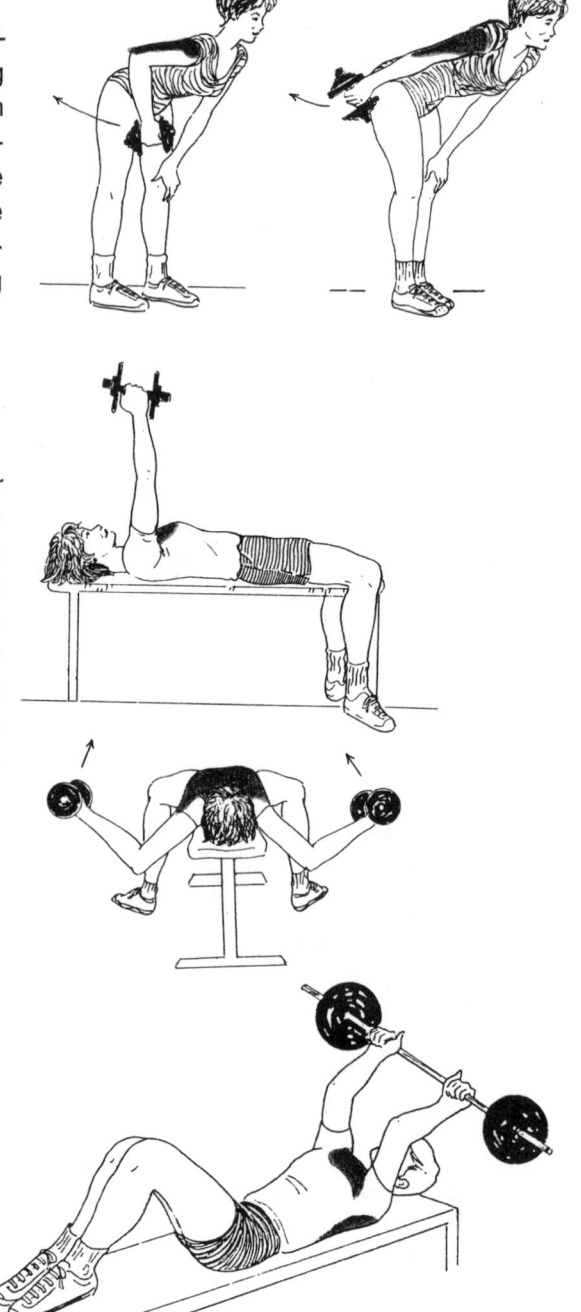

18. **Flies** *(Pectoralis major and Anterior deltoids).* From a position lying with back on a bench and arms extended parallel to the floor even with the chest and elbows slightly bent. Lift clenched hands above the chest with arms straightening on the lift. This is generally performed while holding a dumbbell in each hand.

19. **Pullovers** *(Pectoralis major and Latissimus dorsi).* Seated, standing or lying down position, hold barbell or curl bar behind the neck. Pull weight over the head. Can be performed on pullover machine.

20. **Bent over rowing** *(Latissimus dorsi, Posterior deltoids, Rhomboids and Middle trapezius).* Stand and bend over at the waist with one or both arms extended downward with clenched hands. Pull upward with elbows leading and elbows bending. Can also be performed with one or both hands holding a dumbbell and with both hands holding a barbell.

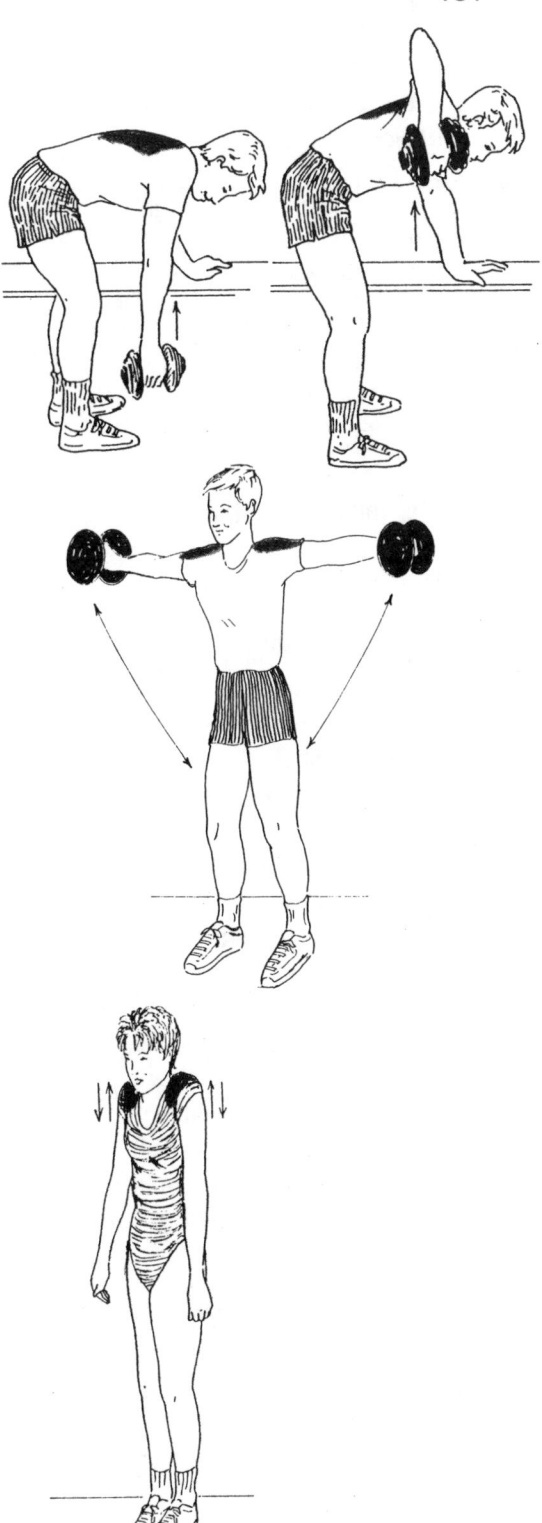

21. **Lateral raise** *(Middle deltoids).* From a standing position with arms at the sides and hands in clenched position, raise arms laterally until shoulder height. Generally performed while holding a dumbbell in each hand.

22. **Shoulder shrugs** *(Upper trapezius).* From standing position with arms at sides, lift and roll (shrug) shoulders backward. Can also be performed while holding dumbbells in each hand.

23. **Bench press** *(Pectorals, Deltoids, Triceps).* Lie down on a machine or free weight bench with both feet resting on the bench. Hold the bar and press upward. (**Spotter needed.**)

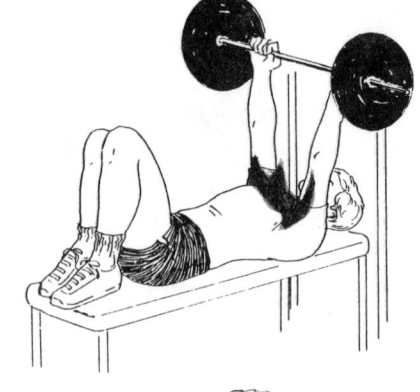

24. **Walking, Jogging, Running Arms** *(Deltoids, Biceps, and Latissimus dorsi).* Hold weights in each hand and position arms for walking, jogging or running. Move arms using the movement involved in walking, jogging or running.

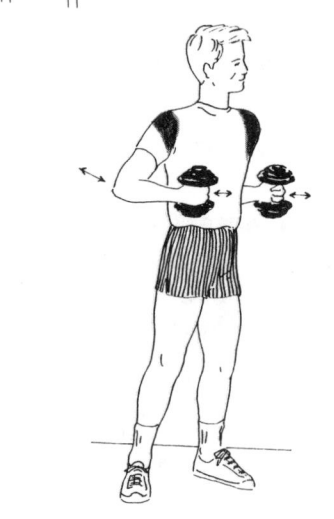

25. **Curl-up series** *(Abdominals).* Lie on back with knees bent, feet resting on the floor or mat and hands across the sternum, or lightly supporting the head by placing the hands over the ears with fingers pointing toward the neck and thumbs resting on the cheek bones. Lift body upward until shoulder blades are off the surface. After resting, establish the same position, but lift shoulder blade on one side off the floor and turn toward the opposite side of the body. Alternate sides and repeat the lift. These may be performed while holding a weight across the chest.

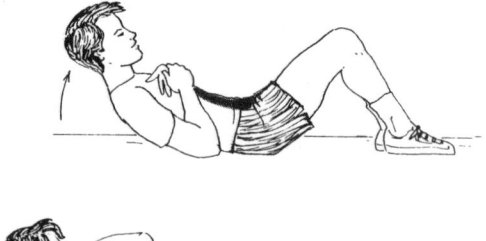

26. Reverse curl-up *(Lower Abdominals).* Lie on back, bend knees and rest bent legs on the chest. Hold onto stationary object above the top of the head. Lift buttocks slightly off the ground and lower.

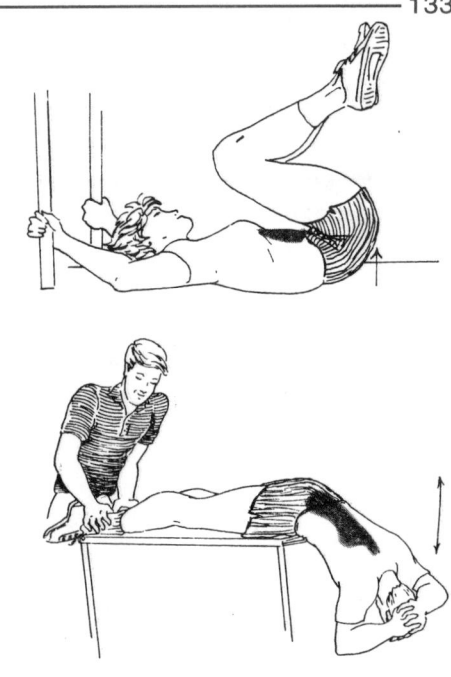

27. Back hyperextension *(Erector spinae).* From a position lying stomach down and hands behind the head, lift chest off the floor several inches. An alternative is to lie stomach down on a table with hands behind the head and upper body hanging down over the table and then lift the upper body until it is parallel with the floor with no back arch. In both exercises, have a partner hold the buttocks and ankles for stability. This may also be performed at a special exercise station or on a machine (caution should be followed if back problems exist).

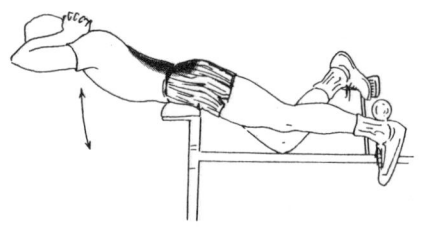

Special Performance Exercises

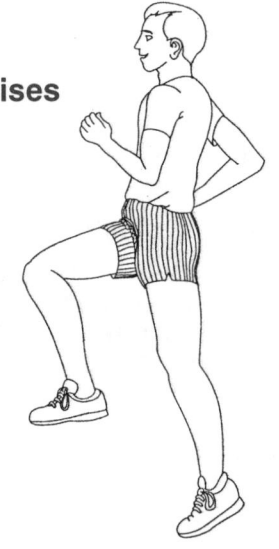

1. Skipping and bounding. Start with relaxed arms and skipping. Gradually increase arm action to simulate a sprinter and try for more air time with each skip for 100 meters. Repeat 2-3 times.

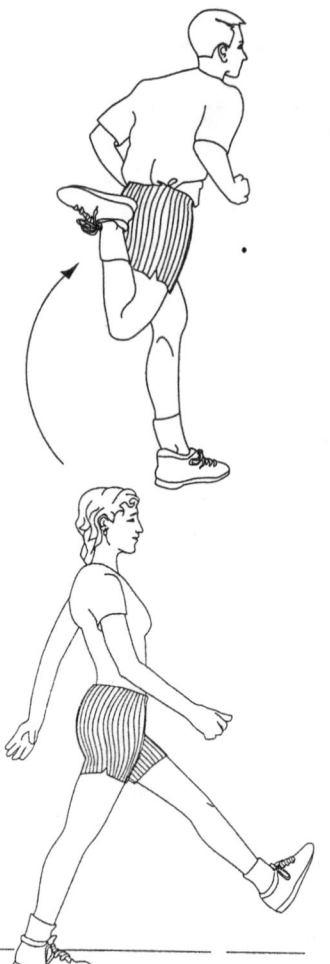

2. **Butt kicks.** At the end of an easy walk, jog, run workout, preferably on a grass or dirt surface, walk, jog or run 60-100 meters, kicking legs back and up with each stride so that heels lightly touch the buttocks. Repeat 8-10 times.

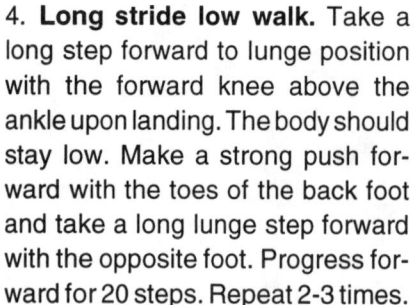

3. **Stiff leg kicks.** With straight (stiff) legs, kick legs forward and land on heels as you walk or run forward for 100 meters. Repeat 2-3 times.

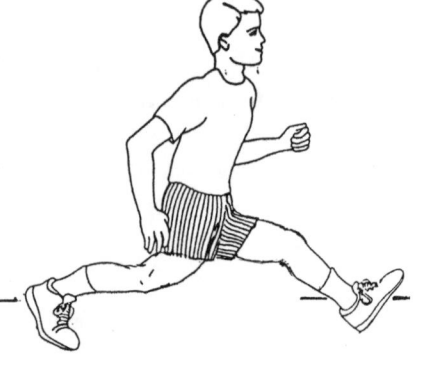

4. **Long stride low walk.** Take a long step forward to lunge position with the forward knee above the ankle upon landing. The body should stay low. Make a strong push forward with the toes of the back foot and take a long lunge step forward with the opposite foot. Progress forward for 20 steps. Repeat 2-3 times.

5. **Single leg long stride low walk.** Use the same long low lunge stride forward. Repeat with the same leg 10 times and switch to the opposite leg 10 times.

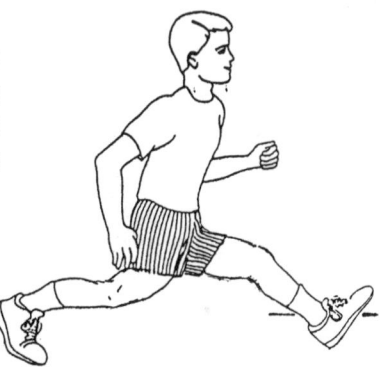

6. **Marching.** Lift knees high and march forward with a strong walk or high knee raise while hopping for 200 meters. Repeat 2-3 times.

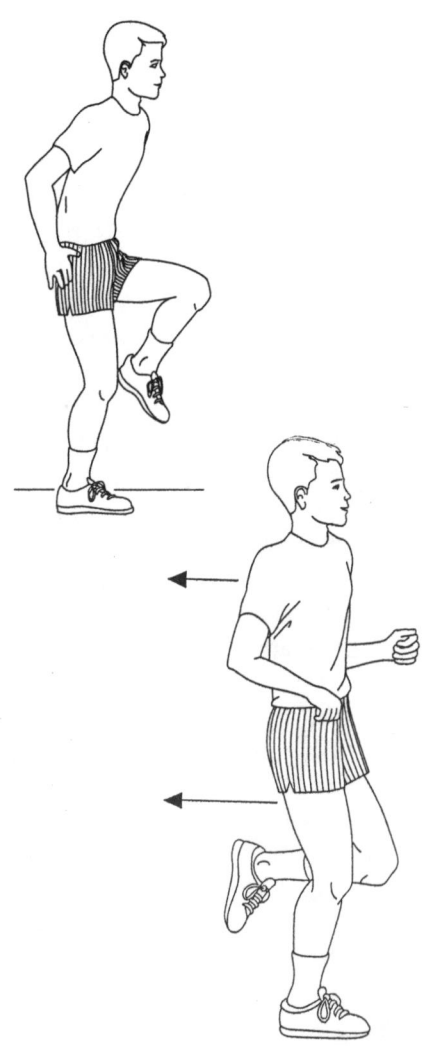

7. **Backward walking or running.** Start slowly and speed up the pace for 100 meters. Be certain to look behind to monitor the surface.

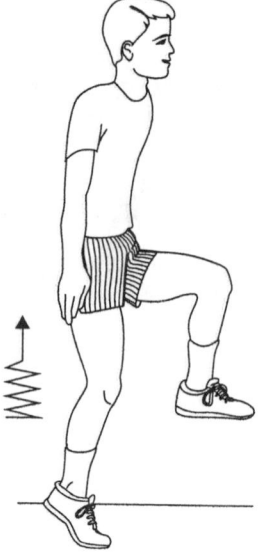

8. **One leg hops.** On grass or soft surface hop 10 times on one leg and 10 on the opposite leg. Repeat 2-3 times for each leg.

General for Overall Conditioning

The following list of exercises may be performed in addition to, or as a replacement for, the previous strength exercises.

1.   **Squats** *(quadriceps, hamstrings, erector spinae, gluteus maximus)*
2.   **Dead Lift** *(quadriceps, hamstrings, erector spinae, gluteus maximus)*
3.   **Front Squat** *(quadriceps, hamstrings, erector spinae, gluteus maximus)*
4.   **Leg Press** *(quadriceps, hamstrings, gluteus maximus)*
5.   **Swingbell Curl** *(biceps)*
6.   **Inclined Dumbbell Curl** *(biceps)*
7.   **Preacher Curl** *(biceps)*
8.   **Reverse Curl** *(biceps)*
9.   **Triceps Curls** *(triceps)*
10.   **Triceps Pull-down** *(triceps)*
11.   **Upright Rowing** *(biceps, middle deltoid, trapezius)*
12.   **Lat Pull-down** *(biceps, pectorals, posterior deltoid, trapezius, rhomboids, latissimus dorsi)*
13.   **Chin Behind the Neck** *(biceps, posterior deltoids, trapezius, rhomboids)*
14.   **Overhead Press** *(triceps, anterior deltoid, trapezius)*
15.   **Inclined Press** *(triceps, pectoralis major, anterior deltoids)*
16.   **Press Behind Neck** *(triceps, middle deltoids, trapezius)*
17.   **Alternate Dumbbell Press** *(triceps, middle deltoids, trapezius)*
18.   **Parallel Bar Dips** *(triceps, latissimus dorsi, anterior deltoids)*

19. **Bent-over Lateral Raise** *(posterior deltoids, trapezius, rhomboids)*
20. **Forward Raise** *(anterior deltoids)*
21. **Push-ups** *(triceps, anterior deltoids, latissimus dorsi)*
22. **Pull-ups** *(biceps, anterior deltoids, forearms)*
23. **Wrist Curl** *(forearm)*
24. **Lateral Wrist Curl** *(forearm)*
25. **Wrist Roller** *(forearm)*

Questionable/Risky Strength Exercises or Positions

As a result of research, several exercises or positions have been cited as risky and potentially damaging. **The authors recommend that the following exercises or positions** *not* **be performed.**

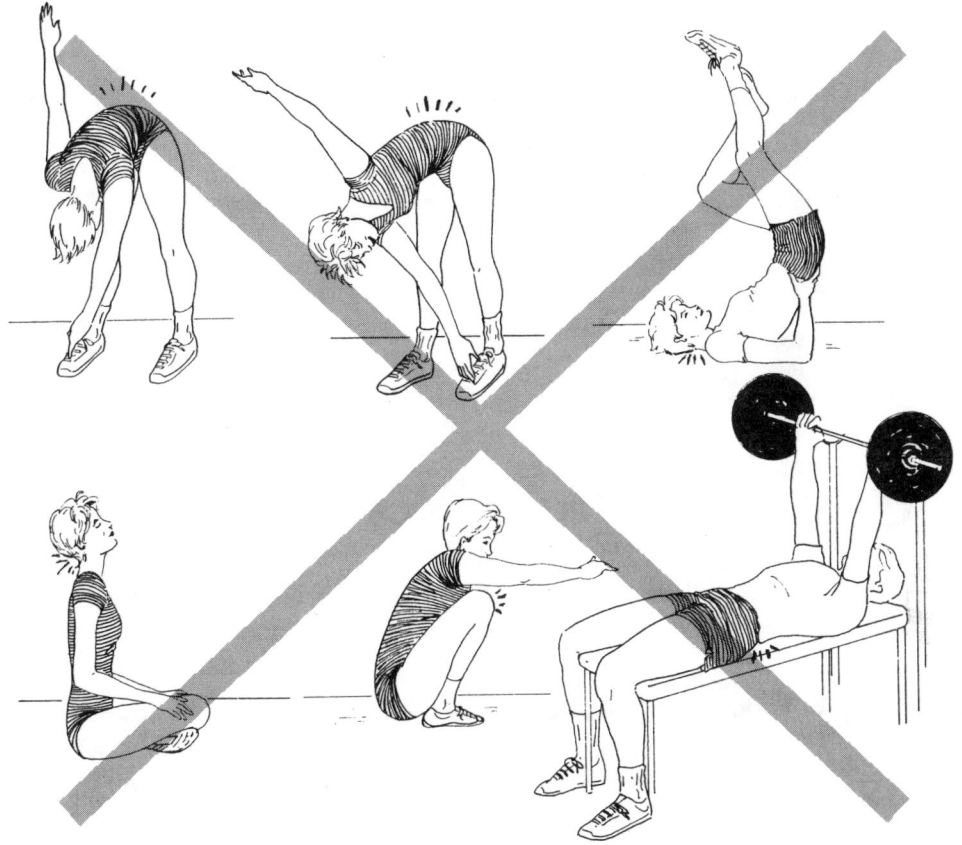

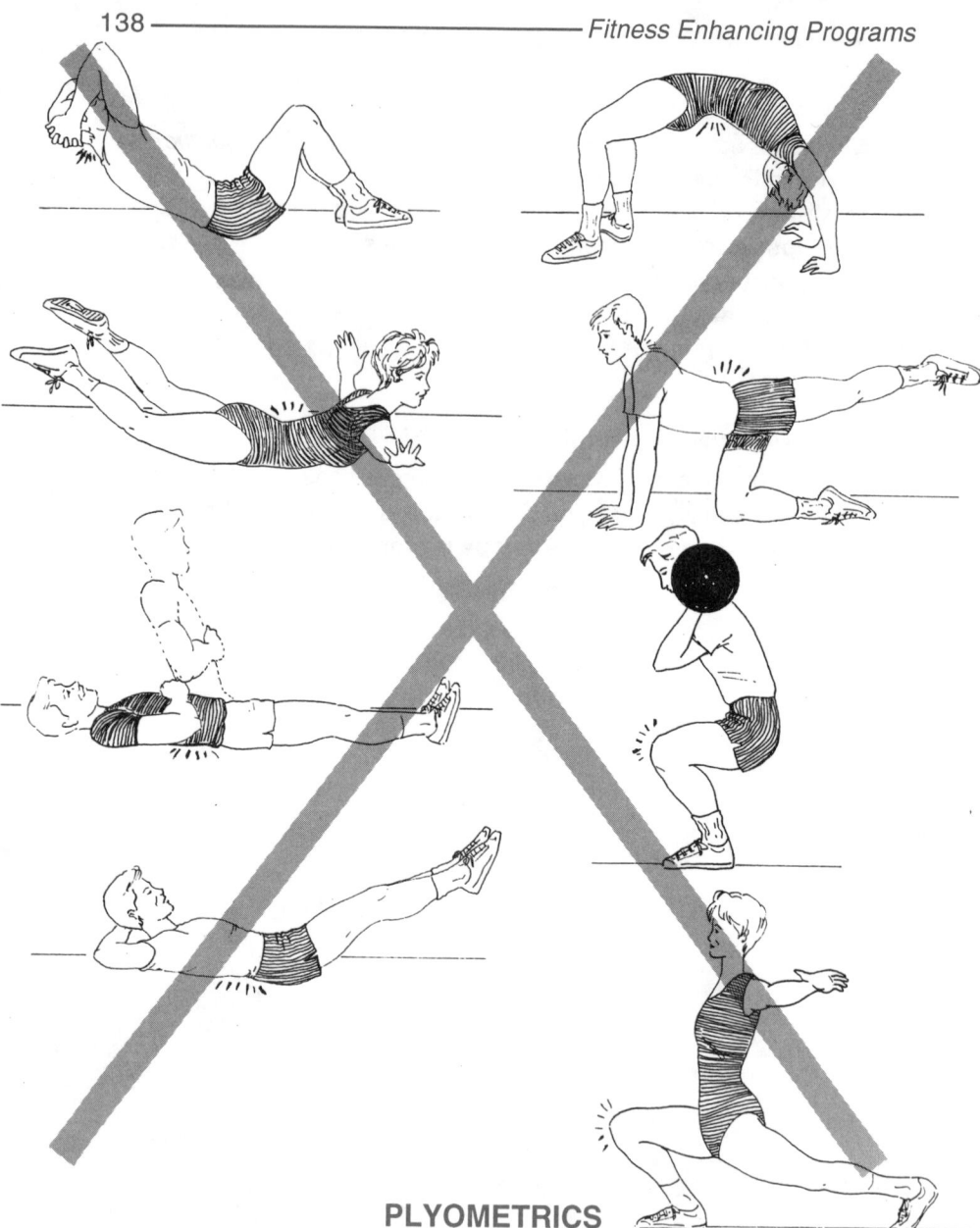

PLYOMETRICS

Principles

Plyometric exercises bridge the gap between strength and power. These exercises involve powerful muscle contractions and help to improve speed by developing muscle power and strength. Plyometrics involve rapid lengthening of a tensed muscle (eccentric contraction) followed immediately by a high velocity shortening of the muscle (concentric contraction). Generally 3-6 sets of 8-10 jumps with 1-2 minutes of recovery between each set. To overload add 1-2 jumps per set. Do not exceed 250 total jumps in one workout. Generally, a different exercise is used for each set. These exercises are of benefit to competitors and, particularly, runners. The fitness walker, jogger or runner will generally not include plyometrics in his/her fitness program.

Since many injuries occur to shins, knees, ankles and lower back, it is important to reduce injury by following these suggestions:

1. **Perform plyometrics only if over 13 years of age**, in excellent physical condition and capable of leg pressing 2.5 times the body weight.
2. **Warm up properly**. Use stretching, jogging, running and sprinting before starting the plyometrics. It would be better to use plyometrics at the end of a running workout.
3. **Perform plyometrics on a soft surface** such as grass or gym mats, and at the end of the workout.
4. **Use these exercises every other day** and on alternate days from weight training. Schedule twice weekly in the early part of the week.
5. **Add heel cups to shoes** if heels are prone to soreness or bruises.

Exercises

These plyometric exercises are suggested for running or racewalking competitors.

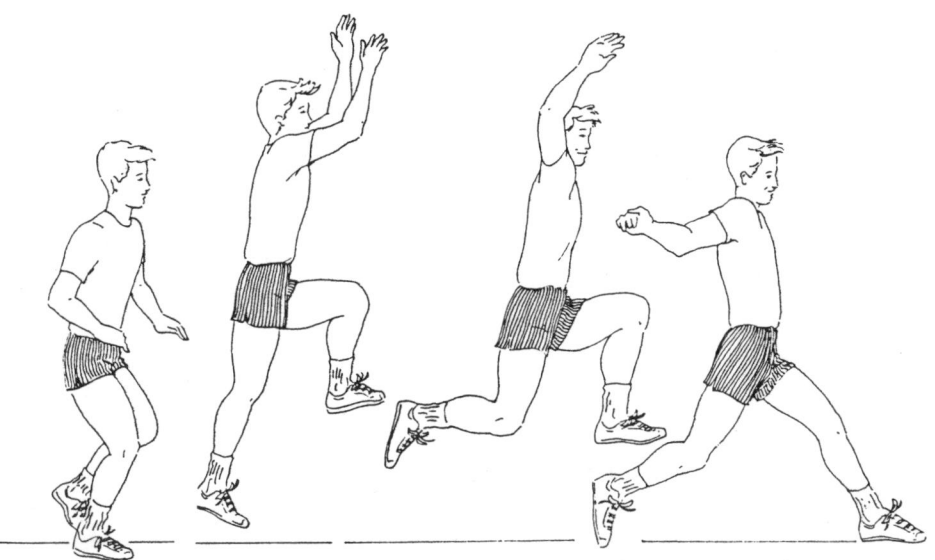

1. **Alternate Leg Bound** — Stand with one foot slightly in front of the other. Lift both arms up as the front knee lifts up and the back leg pushes off. Work for maximum height and distance. When the forward foot lands, attempt to push off immediately and repeat with the opposite knee. Arms should be back as the foot lands to be ready for the upward swing with the next knee lift. Start with 1-2 sets of 8-10 bounds.

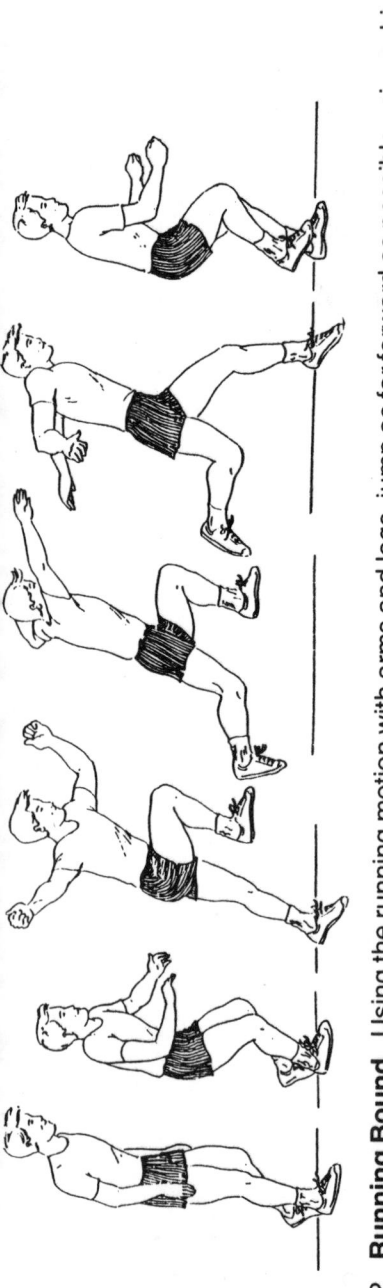

2. **Running Bound.** Using the running motion with arms and legs, jump as far forward as possible using a high knee lift and long stride. Use opposite arm raise to help with height on the knee lift. Although maximum forward motion is desirable, it is important to land with the center of gravity under the body and foot under the bent knee. Start with 1-2 sets of 8-10 bounds.

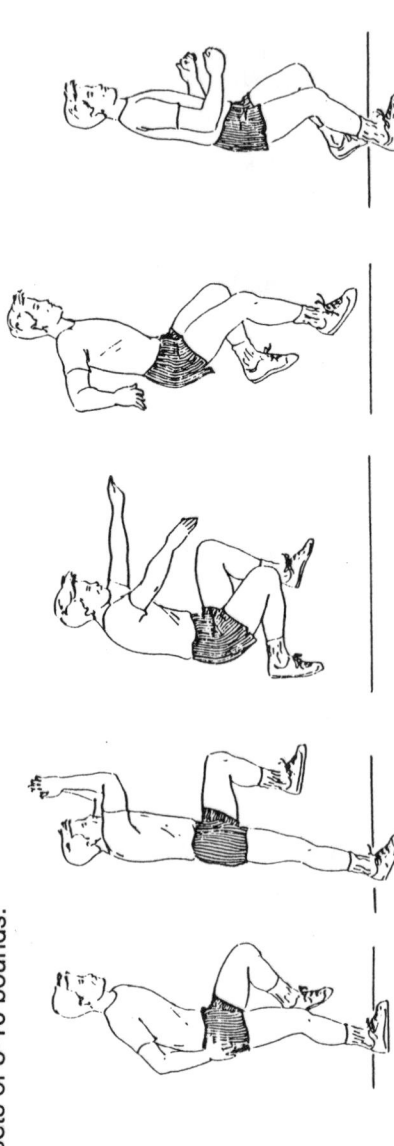

3. **Single-leg Speed Hop.** Start with one foot on the ground and knee slightly flexed while opposite knee is bent and leg is held off the ground. Hop with the planted leg using both arms to lift and attempting to bring the hopping knee up to the suspended flexed knee. Start with 1-2 sets of 10-15 hops.

CROSS TRAINING

Values

Cross training involves substituting one or more alternate aerobic activities for walking, jogging or running on selected days of the workout program. These substitutions can help to prevent injuries which may occur because of the impact from walking, jogging or running, or because of muscle imbalance which results from single activity participation. For instance, walking, jogging and running develop the hamstring muscles more than the quadriceps. By choosing an alternate aerobic activity which builds the quadriceps, a balance will result. These alternate activities not only prevent, but can also rehabilitate injuries when walking, jogging or running are off limits. Cross training may be valuable in helping maintain aerobic fitness during the winter in cold climates and in tropical climates during the summer when walking, jogging and running may be restricted. Finally, a variety of aerobic activities in an exercise program can help prevent boredom, keep interest and enthusiasm high, and be responsible for numerous individuals continuing to work out. However, according to the specificity principle, participation in one aerobic activity will not improve performance in another.

Alternate Types of Aerobic Activities

The most common types of aerobic activities other than walking, jogging or running are aerobic dance, cross country skiing or cross country skiing machines, cycling, rope skipping, rowing or rowing machines, stair climbing or stair climbing machines, swimming, treadmills, water aerobics, and water walking/jogging/running. Recently, step training (also called bench stepping) has gained in popularity.

Aerobic dance can be high impact or low impact. Both involve a variety of exercises to music, which not only improve aerobic fitness but contribute to strength improvement as well. High impact involves more jumping, hopping and bouncing which can lead to injury. Low impact involves stronger arm movements, kicks, knee lifts, various types of fast walking or dance steps. For a relief from walking, jogging or running, low impact would be the better choice for the average walker, jogger or runner. The competitor may not find the low impact workout strenuous enough to tax or enhance his/her aerobic capacity. Because of the strength building movements involved in aerobic dance, walkers, joggers, and runners who have not engaged in a strength program should be cautious and condition slowly with this aerobic activity.

Cross country skiing offers the most dynamic aerobic workout and is rated number one for total aerobic conditioning. It is gentle on the leg joints; however, it builds the upper body muscles as well as leg muscles due to the poling involved. Cross country skiing machines are often difficult to use at first until the coordination is learned and are used typically for 20-30 minute workouts.

Evidence exists that **cycling** will enhance walking, jogging and running. It contributes to the improvement of muscle balance between the quadriceps and hamstrings, the flexibility in the hip and knee joints, and the ability to walk, jog or run uphill. Start with 20-30 minutes and build up to an hour or more using the same 10% weekly increase advocated for walking, jogging and running programs. **Stationary cycling** can be more strenuous than cycling out on the roads, particularly when using the adjustment mechanisms on the bike. Various stationary bikes are available. More recently the computerized bicycles, which vary the degree of difficulty during the workout and provide a calorie expenditure reading, have been popular. Start slowly and work up to a 20-30 minute workout. Pedal speed should range between 80-100 rpm. For the competitor, speed work can be performed on an adjustable speed stationary bike with pedal straps. After a 5-10 minute warm up at 80 rpm, fast pedal on an easy pedaling setting for 30 seconds attempting 100 revolutions during that time, followed by a 1 minute slow pedal recovery. Start with 3-5 repetitions of this sequence and build to 10 or more.

Rope skipping is an excellent cardiovascular activity. However, it stresses the joints due to impact. Use a quality rope of 7-10 feet depending upon the height of the individual. Start with 2 minute sets with one minute recoveries and build to 10 minutes or more of continuous jumping. Try for 160 skips per minute for a good workout.

Rowing, whether in a boat or on a rowing machine, is one of the best supplementary aerobic activities. Start easily for 5-10 minutes and build up to 20-30 at a faster pace. It is important to learn the technique to prevent strain on the back caused by bringing the knees up too soon on recovery.

Stair climbing or exercising on a stair climbing machine is aerobically strenuous and helps to build strong thigh muscles. Start with 5-10 minutes and gradually increase the time. An increase in the climbing speed and number of stairs climbed will also increase the workout intensity.

The freestyle stroke is suggested for a good aerobic workout through **swimming**. This is an outstanding conditioning activity and may be rated higher than running. Several top track coaches include swimming workouts in the training programs of their athletes. A mile or more of swimming should be the goal. However, start with a lesser distance and overload by increasing laps regularly.

Treadmills provide an opportunity to walk, jog or run at a controlled speed in a controlled environment. Intensity can be increased by increasing the speed and/or by inclining the surface. Caution should be followed and the heart rate should be checked regularly to avoid reaching the maximum heart rate. Treadmills can also be used for aerobic testing, but must be monitored by a qualified individual who follows proper precautions.

Water aerobics is similar to aerobic dance. The exercises to music takes place in the water generally at the 3-4 foot level. Special paddles and other water resisting devices may be used.

Walking, jogging or running in water of various depths is gaining in popularity. Deep water workouts with or without vests or special flotation aids have been used for injury rehabilitation and as supplements to training programs for collegiate cross country and distance runners. For an optimal workout, do not lean forward or hold the arms out too far during the water workout. Twenty to thirty minutes is the typical amount of time spent at this activity. Competitors may add or include 5 sets of 2 minute intervals followed by recovery and use the technique of holding on to lane ropes and moving the legs as fast as possible. Research indicates that water walking, jogging or running must be at the same pace as on land to gain the same benefit, but the water exertion will feel harder than the land exertion due to the water resistance.

Step training or bench stepping involves stepping up and down on a bench or platform while exercising the upper body with or without hand weights. This high intensity, low impact workout is usually accompanied by music and includes various stepping patterns as well as upper body exercises. Step training, particularly with hand weights, is recommended for an advanced or ultimate aerobic workout. Intensity may be increased by increasing the platform/bench height within a range of 4-12 inches, amount of the hand held weights, and/or workout speed.

In-line skating is the latest exercise craze. The type of skate, frame, bearings, and number and size of wheels all have an effect on the speed which can be obtained. In order to achieve aerobic fitness, skating must be continuous and at a pace which elevates the heart rate into the desired range.

Comparisons to Walking, Jogging and Running

To include any of the alternate activities in an existing walking, jogging or running program, approximate comparisons of aerobic benefits are helpful. One and one-half miles of walking compares to 1 mile of jogging. To obtain a similar aerobic benefit as one mile of jogging or 1.5 miles of walking, the following approximate comparisons can be used: 1/4 mile free style swimming (Note: The heart rate during swimming will be 10 beats slower per minute because of the horizontal position), 4 miles of cycling, 10 minutes of skipping rope, 1 mile of flat treadmill jogging or 1.5 miles of flat treadmill walking, 22 minutes of aerobic dance, 18 minutes of stationary cycling, 15 minutes of cross country skiing, 30 minutes of water jogging, 9 minutes of step training. These amounts may vary according to the speed at which a person trains and the adjustments used on equipment that may be involved. For a comparable in-line skating workout, one must skate for the identical amount of time and at the same elevated heart rate which one achieves for a 1 mile jog or 1.5 mile walk.

Suggested Programs

If a current walking, jogging or running program is three days per week, substitute one of the cross training activities for one day. For a four day program, substitute the same or two different cross training activities on alternate days from walking, jogging or running. In a five day program, schedule an alternate aerobic activity or two different activities on the 2nd and 4th day. For a 6 day plan, use the same plan as indicated for 5 days and save the 6th day for a long walk, jog, or run. The suggested days for substituting should be those which are designated as easy.

3 Day Week	1	2	3
	Walk, Jog, or Run	Alternate Aerobic Activity	Walk, Jog, or Run

4 Day Week	1	2	3	4
	Walk, Jog, or Run	Alternate Aerobic Activity	Walk, Jog, or Run	Alternate Aerobic Activity

5 Day Week	1	2	3
	Walk, Jog, or Run	Alternate Aerobic Activity	Walk, Jog, or Run
		4	5
		Alternate Aerobic Activity	Walk, Jog, or Run

6 Day Week	1	2	3
	Walk, Jog, or Run	Alternate Aerobic Activity	Walk, Jog, or Run
	4	5	6
	Alternate Aerobic Activity	Walk, Jog, or Run	Long Walk, Jog, or Run

CHAPTER SUMMARY

In order to strive for wellness and also to enhance walking, jogging, and running capabilities, flexibility and strength exercises should be regularly scheduled three or more times per week. Static stretching for 10-60 seconds is recommended. A strength program may involve either calisthenics, weight training, isometrics or a combination of all three types. Weight training is most effective. Plyometric exercises can be performed to help improve speed by developing muscle power and strength. Alternate aerobic activities may be included to supplement a walking, jogging, or running program or to replace 1 or 2 days of walking, jogging, or running.

CHAPTER SIX

Common Injuries:
Prevention and Care

PREVENTION

When developing and implementing a walking, jogging, or running program properly, individuals may experience minor injuries during exercise. Most injuries can be prevented through common sense and knowledge. Most people are unaware how easy it is to injure themselves. In essence, people are not "tuned in" to their own bodies and therefore take unnecessary risks. **The best treatment of injuries is prevention.**

Injuries occur to the ligaments, tendons, muscles, and bones. A continuous stress causes breakdowns, inflammation and pain to these areas. Basically, the two types of injuries are acute and overuse (chronic or stress). The **acute injury** is one that happens suddenly (tripping, spraining the ankle or falling to avoid an object). Applying ice to all new and acute injuries should be done immediately to keep the swelling down and speed recovery. Ice applications relieve pain and slow blood flow, therefore reducing internal bleeding and swelling. Tissue damage is limited and the healing process is faster.

The **overuse** (chronic or stress) **injury** is brought on gradually as a result of wear and tear from a repetitive activity. It consists of nagging pains while training and gets worse each day, until it becomes painful. These injuries need a variety of treatments, such as a change in training routine and healing time. Most of the injuries experienced by walkers/joggers/runners are of the overuse variety. If the overuse injury is not treated properly, the exerciser may be plagued the rest of his/her life.

Contact a physician when there is numbness or tingling, stabbing or radiating pain, significant swelling, or inability to move the injured body part.

The following guidelines should be used to prevent common injuries:
1. **Warm up thoroughly before exercising.** Stretching exercises for the Achilles tendon and groin area are helpful for a walking, jogging, or running program. Cool down afterwards.

2. **Don't overdo.** Start easily and progress slowly in the early stages of the program. Studies suggest that exercising more than five times a week in a high-impact activity such as running may significantly increase the risk of injury. Suddenly intensifying or lengthening the workout may create additional friction in the joints.
3. **Do not follow the "no pain, no gain" plan.** Listen to the body. Instead, train, don't strain. If pain is experienced, lay off or progress slowly.
4. **Avoid hard and uneven surfaces or rough terrain.** Concrete surfaces should be avoided. Persistent impact may cause muscle soreness and foot, tendon and joint injuries. Stress on numerous body parts can result from improper techniques and training such as landing on the balls of the feet (instead of the heels) when jogging.
5. **Wear proper shoes.** Properly-fitting shoes are imperative. Worn-out shoes add stress on the hips, knees, ankles, and feet. Frequently used shoes can lose one-third or more of their shock-absorbing ability in a few months.
6. **Check your feet.** The knees, hips, and ankles sometimes pay the price for foot abnormalities (flat feet), overpronation (feet roll inward too much), or poor leg alignment (knock-knees) which may put greater stress on joints. An orthotic device, such as a custom-made arch support, may help to correct some foot or alignment problems.
7. **Allow an injury to heal before exercising again.** Learn to listen to the body for abnormal sensations and treat an injury as soon as it occurs.
8. **Monitor emotional, behavioral and physical changes of signs of overtraining.** Particularly take notice if the waking heart rate increases by more than five beats per minute, if the heart rate rises abnormally during and after a normal workout, or if the heart rate recovery time increases, and reduce workout time or intensity.

The most common injuries or disabilities that may occur during a walking, jogging, or running program are discussed in this chapter. In addition, some do-it-yourself treatments for common injuries are included.

INJURIES

Achilles Tendonitis

Achilles tendonitis is an inflammation of the thick tendon that connects the heel to the calf (Achilles) muscle which transmits force to the foot and propels an exerciser forward. The injury is easily identified: the big cord that slides into the heel bone hurts when squeezed and there is pain, swelling, warmth, and redness. The pain may bother the individual in the morning or at the start or end of the exercise activity. The pain may be severe when beginning the exercise and diminish as the exercise is continued and the pain may reoccur once the exercise is stopped. In a normal program of exercise, small tears of the Achilles tendon usually heal in a short period of time. The tendon has to be tough, because it absorbs a pull of two to three times the body's weight (1,000 to 1,200 times) each mile. The Achilles injury may be due to the improper cushion of shoes (without thick heels), improper or lack of calf stretching (flexibility), too much activity, landing on toes or hard surfaces, extra stress of hill work or speed. Also, biomechanical problems (tight hamstrings or gastrocnemius, bowed legs, high-arched rigid feet, overpronation and excessive toe-running) may cause Achilles tendonitis.

Recommended treatment for Achilles tendonitis consists of massage (ice) twice a day, a heel lift (2 1/2" heel lifts or soft materials to raise the heel and relax the Achilles tendon), exercise on soft surfaces, and a rest from exercise of 4 to 6 weeks until the inflammation subsides. If the injury doesn't respond to self-treatment in two weeks, seek medical advice immediately. Alternative exercises include swimming, pool running and bicycling (in low gear)—no weight-bearing exercise.

Blisters

Blisters come in seconds and take days to heal. Even a small blister that goes uncared for will be uncomfortable during workouts. The best advice is prevention.

Blisters are caused by friction, a surface of the shoe rubbing against the skin on the foot, a wrinkle in a wet sock, or the excessive use of feet that are not calloused. To assist in the prevention of blisters, lubricate the trouble spot with petroleum jelly and powder the feet before putting on shoes. Purchasing the correct size of shoes and getting the feet accustomed to shoes before any activity is important.

Water Blister Care. Do not open the blister unless there is severe pain, pus or infection. If any of these symptoms are present, wash the skin, swab the blister with iodine or alcohol and make a small incision on the side of the blister with a sterilized razor blade, pin or scalpel. Cover the blister with sterile gauze once it is drained.

Blood Blister Care. The first aid treatment for a blood blister is to ice the area. Do not puncture the blister because the chance of infection is greater due to the connection into the circulatory system. Place a "doughnut-type" compress around the blister until it is reabsorbed or completely healed.

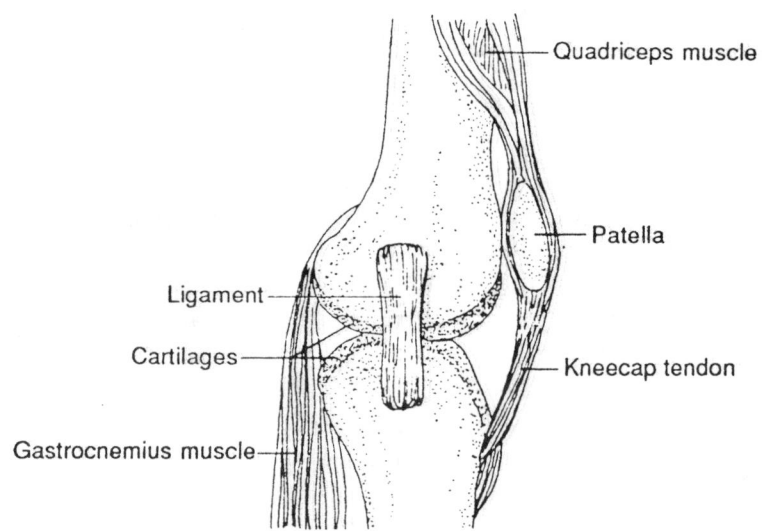

Figure 6-1. Muscles, ligaments and tendons surrounding the kneecap.

Chondromalacia Patella

Pain or inflammation around the kneecap is often called **"runner's knee"** or iliotibial band syndrome. Women runners have more pain because wider hips exaggerate the angle of the upper leg bone which forms at the knee with the lower leg bone. Repeated shock can cause irritation when the knee flexes and extends since it is basically a hinge joint. This pain is frequently experienced by long distance runners, when descending stairs, going downhill or upon standing after sitting. Nearly 30% of runners eventually develop this disorder. Skiers, cyclists, and soccer players are also prone to develop it.

Rest, stretching, application of ice and taking it easy on downhill stretches are important. Extending the leg and gently massaging the kneecap may be helpful. The **"runner's knee"** is aggravated by running or climbing stairs and doing deep knee bends. The patella (kneecap) usually glides up and down in a groove in the femur (upper leg bone) and becomes misaligned, thus rubbing on the underlying surface of cartilage and causing pain. Rotation can occur at the knee joint especially if foot pronation occurs, therefore resulting in a severe irritation along the patella. The muscles which cross the knee (quadriceps and hamstrings) provide less rotation in the area if they are strong. Reducing the ground forces the knee absorbs during a marathon would be helpful, since the average marathon runner takes approximately 25,000 steps. Replace shoes with a better shock-absorbing pair and walk, jog or run on softer surfaces. If self treatment is not helpful after four weeks, see an orthopedic surgeon. Alternative exercises include swimming, pool running, rowing, and any other exercise that does not put pressure on the knee.

Iliotibial Band Syndrome

This syndrome is evidenced by inflammation and pain on the outside of the knee, where the iliotibial band (a ligament that runs along the outside of the thigh) is rubbing against the large leg bone, the femur. After running a mile or two, a dull ache begins and lingers during the run but disappears soon after you stop running. In severe cases, pain may be sharp and the outside of the knee may be swollen or tender.

Treatment for iliotibial band syndrome includes cutting back on speed work, avoiding downhill running, and stretching the band a few times each day. The main thing is to restore the band's flexibility. If your injury is not responding to self treatment after four weeks, see an orthopedic surgeon. Severe cases may need cortisone injections under the band to alleviate the pain. Alternative exercises include swimming, pool running, bicycling, rowing but not stair climbing. Keep press off the outside of the knee.

Muscle Cramps

Muscle cramps are painful spasms of a muscle. Cramping usually affects the gastrocnemius muscle, but it may affect the hamstrings, quadriceps or any voluntary muscle. Cramping may occur during or following a rigorous exercise activity possibly because of two different reasons. Muscle cramping during exercises is primarily due to the body's depletion of essential electrolytes or mineral imbalance and fluid imbalance (sodium, chloride, calcium or potassium, and magnesium) in the system. Also, a breakdown in the coordination between opposing muscle groups. Replacing fluids before and during exercise, particularly in hot weather, is recommended to prevent dehydration (loss of body fluids). Stretching the muscles to be used in walking, jogging or running prior to exercising may help to eliminate muscle cramps.

The most common cramps associated with exercise occur within 24 hours after exercise and may last for several days. These cramps are not associated with electrolyte or fluid imbalance. When a muscle cramp occurs, the muscle squeezes against the artery and partially cuts off the blood flow. A reduced flow of blood to the muscle (ischemia) results in pain.

Treatment for muscle cramping is to statically stretch the muscle in the exact opposite direction. This allows blood to flow to the muscle again, thus reducing the pain and spasm. Massage helps in the dilation of blood vessels close to the skin surface, which may also aid in the return of blood flow to the injury. If stretching or massage do not relieve the cramp, try holding the muscle tightly and pressing your fingertips into the muscle for 10-15 seconds. Release slowly. If the cramp reoccurs repeat the squeezing procedure. If the cramp continues to return, drink fluids and seek medical help.

The lack of calcium and potassium is often the cause of cramping in pregnant and lactating women. Calcium supplements and the consumption of plenty of fruits and vegetables may relieve the problem. Wear loose fitting clothing to prevent a decreased blood flow to the muscle tissue.

Muscle Soreness

Muscle soreness often occurs after a prolonged period of inactivity which is common in weekend athletes who exercise occasionally or frequent exercisers who increase the intensity of workouts too soon (overdoing it). The result is often a **localized delayed-onset muscle soreness (DOMS)**. This discomfort may occur a day or so later but can last a week or longer. DOMS may result from microscopic injury to muscle tissue. The soreness that usually does not appear for 24 to 48 hours and is associated with torn muscle fibers and/or connective tissue. This delayed type needs attention in the form of rest from 5 to 7 days, adequate warm-up and cool-down stretching program, and the incorporation of conditioning and strength activities. Limited activity, usage and gentle stretching is suggested for treating muscle soreness to ease the discomfort. However, recent research suggests that relief from DOMS may be achieved by repeating the activity which caused the soreness at a much lower intensity. If pain continues, consult a physician for appropriate pain relievers.

Tim Noakes, M.D., classifies leg muscle soreness in *The Lore of Running* and makes the following recommendations regarding training or racing:

Grade 0 involves no discomfort—one can continue training.

Grade 1 involves some discomfort on feeling the muscle—one should reduce training for seven days and not race for two weeks.

Grade 2 involves discomfort on walking and inability to squat without discomfort — one should reduce training for fourteen days and not race for one month.

Grade 3 involves severe pain and difficulty with walking — one should reduce training for at least one month and not race for two months.

Plantar Fasciitis

An inflammation of the thick, fibrous band of connective tissue that supports the bottom of the foot (running from the heel to the base of the toes), is called plantar fasciitis. There is a tenderness or pain on the bottom of the foot (near the heel). Early recognition is important. Check shoes and the feet for overpronation (foot pronating inward pulling on the plantar fascia), bone-heel growth (heel spur) or a bursa (inflamed fluid-filled sac) in the bottom of the foot. It is important to reduce running, exercise on soft surfaces, use well-cushioned shoes, check for misalignment of leg and foot bones, go easy on intense workouts, and avoid too little or too much stretching. The **RICES treatment** (discussed later in this chapter), leg stretches, new shoes and heel cups or cushions may alleviate the pain. Reduce the mileage and training on the balls of the feet (speed work/hills). This injury is slow to heal and if it has not healed in four weeks, see a podiatrist, who may prescribe orthotics, ultrasound or friction massage. Alternative exercises include swimming, pool running, cycling (in low gear). After surgery only swimming is recommended during rehabilitation.

Stress Fractures

Stress fractures are microscopic breaks in the bone, usually in the foot, shin, or thigh. They are brought on by stress caused by repeated impact of such activities as walking, jogging, or running on hard surfaces for long periods of time. Often the pain is mild, occurring during or after exercising; it may be a result of exercising too much, too fast and too soon. The area may become tender and painful with possible swelling in the area of the fracture. This fracture may not be detected in an X-ray until two or three weeks after the injury. It is important to not ignore the pain and continue with activity because actual breakage (rarely) can occur in the bone. It is recommended to increase workouts gradually, not dramatically, exercise on soft or resilient surfaces (grass, dirt, not concrete), wear well-cushioned exercise shoes, and adequately stretch before and after exercise.

Sprain

Sprains involve an **injury to a ligament** (a fibrous tissue that connects bones to bones and joint capsules). A ligament has very little elasticity; if it is stretched beyond its elastic limit, permanent injury may occur (see Fig. 6.1). Sprains are often the result of a sudden force or twisting motion, and the surrounding muscles do not have enough strength to control the motion. Also the ligament may even break or rupture.

Sprains are most common in walking, jogging or running exercises. Often they occur in the ankles and knees. The ligament sprain may result in immediate pain, but the degree of pain is not always related to the severity of the injury. Knee injuries may become painless a few minutes after the injury. If a ligament is completely torn, there may be little or no pain, but when the joint is moved an abnormal motion may occur. Some less severe ligament injuries may be painful, while more severe ligament injuries may be painless. Sprains are often more serious than strains since they take longer to heel and a torn ligament can cause the bones to be out of alignment, therefore causing damage to the surrounding tissues. Strong, flexible muscles can help protect a person against sprains. Stretching the calf muscles (ankle) and strengthening the quadriceps (knee) can help prevent sprains. The RICES formula, described later, is the suggested treatment.

Strain

Strains (muscle pulls) involve an injury to a **muscle** or **tendon** which results from overstretching or tearing of a muscle or tendon. The most common strains are quadriceps, hamstring, groin, shoulder, gastrocnemius and soleus muscles. A tendon (tissue that connects muscle to bone) is elastic, but its elasticity is limited, and it may be overstretched and pulled away from the bone (see Fig. 6.1). A strain may be accompanied by swelling and/or bleeding of soft tissue which may increase the severity of the pain.

Two common methods which may be used to treat the injury are: (1) actively stretch the muscle and tendon during the entire healing process to prevent the muscle or tendon from becoming short; and (2) prohibit all activity until the muscle and tendon heals and gradually stretch it to its normal length. Physician assistance is needed for severe strains. Mild strains are often just a nuisance: the tears are microscopic and, with rest, they will repair themselves. In addition, the RICES formula is the suggested treatment for this injury. In the case of chronic muscle tears at specific sites, Tim Noakes, M.D., recommends in *The Lore of Running* that the key to treatment is the vigorous application of a physiotherapeutic maneuver called cross frictions. Cross friction therapy sessions will be painful. However, after 5-10 sessions the individual should be able to exercise pain free. The best prevention for new or recurring strains is to warm up large muscles and stretch all muscles involved in the exercise activity. A light sweat usually indicates that the warm up is sufficient.

Shin Splints

Pain around the front or either side of the **lower leg bone (tibia)** is usually the sign of **shin splints**, the result of inflammation of the thin sheathing (periosteum) that wraps around the tibia, or shin bone. In addition, it can be caused by injury to the muscles that run along the tibia, by inflammation of the tendons that attach these muscles to the tibia, or in some cases by the stress fracture of that bone. Sports medicine specialists don't like to use the term shin splints because it commonly refers to several lower leg injuries which involve minor tears anywhere the muscle attaches to the shin. Shin splints are the most frequent injury experienced by new walkers, joggers or runners, but this injury can affect anyone who engages in physical activity using the legs. Most shin splints occur in the beginning of an exercise program because the lower leg muscles are tight or weak, the exerciser is overweight, exercising on hard surfaces (hard tracks, cement, asphalt, and wooden floors), and speed work, and/or hill training. In addition, muscle fatigue, faulty posture, insufficient stretching of the calf muscles, improper shoes, running on the toes, poor foot biomechanics leading to overpronation (foot rolls to the inside excessively), and fallen arches can cause this injury.

Recommended treatment for shin splints is to wear motion controlled shoes or orthotics to prevent poor biomechanics, avoid overstriding (places more stress on shins), exercise on soft surfaces, taping during activity may be helpful, RICES treatment, and consultation with a physician (one who understands running) for medication if the pain is severe. The icing should be done for 8 to 10 continuous minutes (2 -3 times daily) by means of gently massaging the problem area. A second gentle ice massage, a few hours later, of the same duration of time, should begin to give relief. Continue this procedure for several days. And if necessary, stop exercising and rest if the pain is severe until the shin splints heal, about three days. Toe raises on the edge of a step can help strengthen the posterior muscles which are heavily used in any running, jumping activity. Sitting on a table and raising a small weight (10 times per leg) suspended from the foot is an easy way to build up strength in the tibialis anterior muscles. If icing, rest, elevation, strengthening, and stretching do not create relief within two to four weeks, seek medical assistance to rule out the more serious

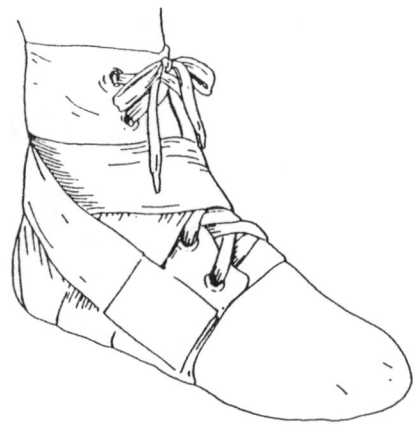

Proper taping or an ankle stabilizer may help in treatment of shin splints.

conditions such as structural imbalances or stress fractures of the tibia. Alternative exercises include nonimpact exercises such as swimming, pool running, walking, and cycling in low gear.

Side Stitch

A **sharp pain** or **stitch in the side** usually represents a **spasm of the diaphragm** (lower portion of the breathing mechanism). Side stitches may occur because not enough oxygen (blood flow) is getting to the respiratory muscles. A decreased blood flow to the location most frequently occurs in those who have recently had a meal or drunk large volumes of fluid. This pain usually occurs in unconditioned beginners or individuals when exercising at higher intensities than accustom.

The preferred treatment is to bend forward from the waist and inhale deeply, therefore making the stomach and intestines push up against the diaphragm, using either a sitting or standing position. Notice breathing and consciously control exhaling. Form the lips as in whistling and exhale through the puckered lips about five to ten times. An additional method is to pull the shoulders up as close to the ears as possible which helps to expand the lungs and take one deep breath. If the pain is not eliminated, slow down and, if necessary, stop exercising.

The conditioned person rarely experiences this pain, so continue programs with regularity, exercise the abdominals with strength exercises and stretching exercises, relax, and regulate speed by using the **"talk test" — can't talk and run, slow down.**

However, conditioned as well as unconditioned walkers, joggers, or runners may experience a side stitch due to the stride position when exhaling. If a person always exhales when his/her right foot strikes the ground, extra pressure is placed on the diaphragm. This extra pressure is caused by the liver when it jolts upward, then falls down onto the diaphragm in the up position. The solution is to change one's breathing pattern in order to exhale when the opposite foot strikes the ground. Also, one may try loud grunting while exhaling to relax the diaphragm.

CARE

Foot Care

Most individuals fail to give feet attention until discomfort or pain occurs. Without proper treatment, injuries may result causing crippling complications for walkers, joggers or runners. Most foot problems can be prevented.

Nails. Nails should be cut or clipped straight across, rounding only slightly at the edges. Cutting deep into the edges may cause ingrown toenails. An instrument specifically designed for trimming nails should be used.

Dry Skin. Regular home care will pamper the feet and also massage tired legs and enhance the circulation. Soaking the feet in a neutral bath oil for 10-15 minutes once per week followed by moisturizing cream will keep feet protected from dryness. Making the feet too soft may make them susceptible to blisters.

Athlete's Foot. A fungal infection which is characterized by redness, burning and itching is commonly called **athlete's foot**. Communal showers, locker-room floors, and sweaty shoes and socks are potential sources of athlete's foot. Wearing clean, absorbent, padded acrylic socks, shoes which allow the feet to breathe, keeping the feet clean and dry, and wearing sandals in the shower or locker room are ways of avoiding this condition.

R.I.C.E.S. FORMULA

Conditioning the muscles is the best way to prevent most sports injuries, but once these injuries occur they must be professionally treated. However, there are minor muscle injuries which can be self treated thus reducing the pain. The standard care for most sports-type injuries includes **"R" for rest; "I" for ice; "C" for compression; "E" for elevation; and "S" for support and stabilization.**

1. **R = Rest.** Restricting movement. When experiencing pain, stop activity. Pain is the body's way of telling you that something's wrong, so listen to the body. Resting the first few days will help stop excess bleeding (internally and externally) and will promote healing of damaged tissues without complications. To prevent movement, splints, tapes, or bandages may be used. Total rest may not be necessary. Additional exercises such as swimming, cycling, and rowing are good physical activities to keep in shape during the injury. Absolute rest should not exceed 48 hours. Muscles can weaken, joints can stiffen and scar tissue may form around the injury and may begin to tighten. Increasing blood flow may assist in the healing process.

2. **I = Ice.** Application of cold compresses (ice or cold whirlpools) to soft-tissue injuries inhibits swelling (caused by "pooling of blood"). Sports medicine literature indicates these compresses should be applied approximately 10-20 minutes after the injury and re-applied every two waking hours for the next 48 hours or until the swelling subsides. Going longer than the 20 minute limit may damage the nerves and skin. Narrowing the blood

vessels by making the body internally (rather than at the surface) supply more blood to the affected area limits swelling and tissue damage. Also, cold compresses may produce relief by blocking (slowing) pain messages to the nerve fibers and preventing pain messages from reaching the brain. Cold may decrease muscle spasms which may accompany severe injury.

The preferred treatment of applying ice to injuries is 10 minutes on and 30 minutes off frequently for 24-48 hours, then 3-5 times per day until the injury heals. Recent research in Belgium by Dr. Romain Meeusen indicates that after 10 minutes of icing nerve activity is depressed, allowing blood vessels to expand and blood flow to rewarm the tissues. When the affected area seems to be the same temperature as the opposite arm and leg, rest of the body, etc. (no longer warm), and a feeling of a burning sensation or aching numbness, the ice compresses can be discontinued. For application to the injured area, the compresses should be wrapped in an absorbent towel/cloth. Water frozen (styrofoam cup) provides a simple means of application. Compresses should not be applied directly (or wrapped in plastic) on the injury since this can cause frostbite plus additional injury. The use of cold compresses (first 24-48 hours), following an injury can reduce pain and swelling and the recovery process will be faster.

3. **C = Compression.** Pressure helps to reduce swelling and blood flow to the injured area. To apply pressure, wrap the injury with an Ace-type elastic bandage or wrap well above and below the injury since swelling may go to other areas. Compression should always be done with icing. The pressure bandages must be tight enough to restrict blood flow and not too tight to cut off blood. If the toes or fingers begin to feel numb or lose their color, the bandage should be adjusted for less restriction.

4. **E = Elevation.** Elevation reduces internal bleeding and "pooling" of blood in the injured area. The injury should be elevated above heart level in order to return the blood to the heart easily and to eliminate pain by reducing the "throbbing" sensation caused by blood rushing to the injured site. Elevation should be combined with icing and compression.

5. **S = Stabilization and Support.** Surround or support the injured area as much as possible to prevent further injury. With a brace, taping or strapping of an injury one can continue to be active. These should stay on the injured area until all of the indications of the injury are gone. The injury should be secured in place, especially when the individual is sleeping. Commercial splints or supports are available from pharmaceutical agencies and/or a medical supply company.

If the injured area is painful or becomes inflamed, stop self-treatment immediately.

HEAT APPLICATION

Heat stimulates blood flow and increases inflammation. Most authorities suggest staying with ice for at least the first 48 hours after an injury and only after the swelling has subsided, try heat (never apply heat to a new injury of any kind). At this point, heat may help relieve pain, relax muscles, speed up healing, and reduce joint stiffness. Apply heat for 20 to 30 minutes, two or three times a day. Consult a physician before using heat on an injury to determine whether to use dry heat (heating pad or lamp) or moist heat (a hot bath, hot-water bottle, heat pack, or whirlpool). Individuals with heart conditions should avoid whirlpools and hot baths. If there is infection or a loss of sensation, do not apply heat.

TEN LAWS OF RUNNING INJURIES

In *The Lore of Running,* Tim Noakes, M.D., lists the following *Ten Laws of Running Injuries:*

1. Running injuries are not an act of God.
2. Each injury progresses through four grades.
3. Each running injury indicates that the athlete has reached the breakdown point.
4. Virtually all running injuries are curable.
5. X-rays and other sophisticated investigations are seldom necessary to diagnose running injuries.
6. Treat the cause, not the effect.
7. Rest is seldom the most appropriate treatment.
8. Never accept as a final opinion the advice of a nonrunner.
9. Avoid the knife.
10. There is no definitive scientific evidence that running causes osteoarthritis in runners whose knees were normal when they started running.

STAYING INJURY-FREE

1. Thou shalt not become a slave to running.
2. Thou shalt not train on legs that are dead.
3. Thou shalt not experiment with a different pair of shoes during a race.
4. Thou shalt not run through any type of muscular or skeletal pain.
5. Thou shalt not attempt to make up miles "lost" due to injury.
6. Thou shalt not increase mileage by more than 10 percent each year.
7. Thou shalt not do more than one hard workout on successive days.
8. Thou shalt not subject yourself to more than one long run per week.
9. Thou shalt not get carried away by an exceptional race and immediately plunge into a higher level of training.
10. Thou shalt not be afraid to rest.

From *Running Injury-free* by editors of *Runner's World,* 1986. Reprinted by permission of *Runner's World.*

CHAPTER SUMMARY

Numerous studies show that the benefits of exercise outweigh the risk of injury. When a person understands the prevention and the care of injuries, the activity will be joyful rather than painful. Accidents do occur even when aerobic activities are carefully planned. An understanding of the basic injuries which may occur while walking, jogging, or running may help to avoid injury, limit the damage done and speed the recovery process. If an injury is suspected, use the **R.I.C.E.S.** formula and, if in doubt, seek professional medical help immediately. Knowing how to handle injuries until professional help arrives can make the difference between a minor fitness injury and a fitness disaster.

CHAPTER SEVEN

NUTRITION

We are creatures of what we eat and we are creatures of what we fail to eat. The typical American diet is too high in calories, fats, sugar, sodium, and alcohol, and too low in complex carbohydrates and fiber. Americans are consuming entirely too much food. Nutrition is used to promote health and prevent diseases.

Proper nutrition signifies that a person's diet is supplying all of the essential nutrients for normal tissue growth, repair, and maintenance of the body. Studies show that six of the ten leading causes of death in North America are linked to poor nutrition. Coronary heart disease, stroke, atherosclerosis, cancer, and adult-onset diabetes are all related to poor nutritional habits and accounted for more than two-thirds of the deaths in the United States.

> "We do not always like what is best for us in this world."
> —Eleanor Roosevelt

Good nutrition and exercise are the foundation to a healthy body and the optimal level of fitness. Without proper nutrition an individual will not have the sufficient energy necessary for exercise or activity. Exercise is as important as nutrition since it is necessary to use energy from the foods consumed, therefore affecting each individual's nutrition and overall health. A nutritious diet is essential to provide sufficient nutrients necessary for cardiorespiratory endurance, muscular strength, muscular endurance, maintaining or controlling body composition, and improving overall performance. Proper nutrition and exercise are preventive medicine and can improve the quality of life.

NUTRIENTS

Nutrients are chemical substances obtained from food during digestion. They meet the body's needs for good health, energy and growth. There is no single food which contains all the nutrients that are needed; therefore, the diet should include a variety of foods. Approximately forty nutrients are needed daily for optimum health. Individuals do not eat nutrients for energy, they eat food for energy. However, the food selection and adequate caloric intake influence adequate nutrient intake.

In 1993 the Food and Drug Administration (FDA) revised food labeling regulations and replaced the U. S. Recommended Dietary Allowances (RDA) with Daily Values (DVs). These recommendations made a significant change on the new food label. The discussion in this chapter will emphasize the DVs.

Calorie

The term "**calorie**" is a measure of heat used to indicate the energy supplied by food and energy expended by the body. A calorie, known as a **kilocalorie (kcal)**, is the main expression of a food's energy-producing value. For simplicity, it is often referred to as a calorie rather than kcal.

Calories can come only from **carbohydrates, proteins, fats,** and **alcohol**. They are nutrients that can be oxidized in the body to yield energy; therefore, they are referred to as the energy nutrients. The energy value of foods primarily depends on the amounts of carbohydrate, protein, fat, and alcohol contained. The values in Figure 7.1 can be used to determine the caloric content of the foods consumed:

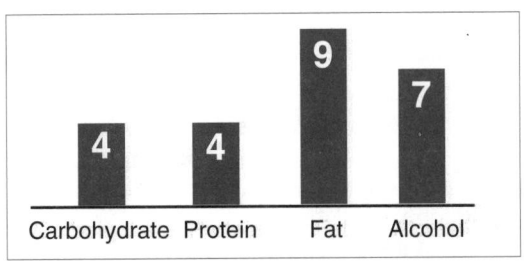

Figure 7.1. Caloric value of major energy foods.

The energy value of a food may be computed by multiplying the number of grams of each energy nutrient in a serving of food by the caloric values per gram of carbohydrate, protein, and fat.

For Example: A food with 12 grams of carbohydrates, 6 grams of protein and 5 grams of fat. The caloric value is calculated as follows:

Nutrient	Total Grams		kcal./g.		Total kcal.
Carbohydrate	12	x	4	=	48
Protein	6	x	4	=	24
Fat	5	x	9	=	45
			Total	=	117 kcal.

Alcohol is not a nutrient because it cannot be used by the body to promote growth, maintenance, or repair. It can serve as an energy source but is high in calories — often referred to as "**empty calories.**"

The number of calories needed per day depends on one's **metabolic rate (MR)**. Metabolic rate depends upon factors such as age, gender, size, muscle mass, climate, glandular function, emotional state, and exercise. The **basal metabolic rate (BMR)** is the number of calories which are burned at rest (heart beating, cellular processes, etc.). MR is a combination of BMR and calories expended in normal daily activities.

In addition, there are activities conducted during the waking hours which utilize calories in addition to the BMR. The more physical activities involved, the more calories needed to sustain body weight. An example of the number of calories (including BMR) needed each day to maintain body weight may be derived as follows:

Formula Used if Presently at Ideal Weight
(If underweight, use present weight.)

Ideal Weight x 14 calories per lb.
(sedentary lifestyle: exercise 0-1 time/week)

Ideal Weight x 15 calories per lb.
(relatively active: exercise 3 to 5 times/week)

Ideal Weight x 16 calories per lb.
(very active: exercise 5+ times/week)

Ideal Weight x 20 calories per lb.
(athlete: vigorous activity)

Note: This formula is derived from actual measurements of numerous individuals; therefore, it is not accurate for each individual. It is only a guideline

Example: The individual is relatively active and weighs 150 pounds (150 x 15 = 2,250). The person should eat 2,250 calories per day. The resulting number is the amount of calories needed to eat each day to maintain current weight.

Knowing the total daily caloric needs, calculate carbohydrate, fat and protein percentages (2,250 x 60%; 2,250 x 20-25%; and 2,250 x 10-15% respectively). **Note:** The National Research Council recommends <30% fat.

THE FOOD GUIDE PYRAMID
A Guide to Daily Food Choices

The Food Guide Pyramid replaces the Basic Four Food Groups. It is a general outline of what to eat each day based on the Dietary Guidelines. An adequate supply of the foods in the Food Guide Pyramid will provide the six basic nutrients for most healthy people. Refer to Figure 7.2. The pyramid calls for eating a variety of foods to get necessary nutrients and the right amount of calories to maintain healthy weight. Start with plenty of

Food Guide Pyramid
A Guide to Daily Food Choices

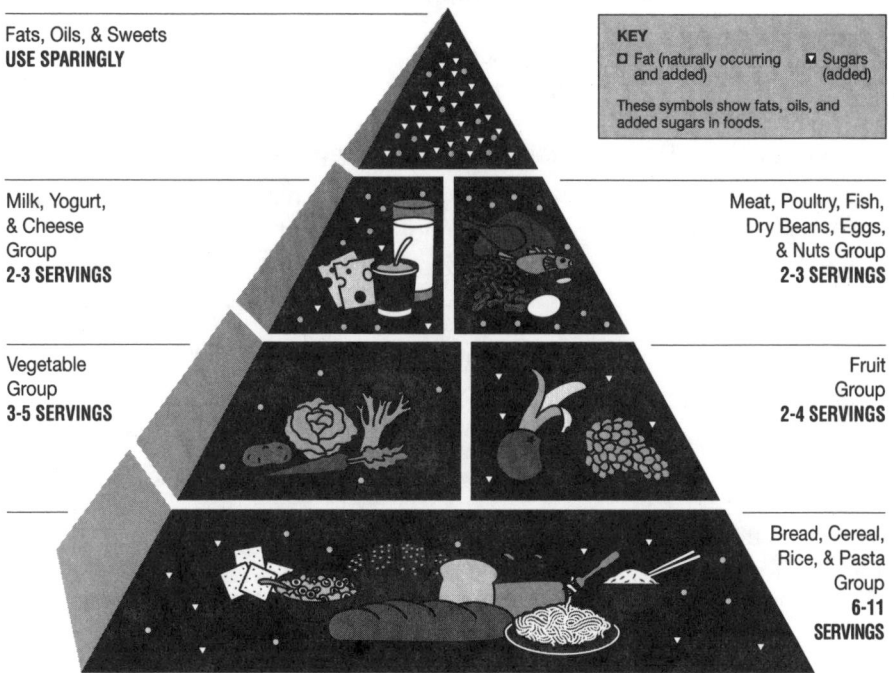

Fats, Oils, & Sweets
USE SPARINGLY

KEY
☐ Fat (naturally occurring and added)   ☑ Sugars (added)
These symbols show fats, oils, and added sugars in foods.

Milk, Yogurt, & Cheese Group
2-3 SERVINGS

Meat, Poultry, Fish, Dry Beans, Eggs, & Nuts Group
2-3 SERVINGS

Vegetable Group
3-5 SERVINGS

Fruit Group
2-4 SERVINGS

Bread, Cereal, Rice, & Pasta Group
6-11 SERVINGS

Figure 7.2. Food Guide Pyramid

breads, cereals, rice, pasta, vegetables, and fruits (complex carbohydrates, which are included in four of the five food groups). Add 2-3 servings from the milk group and 2-3 servings from the meat group. Go easy on the fats, oils, and sweets, the foods in the small tip of the pyramid.

The Food Guide Pyramid does not describe the differences between skim and whole milk or meat and poultry. A cup of skim milk has 88 calories compared to 160 in a cup of whole milk. One ounce of boneless beef has 70-100 calories, while an ounce of boneless chicken has 50-55. While the pyramid tells how many servings of each food to eat each day, it does not specify how much a "serving" is. See Table 7.1 for sample serving sizes.

The number of servings that is right for you depends on how many calories you need, which in turn depends on your age, sex, size, and your activity level. (See Table 7.2.) Almost everyone should have at least the lowest number of servings in the ranges.

TABLE 7.1
WHAT COUNTS AS A SERVING?*

Milk, Yogurt, and Cheese		
1 cup of milk or yogurt	1 1/2 ounces of natural cheese	2 ounces of process cheese

Meat, Poultry, Fish, Dry Beans, Eggs, and Nuts	
2-3 ounces of cooked lean meat, poultry, or fish	1/2 cup of cooked dry beans, 1 egg, or 2 table-spoons of peanut butter or 1/3 cup of nuts count as 1 ounce of lean meat.

Vegetable		
1 cup of raw leafy vegetables.	1/2 cup of other veg-etables, cooked or chopped raw	3/4 cup of vegetable juice

Fruit		
1 medium apple, banana, orange	1/2 cup of chopped, cooked, or canned fruit	3/4 cup of fruit juice

Bread, Cereal, Rice, and Pasta
1 slice of bread
1 ounce of ready-to-eat cereal
1/2 cup of cooked cereal, rice, or pasta

•The amount of food that counts as 1 serving is listed above. If you eat a larger portion, count it as more than 1 serving. For example, a dinner portion of spaghetti would count as 2 or 3 servings of pasta.

Be sure to eat at least the lowest number of servings from the five major food groups listed above. You need them for the vitamins, minerals, carbohydrates, and protein they provide. Just try to pick the lowest fat choices from the food groups. No specific serving size is given for the fats, oils, and sweets group because the message is USE SPARINGLY.

Serving sizes indicated here are those used in the Food Guide Pyramid and based on both suggested and usually consumed portions necessary to achieve adequate nutrient intake. They differ from serving sizes on the Nutrition Facts Label, which reflect portions usually consumed.

TABLE 7.2
HOW MANY SERVINGS DO YOU NEED EACH DAY?

	Many women, older adults	Children, teen girls, active women, most men	Teen boys, active men
*Calorie level**	about *1,600*	about *2,200*	about *2,800*
Bread Group Servings	6	9	11
Vegetable Group Servings	3	4	5
Fruit Group Servings	2	3	4
Milk Group Servings	2-3**	2-3**	2-3**
Meat Group Servings	2, for a total of 5 ounces	2, for a total of 6 ounces	3, for a total of 7 ounces
Total Fat (grams)	53	73	93

* These are the calorie levels if you choose low fat, lean foods from the 5 major food groups and use foods from the fats, oils, and sweets group sparingly.
** Women who are pregnant or breastfeeding, teenagers, and young adults to age 24 need 3 servings.

DAILY VALUES (DVS)

The Daily Values provide the percentage of recommended daily amount of vitamins, minerals, total fat, saturated fat, cholesterol, sodium, carbohydrates, fiber, sugar and protein.

Daily Values are based on 2000 calorie diet with 30% of the calories coming from fat (10% from saturated fat), 58%-60% from carbohydrates, and 10%-12% from protein. Individuals who are ill or unhealthy may require additional nutrients.

BASIC NUTRIENTS

The six essential nutrients required by the human body are carbohydrates, fats, protein, vitamins, minerals, and water. Carbohydrates, fats, protein, and water are called macronutrients because large amounts are needed on a daily basis. Carbohydrates, fats, and proteins are needed to supply energy (measured in calories) necessary for normal body functions and work. Vitamins and minerals are only necessary in small amounts; therefore, they are referred to as micronutrients. These have no caloric value but are still essential for normal body functions and maintenance of good health.

The three major functions of nutrients are:

1. **Provide energy for human metabolism.** Carbohydrates and fats are the prime source of energy (measured in calories), although proteins are burned when carbohydrates are depleted in aerobic exercise.
2. **Nutrients are used to build and repair body tissues.** Protein is the major building material for muscles, other soft tissues, and enzymes, while certain minerals, such as calcium and phosphorus, make up the skeletal framework.
3. **Nutrients are used to help regular body processes.** Vitamins, minerals, proteins and water work closely together to maintain the diverse physiological processes of human metabolism. For example, hemoglobin in the red blood cell is essential for the transportation of oxygen to the muscle tissue via the blood. Hemoglobin is a complex combination of protein and iron; however, other minerals and vitamins are needed for its synthesis and for full development of red blood cells. Refer to Lab 7.1, Dietary Habits Evaluation.

Table 7.3 indicates the percentages of dietary caloric intake recommended by the authors from each of the energy nutrients.

TABLE 7.3
RECOMMENDED RANGE OF DIETARY CALORIC INTAKE
According to Percent

Carbohydrates	**58-60%**
Simple — 10% or less	
Complex — 48-50%	
Fats	**< 30%**
Polyunsaturated — 10% or less	
Monounsaturated — 10% or less	
Saturated — 10% or less	
Protein	**10-12%**
Athletes	10-15%

Carbohydrates

Carbohydrates are the number one **source of energy** used by the body to provide cell maintenance, energy for work, and digestion. The glycogen storage in the body depends partially on the amount of carbohydrates eaten. A high-carbohydrate diet increases glycogen storage, thus allowing the individual to work longer before exhaustion occurs.

The body receives approximately 90 percent of energy from the metabolism of carbohydrates and various carbohydrates are different in their nutritional value. Sugar provides only fat and calories while fruit and potatoes supply essential vitamins and minerals. In addition, carbohydrates play an important role in digestion, regulation of fat and protein metabolism; therefore, they are important in saving body protein as an energy source and allowing fats to be used more efficiently. Carbohydrates are classified into simple and complex carbohydrates.

Simple Carbohydrates

Simple carbohydrates (sugars), are found naturally as part of fruits and vegetables or as a refined product in foods such as cakes, candy, cookies, jellies, white bread, rolls, snack food, and colas. There are over one hundred types of sugars; the most common one in the typical American diet is sucrose (plain table sugar). Sugar does not have to be white; it can be brown such as molasses, brown sugar and honey. After the digestion of honey and white sugar, they are identical; in fact, white sugar contains fewer calories than honey. Sugar is often called "**empty calories**" since it adds calories and is very low in nutritional value. Words ending in "ose" (simple sugars) such as glucose, fructose, galactose, sucrose, lactose, and maltose should be used in moderation. These sugars have been shown to increase the incidence of dental caries and are often low in vitamins and minerals. Processed foods and beverages account for more than two-thirds of the simple sugars consumed. Carbohydrates, with the exception of milk sugar (lactose), are virtually nonexistent in animal foods.

Sugar will not improve performance during exercises such as walking, jogging or running. When consuming sugar within three hours before exercising and before insulin secretion is suppressed, it will increase insulin and hypoglycemia will most likely occur. **Hypoglycemia** occurs when the blood sugar falls below normal due to increased insulin secretion and subsequent increased carbohydrate utilization. Non-diabetics do not spill sugar usually in their urine. Research on runners shows that consuming a sugar drink directly before exercising can reduce athletic performance by 25 percent. Highly concentrated levels of sugar inhibit the absorption of fluids in the body as well as "shunting" blood flow to the stomach to digest the sugar. However, sugar may assist performance during vigorous non-stop endurance activity of more than 1 hour at a time. On a food label, sugars include brown sugar, corn sweetener, corn syrup, fructose, fruit juice concentrate, glucose (dextrose), high fructose corn syrup, honey, invert sugar, lactose, maltose, molasses, raw sugar, table sugar (sucrose), and syrup.

Alcohol is not a true carbohydrate. It comes from carbohydrate foods by natural fermentation (beer, wine) or from the process of distillation to produce hard liquor (whiskey). Generally, alcohol is a source of empty calories; adding a sweet mixer adds additional sugar and calories are included.

Complex Carbohydrates

Two types of complex carbohydrates are **starches** and **glycogen.** **Starches** are commonly found in corn, nuts, grains, roots, seeds, potatoes, and legumes. **Glycogen** is manufactured and stored in the liver. It releases energy and can quickly increase available glucose for exercise. Most dietary carbohydrates are digested and eventually converted to glucose, a simple carbohydrate absorbed into the blood from the intestines. Blood glucose has several metabolic functions. It may be utilized directly by some tissues (brain), to be used for energy, or it may be stored in the liver or muscles as glycogen (a complex carbohydrate). Excess blood glucose may be excreted in the urine or converted into fat and stored in the body's adipose tissue.

Complex carbohydrates are an aid in weight control, since the process of digestion utilizes more energy metabolizing starch than it does metabolizing fat. **It has been stated: "You don't get fat from overeating complex carbohydrates, but from overeating fat."** In addition, complex carbohydrates may be better than fats for informing the body it has taken in enough food; therefore, it is an excellent controller of the appetite. Some complex carbohydrates are an excellent source of **fiber (roughage)**. Potatoes have complete amino acid profile and fiber is low in water. Eating an abundance of complex carbohydrates one can gain weight, but there will be less of a chance than on a diet high in fats and sugar. **The real issue is portion sizes—not food, but the amount of food.**

Scientific research shows that there are naturaly occurring compounds in vegetables and fruits that may help protect against cancer. Beta carotene, Vitamin C and fiber are substances in fruits and vegetables that have protective effects. According to a recent food consumption survey (Cooper), almost 28% of American adults consume no fruit or juice.

Nutritionists usually agree that 58 to 60 percent of the total calories per day should be derived from carbohydrates, and most of these calories should be in the form of complex carbohydrates. Most Americans eat a daily diet of approximately 40-50% or less. During exercise requiring maximal effort for a short period of time (100 yard dash, for example), the main fuel is carbohydrates. During prolonged aerobic exercise, the major fuels are a combination of carbohydrate and fat, with fat being the predominant source of energy after twenty minutes. Complex carbohydrates provide many nutrients (vitamins and minerals) to the body.

TABLE 7.4
HIGH CARBOHYDRATE FOODS

Fruits	Vegetables	Grains/Cereals	Milk Products
Apples	Beans	Bread	Ice Milk
Apricots	Carrots	Biscuits	Skim Milk
Blueberries	Caulifower	Cereal	Yogurt
Blackberries	Corn	Crackers	
Cantaloupe	Eggplant	Corn	
Cherries	Legumes	Flour	
Dried Fruit	Lima Beans	Grits	
Figs	Peas	Macaroni	
Grapefruit	Potatoes	Muffins	
Kiwis	Squash	Noodles	
Oranges	String Beans	Rice	
Nectarines	Tomatoes		
Papaya			
Peaches			
Pears			
Persimmons			
Pineapple			
Plums			
Raspberries			
Star Fruit			
Strawberries			
Tangarines			
Watermelon			

Note: Limit intake of simple carbohydrates (sweets, pastries, sugar and soft drinks) to 10% or less of the total calories.

Fiber

Fiber (roughage or bulk) is often described as indigestible portions of plant foods and found only in plants, never in foods of animal origin. High-fiber foods include whole-grain breads, cereals, pasta, brown rice, fruits, vegetables, dried beans, nuts, and seeds.

There are two types of dietary fiber: **water-soluble** and **water-insoluble**. Certain types of **soluble fibers**, such as those found in oats, fruits, barley and beans (dried, kidney, pinto, navy), have been associated with lowering blood cholesterol levels. Fiber has also been associated with helping to stabilize blood sugar levels in individuals with diabetes. As fiber moves through the digestive system and the colon, it also performs a cleaning action to sweep with it the remains of undigested food and bile secretions. This action contributes to a more thorough elimination of waste products.

Insoluble fiber absorbs water, swelling its size and creating the necessary bulk to stimulate proper functioning of the intestines. It speeds up the movement of food through the intestines and promotes regularity. Water-insoluble fibers, found in whole grain breads, cereals (especially whole wheat products), and wheat bran, vegetables, legumes and fruits (especially those with skins), help retain water and act as natural laxatives. Research evidence indicates an adequate amount of fiber in the diet can help reduce or even prevent many colon problems (second leading cancer), cardiovascular disease, and helps to regular blood sugar of adult-onset diabetes. In addition, other health disorders have been linked to low fiber consumption, including constipation, hemorrhoids, gallbladder disease, diverticulitis, and obesity.

According to the National Cancer Institute an estimated intake of 20 to 35 grams per day of dietary fiber would be a goal to achieve. Americans eat 10 grams or less per day. It takes a concerted effort to increase one's diet to include enough fiber. Eating fruits and vegetables and whole-grain products each day would help to meet this recommendation. Refer to Table 7-5.

TABLE 7.5
HIGH FIBER FOODS

Vegetables	Fruits (Raw)	Additional Sources
Broccoli	Apples	Bran
Cabbage ·	Apricots	Nuts (almonds, peanuts
Celery	Bananas	black walnuts, pecans
Cucumber	Blackberries	Seeds
Dried peas, beans	Cherries	Whole grain breads/cereals
Green peppers	Figs (dried)	
Legumes (kidney,	Grapefruit	
white, pinto, lima	Grapes	Note: Whole grains such as rye,
beans)	Oranges	rice, corn, oats, barley, and whole
Lettuce	Peaches	wheat.
Potatoes	Pears	
Squash, zucchini	Pineapple	
Tomatoes	Plums	
	Tangerine	
	Strawberries	

Lipids (Fat)

Lipids (fats) cushion and protect the internal organs, act as an insulator to control the temperature of the body, carry and store fat-soluble vitamins through the body, and provide the largest reservoir of potential energy for the body due to the use of fats for energy during rest and physical activity. Fats come in solid **(saturated)** or liquid form **(unsaturated)** and both are insoluble in water. Fats are the most concentrated source of food energy and supply essential fatty acids (components of fat) that the body cannot manufacture and must obtain from food sources. (Refer to Tables 7.6 and 7.7.)

Fats consist of more than twice as much energy per unit (9 calories of energy for each gram consumed) of weight as compared to 4 calories per gram for carbohydrates and protein, and are a valuable energy source during moderate physical activity. Americans consume too much fat and fats concentrate a lot of calories into a small amount of food. One table-spoon of fat (margarine, oil, mayonnaise, peanut butter, butter, etc.) contains 100 calories. The average American consumes as much as 40-45 percent of his/her calories as fat. The chief sources of fat in the American diet consist of meats, butter, eggs, cheese and milk. Many fats are invisible fats such as fat in American cheese, 75%; one medium egg, 64%; and one plain doughnut, 41%. Authorities suggest the percentage of fat should be between 20 and 30 % of the total caloric intake and even lower. The authors recommend between 20 and 25% fat intake. Ten percent or less of the fat should come from each of the saturated, monounsaturated and polyunsatu-rated fats. Study the chart "Tips To Cut Fat From Your Diet" in Appendix F.

Fat is slow to leave the stomach. Eating foods high in fat (most fast foods) delays the feeling of hunger, which is the reason that these foods leave a feeling of fullness after consumption. When caloric intake exceeds energy needs, dietary proteins, fats, and carbohydrates are converted into fat, which is stored in the body as adipose (fat) tissue. Once stored, this fat can later be mobilized into the bloodstream to serve as an energy source. Fat can be broken down and used as energy only by aerobic metabolism. Fat cannot supply energy without oxygen being consumed. Approximately twenty to thirty minutes of aerobic exercise, three times per week, stimulates the body to adapt by increasing more fat utilization of enzymes within its cells and, in addition, improving the heart and lungs to deliver oxygen. The key to losing weight (utilizing fat) is steady slow, and long duration activity. We do not burn fat but utilize fat.

Two major lipids in the body will be discussed in this section: **tri-glycerides** and **cholesterol**. Approximately 95% of the fat eaten and stored in the body is in the form of triglycerides (true or neutral fats). There are two types of fatty acids (component of fat): saturated and unsaturated fats.

Saturated Fats

Saturated fats tend to elevate the cholesterol and triglyceride levels in the blood, cause hypertension, cardiovascular disease and many types of cancer. Saturated fats stimulate more cardiovascular disease than cholesterol. These fats appear as a **solid at room temperature** and are found in animal products, chocolate, coconut, palm oils, and hydrogenated vegetable oil products. Saturated animal fats are found in beef, lamb, pork, ham, dairy products and shellfish; poultry and fish have lower levels of fat. Trimming the fat from meats or removing the skin from poultry will reduce the fat content. Fat is found in dairy products: butter, cream, whole milk, and in cheeses made from cream and whole milk. See Appendix F for a chart containing the fat content of various cheeses. While milk contains about 8 grams of fat per cup, skim milk contains about 0.5-1.0 grams which is much less than whole milk.

Saturated vegetable fats are found in **hydrogenated** (hydrogen added, causing them to be saturated) shortenings, mayonnaise, coconut oil, cocoa butter, palm kernels, and palm oil (used in commercially prepared cookies, pie fillings and non-diary milk and cream substitutes). Many foods consumed contain a significant amount of calories in the form of hidden fat (fat content is not obvious). Examples of hidden fat in foods are: cheese, nuts, desserts, crackers, potato chips, peanut butter, doughnuts, whole milk, and commercially prepared foods.

Maximum Total Fat Intake at Different Calorie Levels

Calories	1,600	2,000	2,200	2,800
Total Fat (grams)	53	65	73	93

Here's a handy formula for figuring how many fat calories a day you should have:

Your total calories per day = _____

Multiplied by .30 = _____ fat calories per day

Divided by 9 = _____ grams of total fat
(1 gram of fat has 9 calories) allowable per day

Unsaturated Fats

Unsaturated fats are usually of **plant origin and liquid at room temperature**. There are **two types of unsaturated fats**: **monounsaturated** and **polyunsaturated fats**. (See examples in Table 7.6.)

Monounsaturated fats help to lower total cholesterol but, unlike **polyunsaturated fats**, they have little effect on **HDL ("good" choles-**

TABLE 7.6

Monounsaturated Fats	Polyunsaturated Fats	Saturated Fat
Avocado	Corn oil	Bacon
Canola oil	Cottonseed oil	Butter
Cashews	Fish	Cheese
Peanut oil	Mayonnaise	Chocolate
Peanuts	Nuts	Coconut Oil
Olive oil	(most varieties)	Cream
Olives	Safflower oil	Egg Yolk
	Soybean oil	Hydrogenated
	Sunflower oil	(hard) fats
	Peanut butter	Lard
	Unhydrogenated	Meat
	fats	Milk, Whole
	Tub margarine	Palm Kernel Oil
		Palm Oil
		Poultry
		Shortening
		Sour cream

terol) levels. These oils do contain a percentage of polyunsaturated as well, but the ratio of polyunsaturated to saturated is not as good.

Polyunsaturated fats may help to decrease total cholesterol in the blood by helping the body to eliminate excess newly formed cholesterol. In addition, they appear to decrease the HDL component.

Omega-3 Fatty Acids

Studies indicate the consumption of as little as two to four fish or seafood dishes per week (6 oz.), that contain fish oils rich in polyunsaturated fats called **omega-3 fatty acids**, actually may change the chemistry of the blood to lower the likelihood of heart disease. The oil in certain seafood seems to depress low density lipoprotein (cholesterol), lower serum triglycerides, and raise the amount of high-density lipoprotein cholesterol. However, there are studies that show there is no evidence that by eating fish the participants reversed their underlying coronary artery disease and their cholesterol levels did not change significantly. However, numerous studies have shown that these crucial improvements can only be accomplished by a truly low-fat diet, variety of fiber-rich fruits, vegetables, grains and in combination with other lifestyle changes.

Not all fish contain the same amount of omega-3 fatty acids. Commercially grown fish contain only one-third to one-half as much omega-3 fatty acids as other fish. The commercial feed given to pond-reared fish apparently contains a lower proportion of omega-3s than the natural food eaten by fish in the wild.

TABLE 7.7
PERCENT FAT CALORIES IN SELECTED FOODS

Type of food	Less than 15% Calories from fat	15%-30% Calories from fat	30-50% Calories from Fat	More than 50% Calories from Fat
Fruits and vegetables	Fruits, plain vegetables, juices, pickles, sauerkraut		French fries	Avocados,. coconuts, olives
Bread and cereals	Grains and flours, most breads, most cereals, corn tortillas, pita, matzoh, bagels, noodles and pasta	Cornbread, flour tortillas, oatmeal soft rolls and buns, wheat germ	Breakfast bars, biscuits and muffins, granola, pancakes, waffles, doughnuts, taco shells, pastries, croissants	
Dairy Products	Nonfat milk, dry curd cottage cheese, nonfat cottage cheese, nonfat yogurt	Buttermilk, low-fat yogurt, 1% milk low-fat cottage cheese	Whole milk, 2% milk, creamed cottage cheese	Butter, cream, sour cream, half & half, most cheeses (including part-skim and "lite" cheeses)
Meats		Beef round; veal loin, round and shoulder; pork tenderloin	Beef and veal, lamb fresh & picnic hams	All ground beef, spareribs, cold cuts, bacon, sausages, corned beef, hot dogs, pastrami
Poultry	Egg whites	Chicken & turkey (light meat without skin)	Chicken & turkey (light meat with skin, dark meat without skin), duck & goose (without skin)	Chicken/turkey (dark meat with skin) chicken/turkey hotdogs and bologna, egg yolks, whole eggs
Seafood	Clams, cod, crab, crawfish, flounder, haddock, lobster, perch, sole, shrimp, tuna (in water)	Bass and sea bass, halibut, mussels, oyster, tuna (fresh)	Anchovies, catfish, salmon, sturgeon, trout, tuna (in oil, drained)	Herring, mackerel, sardines
Beans and nuts	Dried beans and peas, chestnuts, water chestnuts		Soybeans	Tofu, most nuts and seeds, peanut butter
Fats and oils	Oil-free and some "lite" salad dressings			Butter, margarine, all mayonnaise (including reduced calorie), most salad dressings, all oils
Soups	Bouillons, broths, consomme	Most soups	Cream soups, bean soups, "just add water" noodle soups	Cheddar cheese soup, New England clam chowder
Desserts	Angel food cake, gelatin, some new fat-free cookies	Pudding, tapioca	Most cakes, most pies	
Frozen desserts	Sherbet, low-fat frozen yogurt, sorbet, fruit ices	Ice milk	Frozen yogurt	All ice creams
Snack foods	Popcorn (air popped), pretzels, rye crackers, rice cakes, fig bars, raisin biscuit cookies, marshmallows, most hard candy, fruit rolls	"Lite" microwave popcorn, Scandinavian "crisps," plain crackers, caramels, fudge, gingersnaps, graham crackers	Snack crackers, popcorn (popped in oil), cookies, candy bars, granola bars	Most microwave popcorn, corn and potato chips, buttery crackers, chocolate

Source: American Heart Association and U. S. Department of Agriculture

Fish Oil Capsules

Fish oil capsules (containing fat extracted from fish whose tissues are rich in omega-3 fatty acids) offer a new approach to warding off heart disease. According to the American Heart Association, the American Medical Association, and clinical research, the proper amount of fish oil capsules which may work has not been determined. It may not just be the oil from the fish that provides protection but a combination of components contained in the fish that work together to bring about beneficial effects.

Consumption of fish oil capsules may cause strokes; decrease blood clotting ability; interfere with the healing of wounds; and may render vitamins A and D toxic. Fish oil capsules may also contain pesticides and contamination. These capsules should not be used—eat fish instead.

Cholesterol (Sterols)

Cholesterol is not a triglyceride; it is a fatty-like substance (solid alcohol) found in the cells of humans and other animals, and is required by the body for metabolism and the production of hormones, cell membranes and other body substances. **Cholesterol is found only in animal products and is not found in fruits, vegetables, grains, nuts and other non-animal foods.** (Refer to Table 7.8.) It is concentrated in the liver, kidneys, spinal cord, adrenal glands and the brain. The liver manufactures about 80 percent of the total cholesterol found in the blood and tissues; the other 20 percent is furnished by dietary sources. Most of the cholesterol needed by the body comes from fatty acids and other products derived from carbohydrate and protein. The amount of saturated fat and cholesterol in the diet determines, to a great extent, how much cholesterol is located in the bloodstream. The American Heart Association recommends that people should limit their daily intake of cholesterol to less than 300 milligrams. The authors recommend the intake of between 200-220 milligrams.

Atherosclerosis is a condition where the inner layers of the arterial wall develop a buildup of yellow plaque consisting of fibrous tissue, calcium, cholesterol and additional lipid material. As the internal channel

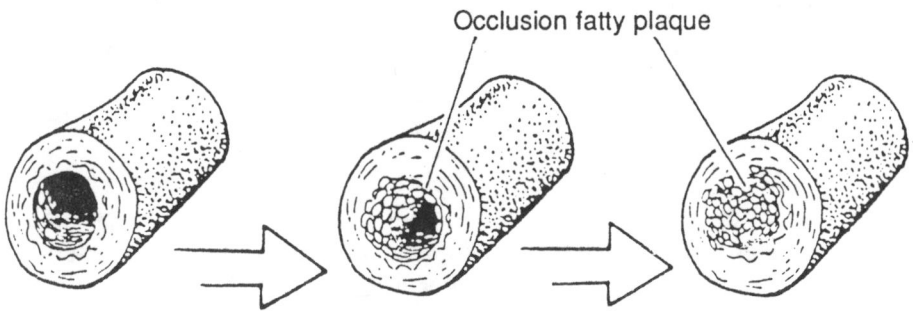

Occlusion fatty plaque

The fatty deposit in arteries: The deterioration of a normal artery (left) is seen as atherosclerosis develops and begins depositing fatty substances and roughening the channel lining until a clot forms and plugs the artery (right), depriving the heart muscle of vital blood, which results in a heart attack.

Figure 7.3. The Development of Atherosclerosis.

TABLE 7.8
CHOLESTEROL CONTENT IN SOME COMMON FOODS

Food	Amt.	Cholesterol (mg.)	Food	Amt.	Cholesterol (mg.)
Meat List			*Bread List*		
Beef	1 oz.	25	Whole grains and nuts contain no		
Pork, ham	1 oz.	25	cholesterol, but cholesterol may be		
Poultry	1 oz.	23	added in the preparation of some foods		
Fish	1 oz.	21	(such as eggs in French toast or other		
Shrimp	1 oz.	45	baked goods).		
Lobster	1 oz.	25	Bread	1 slice	0
Sausage	2 links	45	Biscuit	1	17
Tuna, Salmon	1 oz.	0	Pancake	1	40
Frankfurter	1	50	Sweet roll	1	25
Bacon	1 strip	5	French toast	1	130
Eggs	1	253	Doughnut	1	28
Liver	1 oz.	120	Cereal, cooked	1 cup	0
Milk List			*Fruit List*		
Milk, whole	1 cup	27	Fruits contain no cholesterol.		
Milk, 02%	1 cup	15	*Vegetable List*		
Milk, skim	1 cup	7	Vegetables contain no cholesterol.		
Butter	1 Tsp.	12			
Margarine	1 Tsp.	0	*Source:* U.S. Department of Agriculture		
Cream cheese	1 Tbsp.	18			
Ice Milk	1 cup	10			
Ice Cream	1 cup	85			

(artery) narrows, the blood flow is reduced. When this occurs in the coronary vessels it is known as **coronary heart disease (CHD)** and may cause symptoms from mild discomfort to death. The four primary risk factors associated with CHD are high blood pressure, high serum-cholesterol levels, physical inactivity, and cigarette smoking. Other factors include diabetes, diet, obesity, age, gender, stress and heredity.

Most of the triglycerides and cholesterol are transported in the blood as **lipoproteins**, which are chemical units composed of triglycerides, cholesterol and another lipid called phospholipids. These are attached to a protein carrier that gives the name **lipoproteins**. Fats are not soluble in water and must be combined with some other substance such as protein in order to be transported throughout the body. Most Americans have raised levels of cholesterol because of their high intake of saturated fats, not their intake of cholesterol. However, both sources do increase the cholesterol level.

There are different forms of lipoprotein in the blood as they are classified by their density. Three of the lipoproteins seem to have a relationship with the onset of coronary heart disease and have different amounts of cholesterol in their molecular makeup. The **low density lipoprotein-cholesterol (LDL)**, or **"bad cholesterol"** molecule, contains high amounts of cholesterol and the **high density lipoprotein-cholesterol (HDL)**, or **"good cholesterol"** molecule, has a high concentration of protein. **VLDL**, the largest of the lipoproteins (**very low-density lipoproteins**), consists primarily of **triglycerides**.

Individuals with high levels of HDL-cholesterol (good) have less coronary heart disease when compared to people who have high levels of LDL (bad) cholesterol. It is not known exactly why this occurs but one theory suggests that the HDL cholesterol molecule helps prevent the process of atherosclerosis by blocking the movement of LDL cholesterol into the cells in the artery wall and transporting it back to the liver for reprocessing or removal from the body. **The more HDLs an individual has, the better.** HDLs work like Draino in a sink—it cleans out arteries. Seventy percent of the body's cholesterol is usually LDL cholesterol. Generally, women have higher levels of HDL than men and, in some cases, women may even have a high total cholesterol due to a high HDL level.

Seventy-five percent of all people who have high cholesterol can lower the cholesterol level by diet and exercise. Changing and reducing the type of fat and the total amount of fat in the diet may lower the serum-cholesterol levels. Studies have shown that saturated fats increase blood cholesterol levels. Polyunsaturated and polyunsaturated fatty acids may also reduce the protective form of cholesterol (HDL). Monounsaturated oils have no effect on HDL levels. **Aerobic exercise** can lower total cholesterol, LDL fraction, elevate HDL fraction and lower total cholesterol to HDL ratio.

Total cholesterol in the blood is important, but an analysis of the different types of lipoprotein cholesterol should also be made when blood tests for lipids are conducted. Keeping the cholesterol level below 200 milligrams per deciliter of blood (the unit cholesterol is commonly expressed in), the chances of heart disease are greatly reduced.

An important factor is the ratio of total cholesterol to HDL cholesterol. The ratio can be determined by dividing the total cholesterol level by the value for HDL cholesterol. The lower the ratio the less risk there is for coronary heart disease.

The **finger-stick test,** done at shopping malls, provides faster but less accurate results of the cholesterol level. **The blood profile test done by laboratories is recommended for better results.**

In general, studies indicate that people who are lean, non-smokers (smoking tends to reduce HDLs), regular exercisers, have moderate alcohol consumption, and eat a diet low in saturated fats have higher levels of HDL cholesterol and lower levels of total blood cholesterol. However, heredity plays a major role in HDL levels. After menopause estrogen decreases and women's risk of coronary heart disease is similar to men. Drugs may be recommended for some individuals in lowering cholesterol levels; however, a combination of diet and exercise is beneficial in combating coronary heart disease.

The cholesterol test should include five readings:

1. **Total cholesterol**

   200 mg/dl of blood or less (low risk)
   201-239 mg/dl of blood (moderate risk)
   240 mg/dl of blood or above (high risk)

2. **Low-density lipoprotein (LDL or "bad") cholesterol**
   (130 mg/dl or less of blood)

3. **High-density lipoprotein (HDL or "good") cholesterol**
   (Males 35-50 mg/dl of blood)
   (Females 55-70 mg/dl of blood

4. **The total cholesterol/HDL ratio (most important)**

   The ratio of HDL to total cholesterol less than 4.0 (men) and less than 3.5 (women). If the total cholesterol is more than 4.0 times higher than the HDL count, the risk is greater.

   Example: Total Cholesterol $\dfrac{180}{90} = 2.0$
   HDL Cholesterol

5. **Total triglycerides level** signifies how much cholesterol is being manufactured by the liver and how much is being absorbed from food (should be 150 mg/dl or less of blood).

Proteins

Proteins are chains of **amino acids** which contain nitrogen and are the **building blocks of body tissues**. Protein helps to build and repair tissues such as blood, muscles, internal organs, skin, hair, nails, and bones. In addition, protein helps control chemical reactions in the human body that help build, repair, and regulate the function of the body's cells. They are part of hormones, enzymes, and antibodies and help maintain normal body fluid balance. Also, proteins are stored in muscle tissue and used in very small amounts as a fuel.

TABLE 7.9
TOTAL DAILY PROTEIN NEEDS OF A 70 KG ATHLETE

Authority	Recommendation (g/kg/day)	Protein/Day (g)
Food and Nutrition Board (RDA)	0.8	56
American Dietetic Association	1.0	70
Brotherhood (endurance athletes)	1.0 to 1.2	70 to 84
Brotherhood (power athletes)	1.3 to 1.6	91 to 112
Yoshimura (early training)	2.0	140

Source: Position of the American Dietetic Association: Nutrition for physical fitness and athletic performance for adults, *Journal of the American Dietetic Association.* Smith, M.: *Nutrition for physical fitness and athletic performance for adults.* Copyright The American Dietetic Association, reprinted by permission from *Journal of the American Dietetic Association,* 87:933.

The human body needs approximately 10-12 percent of its daily caloric intake from proteins. Athletes need a slightly higher amount of proteins (10-15%) than sedentary individuals. It is estimated that a person needs about 0.36 grams per pound of body weight (0.8-1.0 gram per kilogram of body weight) per day. To determine individual needs, simply multiply body weight, in pounds, by 0.36 grams. If overweight, use ideal weight for the calculation. The average male needs about 56-70 grams of protein per day, while the average female needs about 44-50 grams. The American Dietetic Association recommends 1 gram protein per kilogram of body weight each day (1 g/kg/day) for the athlete. Other studies recommend even higher protein levels. An athlete weighing 70 kg may choose any level of intake among the recommendations shown in Table 7.9.

The body uses approximately **twenty-two amino acids**, nine **essential amino** acids and the rest nonessential amino acids. The essential proteins cannot be produced in the body and must be provided by the food supplements or beverages. The **complete or "high-quality" proteins** (animal sources) come from meat, fish, poultry, cheese, and eggs. (Refer to Table 7.10.) One of the problems associated with many quick weight-loss programs is a shortage of essential amino acids and, in some cases, death has resulted. See Appendix F for a chart describing food combinations for complete protein.

The rest of the **non-essential** amino acids can be manufactured by the body if sufficient nitrogen is provided from food proteins in the diet. However, if one or more of the essential amino acids is missing, the proteins are referred to as **incomplete or limited** protein.

TABLE 7.10
PROTEIN CONTENT IN SOME COMMON FOODS

Food	Amt.	Protein (grams)	Food	Amt.	Protein (grams)
Milk List			*Vegetable List*		
Milk, whole	1 cup	8	Broccoli	1/2 cup	2
Milk, skim	1 cup	8	Carrots	1	1
Cheese, cheddar	1 oz.	7	Peas, green	1/2 cup	4
Yogurt	1 cup	8	Potato, baked	1	3
Meat List			*Fruit List*		
Beef, lean	1 oz.	8	Banana	1	1
Chicken, breast	1 oz.	8	Orange	1	1
Luncheon meat	1 oz.	5	Pear	1	1
Fish	1 oz.	7	*Starch/Bread List*		
Eggs	1	6	Bread, wheat	1 slice	3
Navy beans	1/2 cup	7	Bran flakes	1 cup	4
Peanuts, roasted	1/2 cup	18	Doughnuts	1	1
Peanut butter	1 Tbsp.	4	Spaghetti	1 cup	5

Protein (grams) may vary slightly from the food exchange lists since these data were derived from food analyses reported by the United States Department of Agriculture.

Intensity exercises (low to moderate intensity) of long duration demand large quantities of fuel, including protein. Short-duration, high intensity anaerobic exercise demands less total protein fuel. However, with the individual that is trained, less protein is used during the exercise activity. Athletes retain more protein and they utilize more protein as fuel. Endurance and power athletes should not neglect carbohydrate needs. If so, they will burn off as fuel the protein that they wish to retain as muscle.

It the diet does not have a sufficient amount of protein, the body immediately begins to break down tissue, usually beginning with muscle tissue, in order to release the amino acids it needs. The body cannot store excess protein for use in times of a deficiency; therefore, daily protein intake is important. Once the body's protein requirement is met, excess protein is stored as body fat. Excess protein places strain on the liver, kidneys, provides extra calories, increases calcium loss, and may be converted to glucose or fatty acids. Protein waste products may be excreted as urea.

Food Choices for the Vegetarian

The vegetarian must obtain sufficient amounts of protein, iron, vitamin B_{12}, Vitamin D and calcium from fewer food sources. A wise selection of food choices is important.

There are four styles of vegetarians:

1. **Lactovegetarian:** One that excludes animal flesh (meat, poultry, fish, eggs) but eats animal products such as milk, milk products, and cheese as well as plant foods (fruits and vegetables).
2. **Ovolacto vegetarian:** One that excludes animal flesh (meat, poultry, fish) but eats animal products such as eggs, dairy products and plant foods (fruits and vegetables).
3. **Vegan:** One that excludes animal flesh and animal products from the diet. This individual eats only plant foods and often takes Vitamin B_{12} supplements.
4. **Partial or Semivegetarian:** One that eats plant food, dairy products, eggs, and a small selection of fish and poultry but not beef or pork.

It is important that vegetarians eat iron-rich foods and find alternative sources of calcium, vitamin D and take a vitamin B_{12} supplement. In addition, foods should be eaten in combinations that provide all the essential amino acids, such as black bean and rice soup, peanut butter and bread, peas and cornbread, cereal and milk, etc.

Protein Supplements

Individuals are constantly looking for a quick solution that will improve their body, and businesses are always ready to profit from these requests. Athletes involved in weight training or strenuous endurance exercise may need more than the RDA for protein in order to maintain or increase protein balance, especially if energy intake (calories) is not adequate to meet daily energy expenditure (daily basis of per Kg of body weight of 0.8-1.2 grams). However, there is a difference of opinion among investigators whether athletes need more protein in the diet. Recreational athletes do not need protein supplements. Expensive protein supplements are not necessary for individuals on a walking, jogging, or running program. The best nutritional advice for good health is to eat a balanced diet of whole foods that emphasize vegetables, grains, low-fat meat and milk.

VITAMINS

Vitamins are **organic substances** essential for **normal growth, metabolism**, and **development of the body**. They are necessary for the body to perform its complex chemical reactions to maintain good health, are not a source of energy, and do not contain calories. There is no food which contains all the vitamins required by the body. The human body needs an adequate supply of thirteen different vitamins. Four of these vitamins are **fat soluble** (A, D, E, K), while the other nine (vitamin C and B-Complex) are **water-soluble.** Vitamins should be obtained through a well-balanced diet of a variety of foods.

Vitamins A, D, E, and K (fat soluble) are those found in foods usually, but not always, associated with fats (lipids). They are not destroyed by ordinary cooking and normally are not excreted in the urine, but tend to remain stored in the body in the liver and fatty tissues until they are needed. The body does not need a day-to-day supply because overdoses of these vitamins can interfere with or disrupt the action or other nutrients. In addition, large doses of fat-soluble vitamins may cause vitamin toxicity in which they cease to function as vitamins and begin to perform like drugs and can be fatal.

Water soluble vitamins, B and C Complex, are transported in the fluids of the tissues and cells, and are not stored in the body in appreciable quantities. These vitamins may be affected by cooking methods and can be lost in varying amounts by discarding the water in which the food was cooked or soaked.

Numerous studies have shown that a deficiency in one or more water-soluble vitamins, especially B vitamins, may be noted in 2-4 weeks. In addition, a decrease in physical performance capacity, fatigue occurring faster, deteriorated work output, and muscular soreness may result. Recent data suggest that daily intakes of less than one-third of the RDA for several of the B vitamins would lead to a dramatic decrease of VO_2 max, endurance capacity, and the anaerobic threshold in less than four weeks.

Symptoms of a **vitamin C** deficiency may include ruptured blood vessels in the skin, muscle cramps and weakness, anemia, and bleeding gums. A deficiency would impair physical performance and anemia would impede aerobic endurance. All functions will return to normal when vitamins are properly restored. Deficiencies of vitamin C do not often occur because of the abundance of fresh and frozen fruits and vegetables.

Smokers should increase their consumption of vitamin C to 100 milligrams, as opposed to 60 milligrams for other adults. Smokers metabolize that nutrient more quickly than non-smokers and are more likely to have less in the bloodstream and body tissues even if they eat the same amount of food. Foods rich in vitamin C are orange juice, broccoli, tomatoes, and strawberries.

TABLE 7.11
VITAMINS

Vitamin	Food Sources	Deficiency Effect	Function	RDA (Adult)
A	Fish-liver oils, liver, butter, cream, whole milk, whole milk cheeses, egg yolk, dark green leafy vegetables, yellow fruits and vegetables	Night blindness, eye inflammation, dry rough skin, reduced resistance to infection	Needed for normal vision. Protects against night blindness. Keeps skin and mucous membranes resistant to infection.	5000 I.U.
B complex B$_1$ (Thiamine)	Pork, liver, organ meats, brewer's yeast, wheat germ, whole-grain cereals and breads, enriched cereals and breads, soybeans, peanuts and other legumes, milk	Beriberi—a disease characterized by nerve disorders and sometimes heart dysfunction. Loss of appetite, nausea, confusion	Promotes normal appetite and digestion. Necessary for healthy nervous system. Maintenance of good appetite.	1.5 mg
B$_2$ (Riboflavin)	Milk, powdered whey, liver, organ meats, meats, eggs, leafy green vegetables, dried yeast, enriched foods	Cracks at corners of mouth, inflamed sore lips, inflamed discolored tongue, dermatitis, anemia	Helps cells use oxygen. Helps maintain good vision. Needed for good skin and vision.	1.7 mg
Niacin	Lean meat, fish, poultry, liver, kidney, whole-grain and enriched cereals and breads, green vegetables, peanuts, brewer's yeast	Pellagra—a chronic disease characterized by gastrointestinal problems, skin eruptions and mental disorders, depression,	Aids metabolism of proteins, carbohydrates and fats. Formation of hormones and nerve regulating substances	20 mg
Pantothenic Acid	Present in most plant and animal tissue, liver, kidney, yeast, eggs, peanuts, whole-grain cereals, beef, tomatoes, broccoli, salmon	(Rare) Gastrointestinal disturbances, depression, confusion, low-blood sugar, leg cramps, headaches	Necessary for metabolism of proteins, carbohydrates, and fats	10 mg
B$_6$ (Pyroxidine)	Wheat germ, meat, liver, kidney, whole-grain cereals, soybeans, peanuts, corn	(Rare) Inflamed mouth and tongue, depression, irritability, convulsions	Maintains normal hemoglobin (carries oxygen to tissues)	2.0 mg
Biotin	Liver, sweetbreads, yeast, eggs, legumes, milk, nuts, dark green vegetables	(Extremely rare) Inflamed skin, hair loss, muscle pain, depression, weight loss	Coenzyme, functions in metabolism of major nutrients	0.3 mg
Folic acid	Widespread in liver, kidney, yeast, dark green leafy vegetables, whole-grain cereals	Anemia, stunted growth, damage to lining of small intestine, less resistance to disease	Maintains normal hemoglobin, cell growth and reproduction	200 mcg (men) 160 mcg (women)
B$_{12}$ (Cyanocobalamin)	Animal protein, eggs, milk, shellfish	Pernicious anemia, stunted growth, impaired balance	Maintains normal hemoglobin	6 mcg
C (Ascorbic acid)	Citrus fruits, tomatoes, strawberries, cantaloupe, cabbage, broccoli, kale, potatoes	Scurvy—disease characterized by weakness, anemia, spongy gums, loose teeth, rough scaly skin, slow-healing wounds	Maintains cementing material that holds body cells together; needed for healthy gums; helps body resist infection	60 mg
D	Fish-liver oils, fortified milk, activated sterols, exposure to sunlight, salmon, tuna	Rickets, osteomalacia (loss of calcium from bones in adults), fractures, spasms	Builds strong bones and tteth; aids calcium/ phosphorus absorpton	400 I.U.
E (Tocopherol)	Plant tissues, wheat germ oil, vegetable oils, nuts, legumes	Unknown in persons eating normal, mixed diet; leg cramps, red blood cell breakdown	Not fully understood; works as an antioxidant	15 I.U.
K	Green leaves such as spinach, cabbage, cauliflower, eggs, peas, potatoes	Excessive bleeding or hemorrhaging	Aids blood clotting	80 mcg (men) 65 mcg (women)

Beta Carotene (pro-Vitamin A) is from a large group of substances called carotenoids, which is often found in fruits and vegetables (orange, yellow and dark green) and may also have anticancer properties. It seems to neutralize the free radicals that damage cells and cause cancer. Too much vitamin A can be dangerous but beta carotene is nontoxic since the body is able to regulate its conversion to vitamin A. Beta carotene comes from plant sources which are high in fiber and other carotenoids. Numerous studies have suggested that beta carotene can defend the body against tumors and enhance the immune system. It has been found that individuals who eat a minimum of vegetables and fruits rich in carotenoids have an increased risk of cancer, especially lung and melanoma (skin) cancer. People should consume 5 to 6 milligrams of beta carotene a day (based on guidelines from the USDA and the National Cancer Institute). The average American consumes less than 1.5 milligrams per day. Foods high in beta carotene are carrots, sweet potatoes, kale, spinach, and cress. Frozen vegetables contain as much carotene as fresh and the longer the food is cooked, the more carotene is destroyed. Anyone who eats the recommended four or more servings of fruits and vegetables a day will probably consume enough beta carotene, vitamin C, and other nutrients.

Antioxidants

Antioxidants are substances which protect the body from oxidative damage as a result of free radical exposure. Free radicals are chemicals produced when the body burns fuel for energy. They have been implicated in the causes of more than fifty diseases, including cancer, cellular damage, emphysema, cataracts, progressive arteriosclerosis, and neurological disorders. In addition, they have a detrimental effect on the immune system and can cause premature aging.

Antioxidant supplements can be taken daily to provide the electron necessary to stabilize free radicals. Foods rich in antioxidants are listed in Table 7.12. Dr. Kenneth Cooper of the Cooper Institute for Aerobics Research, recommends a daily "antioxidant cocktail" consisting of 1000 mg. of Vitamin C, 400 I.U. of natural vitamin E, and 25,000 I.U. (15 mg.) of beta carotene. Due to the known long-term safety of Vitamins C and E and beta carotene, these are the only antioxidant vitamins recommended for daily use. On March 25, 1996, British researchers at the Annual Scientific Sessions of American Cardiology reported that megadose form of Vitamin E reduced heart attacks by 75%.

TABLE 7.12
FOOD SOURCES FOR ANTIOXIDANTS

Beta carotene (Pro-Vitamin A)	yellow, orange, and dark green leafy vegetables and fruits (apricots, asparagus, broccoli, cantaloupe, carrots, mango, peaches, spinach, squash, sweet potatoes, tomatoes)
Vitamin A	dark green, yellow and orange vegetables and fruits, butter, cheese, egg yolk, fish oil, liver, fortified milk, cantaloupes
Vitamin C	asparagus, broccoli, brussels sprouts, cabbage, cantaloupe, cauliflower, citrus fruits, dark green vegetables, melons, peppers, raspberries, strawberries, tomatoes, tomato juice, papaya, kiwi, collard greens, orange juice, brussels sprouts.
Vitamin E	dried beans, egg yolk, liver, nuts and seeds, oatmeal, whole grain cereals and breads, vegetables (yellow and green leafy), vegetable oils (corn, cottonseed, safflower, sunflower), legumes, mayonnaise, sweet potatoes
Selenium	skinless chicken, lean meat, nonfat milk, seafood (swordfish, tuna, oysters), whole grain breads and cereals, garlic, sunflower seeds, nuts
Flavonoids	Purple grapes, berries, apples, peas, beets, onions, garlic, green tea, red wine

MINERALS

Minerals are inorganic substances found in food and in the body. They are important in activating numerous reactions that release energy during the breakdown of carbohydrates, proteins and fats. There are twenty-five known minerals that are essential in the maintenance of water balance, acid-base balance of the blood, blood clotting, normal heart rhythm, nerve impulse conduction, and regulation of muscular contraction. Also, minerals are essential components of respiratory pigments, enzymes and enzyme systems, and are constituents of all cells, especially those found in hard parts of the body (bones, nails, teeth).

Minerals consist of two categories: **six macrominerals** and **fourteen trace minerals**. The six macrominerals are required in larger quantities (**100 mg. or more per day**) than the others. These include **sodium, potassium, chloride, calcium, phosphorous**, and **magnesium**.

TABLE 7.13
MINERAL REQUIREMENTS

Mineral	What It Does	RDA	Good Sources
Calcium	Developing and maintaining strong bones and teeth; normal blood clotting, heartbeat, transmission of nerve impulses and muscle contraction	800 mg.	Milk and milk products; green leafy vegetables, almonds, sardines, salmon
Phosphorus	Utilization of energy, muscle action and nerve transmission. With calcium, essential for formation of bones and teeth.	800 mg.	Meat, poultry, fish, eggs, whole grain foods, nuts, processed foods
Magnesium	Essential for energy conversions in the body. Helps control muscle contractions.	300-350 mg.	Dark bread, nuts, green leafy vegetables, dairy products, soybeans, seafood, legumes
Potassium	With sodium, helps regulate the balance and volume of body fluids. Influences contractiblility of muscles.	1875-5625 mg.	All fruits and vegetables, pecans and walnuts, wheat germ, soybeans, molasses
Sodium	Found in blood plasma and other fluids outside cells; helps to maintain normal water balance.	500-2400 mcg.	Meat, fish, pouultry, eggs, milk
Chloride (Mainly in compound form with sodium or potassium)	Regulates correct balance of acid and alkali in blood. Stimulates production of hydrochloric acid in stomach for digestion.	1700-5100 mg.	Table salt, kelp, ripe olives, rye flour
Iron	Red blood cell formation. Aids in energy utilization.	15 mg.-F 10 mg.-M	Eggs, liver, whole grains, dried fruits, dried legumes
Zinc	Protein synthesis, growth and development, hormones, insulin, enzymes	15 mg.	Fish, beef, chicken, whole grains, vegetables, oysters
Iodine	Functioning of thyroid gland (breathing rate of tissues)	150 mcg.	Seafoods
Copper	Action of enzyme systems; normal functioning of central nervous system; involved with storage and release of iron to form hemoglobin.	2.0-3.0 mg.	Organ meats, shellfish, nuts, dried legumes
Selenium	Functioning of kidneys, pancreas, and liver	55 mcg.-F 70 mcg.-M	Organ meats, muscle, seafoods
Manganese	Normal tendon and bone structure.	2.5-5.0 mg.	Peas, beans, nuts, fruits, whole grains

The **fourteen trace minerals (microminerals)** are required in smaller quantities of **100 mg. or less**. Iron, zinc, manganese, copper, iodine, and cobalt are just a few of these. A deficiency of minerals have been linked to anemia, high blood pressure, cancer, diabetes, tooth decay, and osteoporosis. A well-balanced diet of sufficient caloric content should supply enough of the essential minerals.

The macrominerals, **calcium** and **phosphorus**, are located in the teeth and bones, and account for 5-8 percent of the body's mineral content. (Refer to Table 7.13.) Dairy products (milk is the best source) provide a high content of calcium. Fish (sardines and salmon), dark green leafy vegetables (broccoli and turnip greens), tofu, legumes and nuts are excellent sources of calcium. (Refer to Table 7.15.) Vitamin D, lactose, and adequate protein may help to absorb calcium from the intestines; however, excessive amounts of protein, dietary fat, phosphorus, caffeine, and fiber may decrease the amount absorbed. As a result of low calories, females are at a greater risk for micronutrient inadequacies, especially calcium and iron.

Ninety-eight percent of the body's **calcium** is found in the skeleton. A health condition associated with calcium intake and limited physical activity is the development of osteoporosis (reduced bone mass). **Osteoporosis,** a brittle bone disease, increases the susceptibility to stress fractures occurring in the hip, spine and wrist. The main cause of

TABLE 7.14
RECOMMENDED CALCIUM INTAKES*

	Amount	Equals
Men and Women	1,000 mg/day	Three 8 oz. glasses of skim milk.
Post-menopausal Women		
• On Estrogen replacement therapy	1,000 mg/day	
• Not on Estrogen replacement therapy	1,500 mg/day	Five 8 oz. glasses of skim milk

*Source: National Institutes of Health and National Osteoporosis Foundation.

TABLE 7.15
CALCIUM CONTENT
OF SELECTED FOODS

Food	mg
Navel or Valencia orange (1)	50
broccoli (1/2 cup)	90
navy beans (1 cup)	128
sardines (2 x 3")	100
salmon (3 oz.)	200
tofu (1/2 cup)	150
cheese (1 oz.)	204
skim milk (8 oz.)	302
yogurt (8 oz.)	400
frozen yogurt (8 oz.)	200

Osteoporosis Risk Factors

Some women are at a greater risk than others. This checklist will indicate how many risk factors a person may have.

Yes No

____ ____ 1. family history of osteoporosis?

____ ____ 2. fractures or lost teeth recently?

____ ____ 3. thin, small-boned frame?

____ ____ 4. physically inactive

____ ____ 5. post-menopausal?

____ ____ 6. early or surgically-induced menopause?

____ ____ 7. diet high in salt, fat or caffeine?

____ ____ 8. daily alcohol consumption?

____ ____ 9. smoker?

____ ____ 10. eliminated dairy products as a child?

____ ____ 11. diet low in dairy products and other sources of calcium?

____ ____ 12. reduction in height in past few years?

____ ____ 13. never been pregnant?

____ ____ 14. taking excessive thyroid medication or high doses of cortisone (such as drugs for asthma, arthristis, or cancer)?

Each "yes" means you are at a greater risk for developing osteoporosis.

osteoporosis in older women is the diminished production of estrogen which leads to a negative calcium balance and a rapid onset of bone demineralization. Evidence suggests that peak bone density and strength are reached between ages 25 and 35. At some time after that peak is reached, calcium begins to be lost from the bones as a natural process of aging. The current treatment for osteoporosis is estrogen replacement, calcium supplements and moderate endurance exercise consisting of walking, jogging, weight-bearing and weight lifting activities. Vigorous exercise may be detrimental to bones. Although osteoporosis affects more than half of all women over age 65, one out of every five persons with osteoporosis is a man.

Osteoporosis can be prevented and treated with adequate calcium and Vitamin D intake in the diet and regular weight-bearing exercise. Adequate daily calcium, coupled with at least 400 I.U. of Vitamin D and 30-60 minutes of weight-bearing exercise four to five days per week not only stabilizes osteoporotic bone degeneration but in some people produces an increase in bone density, according to the Cooper Institute for Aerobics Research.

Phosphorus is the second most abundant macromineral mineral in the body after calcium. Excellent sources include meat, eggs, milk, cheese, nuts, dried beans and peas, seafood, grain products, variety of vegetables and soft drinks. Excess amount of phosphorus is excreted by the kidneys. However, if the ratio of phosphorus to calcium greatly exceeds a 1:1 ratio, such as a diet low in calcium foods and excessively high in phosphorus foods such as meat protein and soft drinks, then calcium may be lost from the bones. In addition, phosphorus may interfere with the absorption of iron, zinc, and copper.

Current RDA of **iron** (trace mineral) is 10 mg daily for men and 15 mg daily for (healthy, non-pregnant, nonlactating) women and teenagers of both sexes. Shortness of breath, loss of vision, loss of appetite, chronic fatigue, faintness, depression, constipation or diarrhea, sleeplessness, sensitivity to cold, pallor (in light-skinned individuals), and shortened attention span may be the result of low iron (anemia). As the result of excessive iron, severe constipation, infections, tissue and liver damage may occur.

Iron is essential to the transportation of oxygen. The majority of iron is used to form hemoglobin, a protein-iron compound in the red blood cells which transports oxygen from the lungs to the body tissues. Another iron component includes myoglobin which helps use oxygen energy system, therefore being essential for endurance athletes to have adequate iron in the diet to maintain optimal performance. The concern is especially important to endurance athletes in exercises such as running which may contribute to iron loss. Iron loss may be caused by the repeated foot (soles of the feet) contact with the ground (unyielding surface) causing red blood cell destruction thus releasing hemoglobin. This hemoglobin is then excreted by the kidneys. In addition, prolonged running could lead to ruptured muscle cells, thus releasing myoglobin, therefore having the same effect. An irritation of the inner lining of the urinary bladder may also be a source of red blood cell loss. Several studies have revealed an increased loss of blood in the feces of endurance runners, which may be due to the loss of intestinal wall cells. In addition, small amounts of iron may be lost in sweat. Sweat of trained athletes contains less iron than the sweat of others (adaptation of conditioning). Vegetarians may be at a higher risk of having low iron. Avoid coffee and tea (they inhibit iron absorption). Careful selection of the proper foods is important for vegetarians.

Iron-deficiency anemia and, with high-mileage runners (**runner's anemia**), is another concern of the endurance athlete. Studies have shown that anemia will cause a significant reduction in the ability of the athlete to perform prolonged high level of exercise. The donation of blood causes a drop in hemoglobin which may decrease performance capacity, therefore decreasing the ability of transportation and usage of oxygen in the body. Medical testing is necessary to correct this deficiency of iron.

Sports anemia which is caused by a temporary low hemoglobin concentration in the blood after sudden increase in aerobic exercise and other strenuous activity. Vigorous aerobic exercise promotes the destruction of fragile, older red blood cells and increases the blood plasma volume. Sports anemia tends to be a temporary response to endurance training and will usually disappear by itself.

Heme (animal) **foods** such as lean red meats, iron-rich organ meats, fish, and skinless poultry are the best iron sources. Good plant sources include beans, bran flakes, soybeans, red kidney beans, legumes, whole grain cereals, as well as broccoli. The iron in these plant foods is not as available to the body as is the iron in animal food, but its ability to be absorbed into the system is increased when it is taken in with foods rich in vitamin C. Cooking foods in cast iron pots will also increase iron intake that the body can utilize. Female distance runners who may experience heavy menstrual blood flow and athletes who are on restricted caloric intake may need iron supplementation in their diets. However, consuming too much iron will not improve the quality of red blood cells but may cause problems in the liver.

TABLE 7.16
SOME GOOD SOURCES OF IRON

(Note: This is not a complete list of examples. You can obtain additional information from "Good Sources of Nutrients," USDA, January 1990. Also read food labels for brand-specific information.)

- Meats—beef, pork, lamb, and liver and other organ meats*
- Poultry—chicken, duck, and turkey, especially dark meat; liver*
- Fish—shellfish, like clams, mussels, and oysters; sardines; anchovies; and other fish*
- Leafy greens of the cabbage family, such as broccoli, kale, turnip greens, collards
- Legumes, such as lima beans and green peas; dry beans and peas, such as pinto beans, black-eyed peas, and canned baked beans
- Yeast-leavened whole-wheat bread and rolls
- Iron-enriched white bread, pasta, rice, and cereals. Read the labels.

*Some foods in this group are high in fat, cholesterol, or both. Choose lean, lower fat, lower cholesterol foods most often. Read the labels.

Vitamin/Mineral Supplements

Exercisers who select proper foods with care can be sure of meeting vitamin and mineral needs without additional supplements. Individuals who take supplements gain no competitive advantage but studies consistently show that compromised nutrition status impedes performance.

According to the National Research Council's recently released *Diet and Health* report, "the desirable way for the general public to obtain recommended levels of nutrients is by eating a variety of foods." The report also lists several instances in which supplements may be appropriate. Those who may benefit from nutrient supplements include:

1. Pregnant or breast-feeding women, who have hard-to-meet needs for nutrients such as folic acid, iron, and calcium.
2. Individuals not consuming 75% of RDAs in daily calorie diets.
3. Women who suffer from excessive menstrual bleeding and need extra iron to help replenish stores of that mineral lost in the blood.
4. Individuals on very low-calorie diets or strict vegetarian regimens, which often lack sufficient zinc, calcium, iron, and vitamin B_{12}.
5. Individuals who suffer from a disease, or take drugs that interfere with appetite or the way the body handles certain nutrients.
6. Practices such as smoking, alcohol consumption, use of drugs such as aspirin and oral contraceptives.

There is no difference between the **synthesized vitamin** and the **"natural" vitamin**, except expense, for proper bodily functions. They have the same chemical composition and are no different from vitamins found in generic vitamin tablets. If concerned about getting insufficient vitamins in the diet, the least expensive or a one-a-day brand should be enough. Vitamins need proper food for adequate absorption.

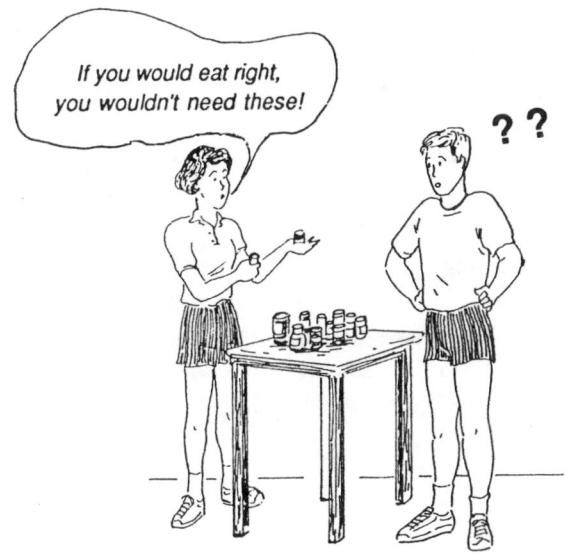

Electrolytes

Electrolytes (**water, sodium, potassium, magnesium, chloride**, and **calcium**) lost through sweat and water vapor from the lungs should be replaced as quickly as possible. Individuals beginning an exercise program will lose electrolytes to a greater degree than trained individual except for magnesium loss through sweat which is the same for both trained and untrained individuals. As the body adapts to the exercise it becomes better at conserving electrolytes. Proper balance of these elements prevents dehydration, heat cramping, heat exhaustion, and heat stroke. Refer to Chapter Four (Drinking and Eating Section) for additional information on electrolytes.

Sodium

Individuals eat more sodium than is needed in the daily diet. Excessive sodium is linked to high blood pressure which can lead to strokes. **Salt** is 40% sodium and 60% **chloride**, and an abundance of salt without adequate water actually draws fluids from the cells and increases urination and potassium loss. Foods with excessive sodium which should be avoided include salt, canned soups, MSG, pickles, ham, cold cuts, fast foods, snack foods, cheese, processed and packaged foods. Foods lowest in sodium, cholesterol, fat and animal fat are potatoes, pasta, rice, beans, oats, peas and fresh fruit and vegetables. Sodium is found naturally in foods and manufacturers use it as a food preservative. Sodium is useful to retain fluid inside blood vessels in order to maintain blood pressure and is essential for muscle function and nerve conduction. Many individuals are "salt sensitive," especially African Americans; fluids are drawn into the circulatory system which produces high blood pressure problems. Limiting salt intake (1 teaspoon or less) reduces hypertension, heart attacks, and kidney disease for these "salt-sensitive" individuals as well as other individuals. The American Heart Association recommends less than 3000 mg of salt per day. The authors recommend 2400 mg or less per day, equivalent to approximately one teaspoon of salt.

Salt supplements are not needed because table salt and the salt in food will provide sufficient sodium for active individuals. Salt is not recommended before or after an activity because it causes interference with the absorption of water from the gastrointestinal tract.

Chloride

Loss of too much chloride upsets the acid-base balance of the body (stomach). Chlorine is added to public water and it provides humans with this valuable element and makes water safe for human consumption.

Potassium

Potassium is essential for the maintenance of body fluids and in the generation of electrical impulses in the nerves and muscles, such as the heart muscle (heart beat). In addition, potassium has an important role in carbohydrate and protein metabolism. Low potassium levels lead to muscle weakness and fatigue. Sudden death from heart failure may occur when potassium storage drops to very low levels. Diarrhea, certain diuretics, heavy sweating, and vomiting reduce potassium levels. Potassium should be replaced daily by consuming a diet of oranges, bananas, cantaloupes, raisins, prunes, dates, nuts, potatoes, sweet potatoes, grapefruit, meat, fish, fresh vegetables, spinach, Swiss chard, broccoli, winter squashes, dried peas, dried beans, lentils, dried apricots, milk, yogurt, orange and grapefruit juices.

Water

People can live for weeks without food but can survive only days without water. Water is a clear, odorless, and tasteless fluid. Water needs depend upon the individual and factors such as body weight, activity patterns, sweat loss, loss through expired air and urine, and the amount of liquid consumed through other foods and drinks.

Three major sources supply water to the body: foods, fluid intake, and as a by-product of metabolism. Fruits and vegetables are the major sources of water (fluids). For example, oranges contain approximately 86% water; lettuce, 96%; tomatoes, 94%; and apples are 84% water. Most foods have some amounts of water. Fluid intake should not count

---

ENERGY REPLACEMENT OPTIONS:
Water (H20), Sports Drinks, Energy Gels and Energy Bars

Water is the ideal fluid replacement for most exercisers. During strenuous activity lasting more than an hour, slightly sugared beverages may help the body conserve its carbohydrate stores, maintain normal blood sugar levels, and delay fatigue. Nutritional sports drinks are similar to diluted juice or soft drinks but more expensive. Sports nutritionist Nancy Clark suggests a homemade recipe:

In a glass dissolve 1 tablespoon of sugar and a pinch (1/6 teaspoon) of salt in a little hot water. Add 1 tablespoon orange juice or 2 tablespoons lemon juice and 7.5 ounces ice water.

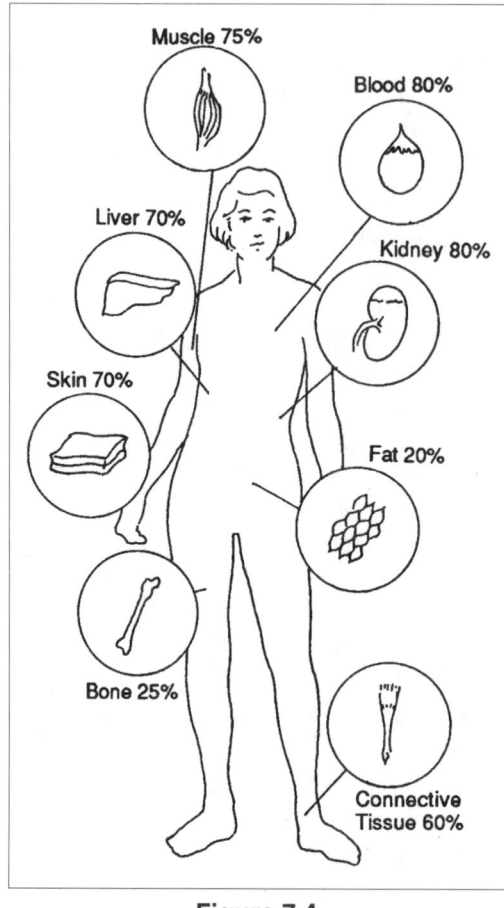

Muscle 75%

Blood 80%

Liver 70%

Kidney 80%

Skin 70%

Fat 20%

Bone 25%

Connective
Tissue 60%

Figure 7.4

caffeinated drinks, coffee, tea, etc., due to diuretic properties. The breakdown of carbohydrates, proteins and fats (food) during the metabolic process provides water to the body. Water loss is caused by air travel, exhalation (lungs), perspiration (skin), urine and body functions. Water loss, not salt or sodium loss, impairs an athlete's performance.

The adult body contains about 10 gallons of water, approximately 55-60 percent of total body, and is found in muscle, blood, brain, bone, etc.. The percentage of water may be as low as 40 percent in obese individuals and as high as 70 percent in muscular individuals. The reason is that fat tissue is low and muscle tissue is high in water content.

The first symptom of **dehydration (water loss)** is fatigue. Water loss of 5 percent of the body weight can reduce muscular work capacity by 20-30 percent and a 15-20 percent loss of body water can be harmful and even cause death. A loss of 7 pounds for a 150 lb. person equals a 5% loss. Actually, second to oxygen, water is the most vital substance required. It is involved in almost every vital body process. Water is used in digestion and absorption of food, in the circulatory process, regulates body temperature particularly during exercise in the heat, acts as a cushion for nerves, lubricates the joints, removes waste products, transports other nutrients, building and rebuilding cells. Refer to Chapter 2 for discussions on heat cramps, heat exhaustion, and heatstroke due to dehydration or water loss.

Under normal temperatures and activity levels, the average adult needs a minimum of eight glasses of water (2 quarts) per day to maintain adequate water balance in the body. Athletes require eight to ten glasses or more of water during exercise. During prolonged exercise in the heat, people can become dehydrated at a rate of 1-2 liters every hour (about 2-4 lbs. of body weight loss per hour). Each pound of weight loss corresponds to 450 ml (15 fluid ounces) of dehydration. Additional water is needed if the color of the urine is darker than the color of a manila folder. **Note:** Many medications alter the color of urine. Also, more water is needed in the body by walkers, joggers and runners (12 glasses per day) and in hot and humid weather. Athletes can lose 2 to 4 quarts of fluid in every hour of vigorous exercise during warm weather. During warm weather, consumption of cool water is better since it cools the body and rapidly leaves the digestive tract to enter tissues where it is needed. For information on hydrating for exercise, refer to Chapter 4. During cold weather, the water consumed should be warm or at room temperature. Drinking an over-abundance of water generally poses no problem since the kidneys merely excrete the excess water.

During hot and humid weather, thirst sensations will underestimate the need for water. Drink before becoming thirsty. A water deficit is created and cannot be undone for several hours when a person becomes thirsty. Forced drinking, even when no thirst sensation exists, will minimize water deficit and will result in better performance, therefore delaying fatigue. Caffeine and alcohol have a dehydrating effect and decrease body fluids.

Spring water (according to the law) must actually have come from a spring and water labeled **"natural spring water"** must be bottled exactly as it came from the ground. The mineral content of **natural spring water** is dependent on the spring it comes from and may contain calcium, magnesium, potassium, and sodium. When minerals are added to the water, it is the manufacturer who decides what is put in the water. **Distilled water**, which is usually sold in drugstores, is tap water processed to remove all minerals. It is tasteless (minerals give water taste) and pure; that is, if it has been properly bottled and handled. Distilled water and drinking water may be expensive and do not contain fluoride which helps prevent tooth decay. Some bottled water is artificially carbonated with carbon dioxide gas, artificially added minerals, dissolved minerals, relatively poor in mineral content, alkaline, process water from local taps, while many are not natural mineral water at all. Water from the faucet should be monitored by the local health department or municipality. This water is safe to drink and is the cheapest source of water. It is suggested that the government usually monitors the public water supply more carefully than it monitors commercially bottled waters. To minimize water loss: increase fluids in hot, humid weather; increase fluids with increased fiber consumption to prevent constipation; drink plenty of water to prevent dehydration when flying since one pint of water is lost for every one hour of air travel. Water consumption prior to, during, and after a walking, jogging, or running workout or competition is discussed in Chapter 4 in the section Drinking and Eating. Refer to Lab 7.2, Daily Nutritional Evaluation, to record results.

CAFFEINE AND ALCOHOL

Caffeine and **alcohol** are diuretics and promote the excretion of water, vitamins and minerals (thiamin, riboflavin, calcium, magnesium and potassium). Caffeine and alcohol are the equivalents of taking a diuretic (water pill) as far as their effect on the body's fluid balance. Alcohol and caffeine can make heatstroke more likely, especially when exercising in a hot, warm, or humid environment.

Caffeine is a stimulant which occurs naturally in nonherb teas, coffee, cocoa, and chocolate. In addition, caffeine is an additive in certain kinds of aspirin, cold remedies, carbonated beverages, and diet aids. Caffeine is medically classified as a drug and too much may be poisonous.

Caffeine stimulates the central nervous system that can increase alertness and stamina, and some studies indicate it may enhance performance in endurance events of an hour or more. Caffeine takes about 30 minutes to reach the brain after it is ingested. It continues to simulate the nervous system for up to eight hours. Studies reveal that caffeine will not improve performance in events characterized by speed, power, strength, or local muscular endurance, nor in endurance events of less than 30 minutes. It also appears to increase the use of fat as a fuel during long endurance exercise of 45 minutes or longer. Caffeine can reduce muscle tension by increasing blood flow to the muscle cells and is known to relieve certain types of headaches. Caffeine has been found to decrease the body's absorption of iron and calcium, cause mood changes (anxiety, irritability, and depression), and stomach upsets. Irregular heartbeats and temporarily increased blood pressure have been documented with caffeine consumption.

Alcohol has no nutritional value (7 calories per gram). Evidence suggests that alcohol is not utilized in improving performance to any significant extent during exercise. In addition, alcohol impairs athletic performance by slowing down reaction time, altering perceptions and judgment, and, in fact, compromises the safety of the individual involved in the activity. Many accidents are related involving the usage of alcohol during activity. When males and females drink alcohol, in proportion to body weight, the blood levels of females are higher than males. This result is due to the decreased stomach enzyme activity which breaks down some of the alcohol in males. Therefore, females tend to feel the greater effects of alcohol.

AIRPLANE FOOD

Due to changing lifestyles, airplane food is now an important dietary consideration. Call the airline at least 24 hours before your flight and order a "special meal." Popular meals include Kosher, low-cal, low cholesterol, low salt, vegetarian, fruit plates and seafood platters. Tell the flight attendant that you have ordered a special meal.

FAST FOODS

It is estimated that one-fifth of all Americans eat in fast food restaurants on a typical day. **Fast foods have three major problems: high calories, fat and salt.** Forty to fifty-five percent of the calories in some fast food come from fat, and much of the fat is highly saturated which means it helps to raise blood cholesterol levels. Hamburgers, chicken and fish are sometimes fried in beef tallow. Chicken nuggets and sandwiches often contain ground chicken skin (high in fat). Fast foods are high in sodium, usually 700 to 900 milligrams per meal; special items such as bacon cheeseburgers may have 1300 to 1950 mg. Additional foods added may result in an entire day's sodium in just one meal. Fast foods are generally low in fiber. However, salad bars are becoming popular and can help increase daily fiber in the diet. Most fast foods are low in calcium because of the selection of coffee and colas, although milkshakes and skim milk are being offered in some fast food restaurants. Eating in a fast food restaurant, a person will eat a large number of calories in order to obtain adequate nutrition. Due to consumer pressure, restaurants are now offering salad bars, low-fat salad dressings, low-fat or skim milk, whole grain buns and fruit juices. Many states require fast food restaurants to provide nutritional information about their foods.

When eating fast food consider the following:
1. Avoid fried foods, foods prepared with sauces, gravies, or sauteed in butter.
2. Choose roast beef, leaner than hamburger. Skip the mayonnaise (save 100-150 calories, nearly all from fat), bacon and cheese (save 200 calories, saturated fat and cholesterol).

TABLE 7.17
SELECTING THE BEST SALADS

Salad Ingredients (1/8 cup unless otherwise noted)*	% Calories from fat	Calories	Fiber (grams)
cauliflower, 1/3 cup	less	4	.5
carrot, grated	than	5	.5
strawberries, 1/3 cup	10%	15-50	1
pineapple, 1/3 cup		15-50	1.3
melon pieces, 1/3 cup		20	.5
kidney beans		27	2
green peas		12	2
tomato, 1/2 whole		12	1
cucumber, 6 slices		2	.2
broccoli, 1/3 cup		8	2
green pepper		4	.2
crab meat, 1/3 cup		40-60	0
shrimp, 1/3 cup	less	40-60	0
mushrooms	than	2	.5
garbanzo beans	20%	30	1.3
turkey breast, 1/3 cup		70-80	0
chicken breast, 1/3 cup		70-80	0
lean ham, diced, 1/3 cup	37%	68	0
fried noodles	43%	28+	0
croutons	43%	28-30	0
coleslaw, 1/3 cup	55%	120	.5
Parmesan cheese	60%	44	0
chopped egg	65%	26	0
potato salad, 1/3 cup	67%	128	1
sunflower seeds	71%	97	1
macaroni salad, 1/3 cup	74%	118	.4
cheddar cheese, grated	74%	55	0
bacon, crumbled, 1 Tbs.	78%	18	0
avocado, 1/4 whole	79%	81	1.5
black olives	93%	25	1

Dressings (2 tablespoons)*	% Calories from Fat	Calories
non-fat yogurt, plain	3%	16
low-fat yogurt, flavored	9%	29
low-fat yogurt, plain	22%	18
light sour cream	60%	45
reduced-calorie mayo-type	73%	70
thousand island	83%	118
French	84%	134
Italian	91%	137
blue cheese	91%	154
ranch	92%	109

*based on average values

3. Request no added salt in the preparation of food.
4. Include dairy products for additional calcium.
5. Include fresh fruits/vegetables for vitamin A and C, and fiber.
6. Eat chicken (not fried chicken, high in fat) and fish in order to cut down on total calories from fat.
7. Eat salads and request that the dressing be served on the side. (Use dressing with moderation—two small ladles can contain nearly as much fat as a large burger, although fat is largely unsaturated.) (Refer to Table 7.17.)
8. Avoid frosted desserts and cakes. Instead, choose fruit, sherbet or plain ice cream.
9. Eat a baked potato. Go easy on the French fries and skip the toppings made with sour cream, melted cheese, or butter.

SUPERMARKET SHOPPING

Due to busy schedules and families working outside the home, it is not always easy to find time to shop or to take the time to look for good, nutritional foods. Keeping a shopping list can assist the shopper in buying only items that are needed. Studies show that, when shopping on an empty stomach, hungry shoppers buy more junk food. Fresh produce and dairy products are generally located around the perimeter of the store, whereas processed and packaged foods are usually displayed in the inner aisles. The healthiest and least expensive foods are put on the top and bottom shelves Less healthful and more expensive foods often are positioned at eye level. For healthy grocery shoping, look high and look low.

Shopping Suggestions

1. Check expiration and "sell" dates on perishable foods (dairy products, breads, cereals). **Purchase products with the distant date.**
2. Choose **whole grain products** for greater nutritional content, rather than "enriched" breads. Larger stores or health food stores may carry the hard-to-find nuts and seeds and whole-grain products.
3. Plan to shop for fresh produce twice a week (vegetables and fruits lose their nutrients during prolonged refrigeration).
4. Avoid wilted vegetables and bruised fruits, even if less expensive. They do not contain the same nutritional value as fresh products.
5. **Select fresh or frozen produce, avoid prepackaged fruits and vegetables.**
6. Choose small, young vegetables and remove the leafy tops to prevent wilting.

DIETARY GUIDELINES FOR AMERICANS

(Source: U.S. Department of Health and Human Services, *Nutrition and Your Health: Dietary Guidelines for Americans,* Fourth Edition, 1995)

○ Eat a variety of foods.

○ Balance the food you eat with physical activity—maintain or improve your weight.

○ Choose a diet with plenty of grain products, vegetables, and fruits.

○ Choose a diet low in fat, saturated fat, and cholesterol.

○ Choose a diet moderate in sugars.

○ Choose a diet moderate in salt and sodium.

○ If you drink alcoholic beverages, do so in moderation.

1. ***Eat a variety of foods.*** Choose the recommended number of daily servings from each of the five major food groups displayed in the Food Guide Pyramid.

2. ***Balance the food you eat with physical activity— maintain or improve your weight.*** Increase physical activity of 30 minutes or more of moderate activity on most days of the week; reduce calories by eating fewer fatty foods and sweets and less sugar, and by avoiding too much alcohol; lose weight gradually.

3. ***Choose a diet with plenty of grain products, vegetables, and fruits.*** Substitute starches for fats and sugars; select whole-grain breads and cereals, fruits and vegetables, dried beans and peas, and nuts to increase fiber and starch intake.

4. ***Choose a diet low in fat, saturated fat, and cholesterol.*** Choose low fat protein sources such as lean meats, fish, poultry, dried peas and beans; use eggs and organ meats in moderation; limit intake of fats on and in foods; trim fats from meats; broil, bake, or boil — don't fry; read food labels for fat contents.

5. ***Choose a diet moderate in sugars.*** Use less sugar, syrup, and honey; reduce concentrated sweets like candy, soft drinks, cookies, and the like; select fresh fruits or fruits canned in light syrup or their own

juices; read food labels — sucrose, glucose, dextrose, maltose, lactose, fructose, syrups, and honey are all sugars; eat sugar less often to reduce dental cavities.

6. ***Choose a diet moderate in salt and sodium.*** Reduce salt in cooking; add little or no salt at the table; limit salty foods like potato chips, pretzels, salted nuts, popcorn, condiments, cheese, pickled foods, and cured meats; read food labels for sodium or salt contents, especially in processed and snack foods.

7. ***If you drink alcoholic beverages, do so in moderation.*** For individuals who drink, limit all alcoholic beverages (including wine, beer, liquors, and so on) to one (women) or two (men) drinks per day. Count as a drink: 12 ounces of regular beer (150 calories); 5 ounces of wine (100 calories); 1.5 ounces of distilled spirits,80 proof (100 calories). (*Note:* Use of alcoholic beverages during pregnancy can result in the development of birth defects and mental retardation called fetal alcohol syndrome.)

NUTRITION LABELS

Food manufacturers often distort nutritional facts and some have made rather extravagant claims for their particular products. On October 24, 1990, Congress passed the Nutrition Labeling and Education Act of 1989, which requires most foods under the FDA to meet labeling guidelines. However, this Act of 1989 does not pertain to foods that are under the USDA such as meat and poultry. Foods under FDA that would be exempt include spices, infant formulas, and foods that have negligible amounts of nutrients. However, since May 8, 1993, the federal government requires food manufacturers to provide accurate nutritional information on their product labels. The term "Nutrition Facts" signals the new label. (See the next page.) It is not necessary to be placed by small food manufacturers with low profits or food packages too small for labels.

Labeling Tips

Remember to multiply carbohydrates and protein grams by 4; and fats by 9 calories for each gram consumed to determine the percentage of daily caloric intake.

| *An Example of Fat:* |
| Multiply the grams of fat by 9 (there are 9 calories in a gram of fat). Then divide that number by the total calories. The formula is:

$$\frac{(\text{grams of fat} \times 9)}{\text{total calories}}$$ |

The Nutrition Label
Plain Lowfat Yogurt

Nutrition Facts

Serving Size 1 cup
Servings Per Container 1

Amount Per Serving

Calories 140   Calories from Fat 35

	% Daily Value*
Total Fat 4g	**6%**
Saturated Fat 2.5 g	**11%**
Cholesterol 15 mg	**5%**
Sodium 160 mg	**7%**
Total Carbohydrate 16 g	**5%**
Dietary Fiber 0g	**0%**
Sugars 12 g	
Protein 12 g	**24%**

Vitamin A 4%	•	Vitamin C 4%
Calcium 40%	•	Iron 0%

* Percent Daily Values are based on a 2,000 calorie diet. Your daily values may be higher or lower depending on your calorie needs:

	Calories:	2000	2,500
Total Fat	Less than	65g	80g
Sat Fat	Less than	20g	25g
Cholesterol	Less than	300 mg	300 mg
Sodium	Less than	2,400mg	2,400mg
Total Carbohydrate		300g	375g
Dietary Fiber		25g	30g

Calories per gram:
Fat 9 • Carbohydrate 4 • Protein 4

Ingredients: Cultured grade A lowfat milk and pectin. Contains active L. Acidophilus cultures.

For example: A tablespoon of peanut butter has 8 grams of fat and 95 calories. So 8 x 9 = 72, divided by the number of calories (95) = 0.76, or 76% of calories from fat.

An easier way to estimate this number is to multiply the grams of fat by 9; if the result is more than a third of total calories, the food is relatively high in fat. Limit the intake of fat, especially if it is high in saturated fat.

Items labeled "lite," "reduced fat" or "low fat," "natural," "whole wheat," "oat bran," etc., should be read cautiously. Refer to labels for accurate ingredients.

Example: 5 grams of fat is not low fat but may be lower than the original item. Lunch meat labeled as 82% fat free (18% fat) means that only 18% of weight of the product is from fat.

Using the above formula, calculate the percentage of fat in this lunch meat:

Fat 5g   Calories 60   Sodium 180 mg   Protein 4g
5g fat x 9 = 45 calories from fat
45 ÷ 60 calories per serving = 75% calories which come from fat
Note: Labels can be confusing so read the fine print and calculate the percentage before making a selection.

The food label bases its % daily values on a 2,000-calorie diet. Use this chart to compare your intake and daily values with the ones the label is based on.

Nutrient Needs for Different Calorie Levels*

Food Component	Calories Per Day					
	1,400	1,800	**2,000**	2,500	3,000	3,500
Total Fat(g)	47	60	**65**	80	100	116
Saturated Fat (g)	16	20	**20**	25	34	39
Cholesterol (mg)	300	300	**300**	300	300	300
Sodium (mg)	2,400	2,400	**2,400**	2,400	2,400	2,400
Total Carbohydrate (g)	210	270	**300**	375	450	525
Dietary Fiber (g)	20	20	**25**	30	35	42
Protein (g)	46	48	**50**	65	75	87
Total % Daily Value	70%	90%	**100%**	125%	150%	175%

* Numbers may be rounded

A diet:	May reduce risk of:
High in calcium	Osteoporosis (brittle bones)
High in dietary fiber from grain products, fruits, and vegetables	Cancer and heart disease
High in vitamins A or C from fruits and vegetables	Cancer
Low in fat	Cancer
Low in saturated fat and cholesterol	Heart disease
Low in sodium	High blood pressure

COMMON FOOD LABEL TERMS

diet — Must either meet "low calorie or "reduced calorie" requirements or state actual content

low-calorie — 40 calories or less per serving

reduced calorie — At least 1/3 less calories

extra lean — 95% fat free by weight

lean or low fat — 90% fat free by weight

low sodium — 140 mg or less per serving

reduced sodium — Reduced usual sodium content by 25%

low salt — Made with less salt than the regular food item

health or organic food No legal definition

enriched — Nutrients that are added to a processed food. For example, during the milling of wheat many of the B vitamins and iron are lost. These are added back, usually in greater quantities, during enrichment.

fortified — Nutrients that are added to a food to prevent nutrient deficiencies. These nutrients may or may not have been present in the original product.

CHAPTER SUMMARY

Before starting that walking, jogging, or running program an individual should remember that eating a well-balanced diet is the foundation to any exercise activity. The individual who wishes to excel physically will exercise and make the right food choices, therefore enhancing appearance and performance.

A proper nutritional diet must contain an adequate amount of the forty plus essential nutrients to sustain growth and repair of body tissues during the various stages of life. In addition, it must be balanced in caloric intake for the control of body weight (weight maintenance, gain or loss, depending upon the individual). **The six essential nutrients (carbohydrates, fat, protein, vitamins, minerals, and water) should be consumed in moderation and included on a daily basis.** Eat more nutritious food and less of the other foods. You do not have to avoid foods—just eat them in moderation. The amount of portion sizes counts. Choose healthy calories and enjoy a variety of foods for a lifetime of good health. Variety is dietary insurance. Being aware of fast foods, caffeine and alcohol also can be advantageous to the individual's performance. When shopping for a nutritious food plan, one should read labels cautiously and watch for misconceptions advertised by manufacturers.

You are what you eat. In order to maintain a healthy body and live life to its fullest, **eat to live rather than live to eat. Remember: Food for fuel to function.**

CHAPTER EIGHT

Weight Management

America is known as the fattest nation on earth. Fifty percent of U.S. women and thirty-three percent of men have, at some time, trimmed food intake in an effort to lose weight. The past ten years the average weight of American adults has increased by approximately 15 pounds. As much as 90-95 percent who diet regain the weight lost in five years; only approximately 10% remain thin. Sedentary lifestyles, excessive food, accessibility to fatty snacks, and, in some cases, genetics contribute to weight problems. Thirty-three billion dollars are spent each year on diets or the war against fat.

> "It isn't what we ate when we were twenty that kept our weight down. It was what we were doing with our bodies." —George Sheehan

Obesity (excess body fat) is associated with the increased incidence of mortality and cardiovascular diseases (high blood pressure, atherosclerosis), type II diabetes, cancer, varicose veins, bone and joint diseases, and cerebral hemorrhage. In less than two percent of the cases, glandular problems cause over-fat condition. America is a push-button society, resulting in limited activity and, without adequate knowledge in regard to controlling weight, obesity is evident.

A diet is something which is done the rest of one's life. **A food plan, simple course of low-fat eating combined with daily exercise, is something participants can rely on for the rest of their lives.** The emphasis of this chapter will be on permanent weight control (food plan) rather than dieting for good health.

THEORIES OF OBESITY

The *genetic predisposition theory* states that the genes inherited do influence weight. Children inherit their body type from their parents. The ectomorph has a slender body frame and less capacity for storing fat. The endomorph has a soft, rounded appearance and a greater tendency for storing fat. The mesomorph has a muscular body frame and tends to be less likely to have a weight problem. It is important to understand the

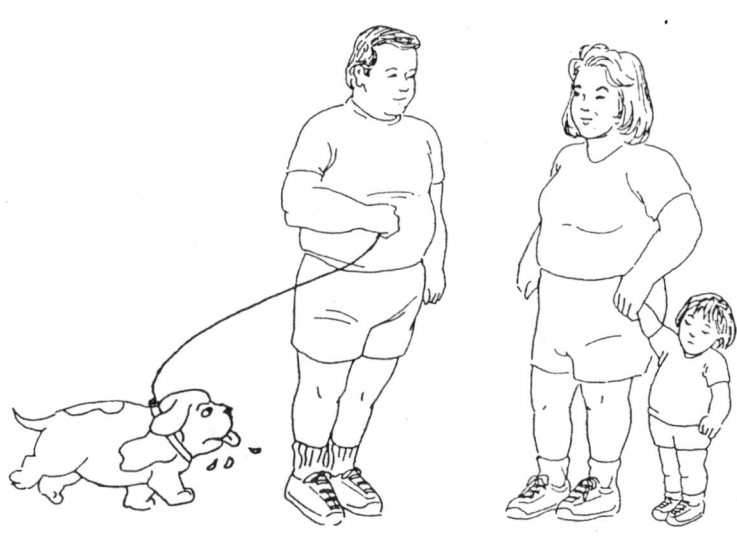

A "typical" American Family

different body types. Consider, for example, a stocky bulldog and a lean, sleek greyhound. Starving a bulldog to death will never make him look like a greyhound and vice versa. The body type cannot be changed but the percent of body fat can be altered. Children with both parents overweight or obese have an 80% chance of being overweight or obese; with one parent, 40%, and with neither parent, 7% chance of being overweight or obese. This suggests a hereditary tendency toward being overweight but it doesn't prove it. The family environment, parents' eating and exercise habits, could be a factor in such statistics. Individuals with one or both parents overweight may have to work harder than others to prevent obesity. **Genetics may be the foundation for obesity but environment determines the outcome of the foundation.** Several studies have shown that fat people are more likely to have fat pets. Fat foods and snacks, large portions, and inactivity can affect humans and beast alike. By establishing good eating habits and exercising regularly, obesity can be avoided.

The *fat-cell theory* states that the number of fat cells in the body predispose an individual to obesity. Obese people do not necessarily eat more than thin people; however, they have more fat cells. There are **three stages of development which increase the number of fat cells.** The **first stage** begins in the **last trimester of prenatal care**: If the mother gains an excessive amount of weight, the infant will acquire more fat cells. The **second stage**, the **first three years** of the **child's life,** has significant

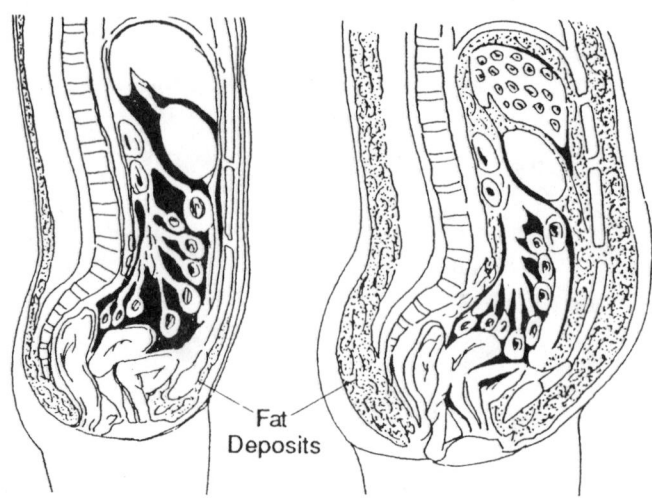

Figure 8-1. Distribution of body fat: Approximately 50% of fat deposits are directly under the skin and 50%surrounding internal organs.

impact; and the **third stage** is during **adolescence**. Researchers believe that individuals are born with a certain number of fat cells, which can swell or shrink. People who are obese have enlarged or more fat cells. The greater the number of fat cells, the greater the capacity to store more energy in the form of fat. However, the environment is still important. Daily eating/drinking habits and exercise can overcome the genetic tendency to be thin or fat.

The *white fat versus brown fat* activity theory states that people who have weight problems have little brown fat activity. The body has **two types of fat tissue**: white fat tissue and brown fat tissue. White fat, or fat stored in the cells, is pink in color because of the blood flowing in it. It mainly accumulates in the subcutaneous tissue, the abdominal cavity (around the internal organs), and the intramuscular tissue. The brown fat accounts for approximately one percent of body weight. It is located in the back, shoulder region and the back of the neck. Brown fat has a high metabolic activity potential. The younger the individual the more brown fat is available. Obese individuals may have more brown fat tissue.

The *set-point theory* states that body weight is controlled by a weight-regulating mechanism located in the hypothalamus, a gland in the brain responsible for stimulation of hormones of the pituitary, a master gland which is responsible for the process of fat mobilization during exercise. Each individual appears to have an ideal biological weight (set point) and will defend it against pressure to change. Within a 24 hour period of beginning a low-calorie diet, the metabolic rate (amount of calories burned at rest) slows by 5-20% as a means of conserving energy, therefore making it more difficult to lose weight. The body thinks it is starving and conserving calories is the only way of surviving. An internal **"thermostat"** regulates body fat and weight, and triggers an increase in food intake when fat and weight are too low. The combination of regular aerobic exercise, reduced consumption of caffeine (stimulates production of insulin), a diet high in complex carbohydrates and low in fat and sugar (simple carbohydrates) seems to be the only practical and effective way to lower the setpoint and lose fat weight.

HEALTH PROBLEMS

Gaining or losing body weight for improved performance, appearance and self-concept may provide some health benefits but it can lead to deterioration of health if done improperly. A body fat level too low can be just as dangerous as having a body fat level that is too high. A nutritious food plan and exercise are the foundations of a sound weight management program. Dieticians and psychologists are excellent contacts if assistance is needed in dealing with the problems discussed in this section.

Individuals, especially young women, use starvation, diuretics, and diet pills to achieve a rapid weight loss. This may cause serious medical disorders such as electrolyte imbalance and altered excretory and digestive systems which can lead to heart and kidney dysfunction and even death. A quick weight loss over a period of a few weeks is usually achieved by dehydration and starvation-type diets. Certain physiological changes can occur during these diets that may be potentially harmful to some individuals. Health problems may include, but are not limited to, the following topics.

Anorexia Nervosa

Anorexia nervosa (fear of fatness) is characterized by little or no eating in an attempt to limit or reduce body weight. It is considered a symptom of mental illness, that results in self-induced starvation which could result in death. The cause of the obsession to be thin is not known. Most of the individuals are female (90-95%), typically in the upper teens or twenties, and come from an upper-middle socioeconomic status. The typical person starves herself on 50-100 calories per day. The anorexic is often times a perfectionist and self-critical. This condition is marked by a loss of appetite and skipping meals, leading to various degrees of emaciation. Various techniques are used by the anorexic including exercise, laxatives, starvation and regurgitation.

Bulimia Nervosa

The **bulimic**, who suffers from morbid hunger, is of the same general age and background as the anorexic. This condition is often associated with a **loss of control over the impulse to binge**. The person continuously ingests large quantities of food and induces vomiting, uses laxatives, fluid reduction pills, and weight reduction in order to avoid weight gain. Bulimia is also known as the binge-purge syndrome.

Amenorrhea

Excessive weight loss can also lead to the **cessation of menstruation, amenorrhea**. The precise cause has not been determined; however, there are several theories: decreased intake of calories, protein, fat; increased exercise intensity; a vegetarian diet; psychological stress; and excessive losses of body weight and body fat. Research conducted over the past ten years reveals that even moderate losses of body weight during exercise may be associated with a disturbance of the normal menstrual cycle; hormone levels decrease estrogen, thus ceasing blood flow. Research also indicates an increased risk for the development of osteoporosis. Often a decrease in the intensity and duration of exercise will restore normal menstruation.

Binge Eating

Binge eating has been recently recognized as an eating disorder. The binge eater is often overweight and diets. Characteristics of a binge eating disorder include feeling unable to stop eating, eating rapidly, eating large amounts of food when not hungry, eating a lot of food when alone, eating with no planned meal times. Some binge eaters develop bulimia nervosa while others continue to overeat or binge.

Anorexia Athletica

Anorexia athletica is a term applied to individuals who become overly concerned about their weight, exercise excessively and who also exhibit some of the diagnostic criteria associated with anorexia nervosa. Studies indicate that approximately 20-40% of female athletes may exhibit these symptoms. The condition may begin as a means of weight control for competition on a short-term basis but may develop into a long-term medical problem. The condition generally improves when the athletic season is completed and the athlete resumes normal dietary habits.

TABLE 8.1
GUIDELINE TO ESTIMATE IDEAL BODY WEIGHT

Men:	106 pounds for the first five feet +06 pounds for each additional inch + or - ten percent to account for individual differences (small or large frame)
Women:	100 pounds for the first five feet +05 pounds for each additional inch + or - ten percent to account for individual differences (small or large frame)

Modifications for African Americans*
Men: 110 lbs. for the first 5 feet of height.
Women: 104 lbs. for the first 5 feet of height.

*Barbara Dixon, *Good Health for African Americans* (New York, Crown, 1994) p. 89.

Refer to Lab 8.1, Estimation of Ideal Body Weight, to record results.

DESIRABLE BODY WEIGHT

The important factor is not how much one weighs, but how much of the body weight is fat. It is more important to know the percentage of body fat than to know one's weight. Therefore, it is essential to differentiate between the terms "overweight" (how much a person weighs on a scale) and "overfat." An **overweight** individual is generally defined as someone who weighs more than the average person for that age, sex and height. Being overweight is not a problem as long as the excess weight is lean body tissue or muscle. A muscular person could have body composition of almost entirely muscle, making him/her overweight but certainly not overfat.

Overfat **(obesity)** is commonly defined as anything above **25% or over body fat in men** and **30% or over body fat in women**. When a person consumes more food than is used for activity, this energy is put into storage in the form of fat tissue. Eating less food and exercising more, and doing it for the rest of one's life, can assist the individual in obtaining the desirable body weight.

Height-Weight Tables

One of the most abused and most used methods of determining body weight in the past is the height-weight tables developed by life insurance companies. Height-weight tables are based on averages of measurements obtained from large populations of people. They are meant as guides to weight control, and are based on studies of lowest mortality. As the population becomes heavier the averages on the tables increase. These tables do not take into consideration the levels of body composition. Two individuals may be the same height and weight, and based on these tables, one may be considered obese while the other may be considered muscular because of the distribution of their body weight. Even though they have limitations, these tables should only be used to determine a general weight range for the average adult. The charts do not identify low, average, or high levels of body fat.

Apple or Pear?

Where the fat is on your body makes a big difference, research shows. Individuals who are shaped like apples (round in the middle with relatively slim hips and thighs) seem to be more at risk for developing chronic diseases. Abdominal fat is associated with inefficient insulin metabolism and elevated triglycerides and cholesterol. In contrast, their heavy-hipped counterparts, the pears, have fewer health problems. It is the waist-to-hip ratio that can tell you if you are in the higher risk, apple group. See the box below. Tables 8.2 and 8.3 are based on the Dietary Guidelines for Americans and indicates the weight you should be in the healthy weight ranges to reduce your risk for health problems. These tables covers all people—women have less muscle and smaller bones than men the same size, so they should be at the lower end of the ranges while large-boned men will be at the higher end. If your weight is above the recommended range, you may be at risk for developing heart disease, diabetes, high blood pressure, and certain types of cancer.

WHICH FRUIT DO YOU SUIT?

Your tape measure can tell you whether you're apple- or pear-shaped. Measure around your waist at its smallest point without sucking in your stomach. Take your hip measurement across your buttocks where you are the widest. Divide the waist measurement by the hip measurement to get the waist-to-hip ratio.

$$\frac{waist}{hip} = ratio$$ For men this ratio should be less than .95; for women, the ratio should be less than .8

TABLE 8.2
HEALTHY WEIGHT RANGES

HEIGHT	WEIGHT*	HEIGHT	WEIGHT*
4'10"	91-119	5'9"	129-169
4'11"	94-124	5'10"	132-174
5'0"	97-128	5'11"	136-179
5'1"	101-132	6'	140-184
5'2"	104-137	6'1"	144-189
5'3'	107-141	6'2"	148-195
5'4"	111-146	6'3"	152-200
5'5"	114-150	6'4"	156-205
5'6"	118-155	6'5"	160-211
5'7"	121-160	6'6"	164-216
5'8"	125-164		

*No shoes or clothes

TABLE 8.3
ARE YOU OVERWEIGHT?

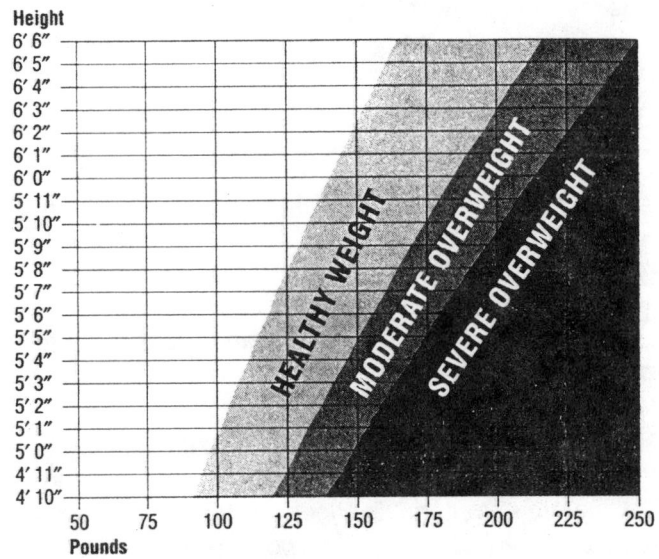

SOURCE: Dietary Guidelines for Americans, 1995

ASSESSING BODY FATNESS

Fat cannot be measured with absolute accuracy; however, there are several methods of estimating body fat that are fairly reliable and accurate. These include **hydrostatic or underwater weighing** (measuring water displacement), **bioelectrical impedance analysis, skinfold measurements, circumferences, X-rays, ultrasound**, and **Body Mass Index (BMI)**. Of these, the skinfold measurement is one of the least expensive, most available methods. Hydrostatic, electrical impedance, skinfold, circumference measurements, and the use of a mirror will be discussed. Some of these methods are not as valid or reliable as others; therefore a standard error from 2.0 to 3.5% may result.

Body Mass Index (BMI)

The body mass index (BMI) is a statistical method that correlates a person's weight and height with disease risk. The old government table used to permit a BMI between 19 and 27 for people over age 35, but since research shows that gaining weight as you age increases risk of early death, the new guidelines cap the BMI at 25. Weight Watchers International is using the BMI of 20 to 25.

To calculate your BMI use this formula:

Your weight (in pounds): _____ x 700 = _____	(a)
Divide (a) by your height (in inches) = _____	(b)
Divide (b) by your height (in inches) = _____	(BMI)

Hydrostatic (Underwater) Weighing

Underwater weighing is one of the most common **research techniques of determining body density**. This method is a more accurate body composition assessment for older persons (or any age) because after middle age body density changes. The procedure is expensive, time-consuming, requires special equipment, and specialized training. It may not be practical except for special laboratories. The procedure of the test requires a submersible scale upon which the individual sits and is lowered in a tank of water. While completely submerged, the person must totally exhale and then the body weight is measured. The procedure is repeated. Few individuals feel comfortable enough in the water to completely exhale all of the air out of the body. Fat has a lower density than water and the more body fat in a person the greater the buoyancy in water. When the person has a small amount of fat and a high amount of muscle (higher density than water), the person will have difficulty staying afloat or will sink in water.

Bioelectrical Impedance Analysis

A recent technique (commercially available in 1982) known as **bioelectrical impedance** is used to **measure fat and body density**. The procedure for using this technique is by attaching electrodes to the right wrist and right ankle while the person is lying down. A harmless undetectable current is transmitted from electrode to electrode at 800 microamps through the body and the areas of lean body mass and fat can be measured by the degree they "impede" this electrical current. The measurement of total body water is accomplished by using a computer-like analyzer and a two-page computer printout of individualized information is available. The accuracy of equations used to estimate percent of body fat is debatable because the test results may not be completely accurate but could serve in assessing changes over a period of time.

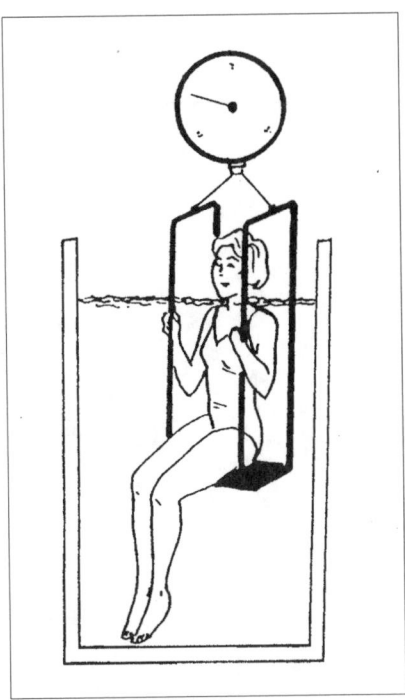

Figure 8.2. Hydrostatic or Underwater Weighing

DEXA Technique

The use of dual energy x-ray absorptiometry (DEXA) has been approved by the FDA. DEXA was created to measure bone density and is readily applicable to body composition measurement. DEXA uses an actual reading of bone rather than predetermined standards and is ideal for people who are losing weight and want to check from time to time to be sure the fat component is decreasing and the lean tissue is increasing. DEXA is not as accessible as the skinfold since the equipment is not available in most labs.

Skinfold Measurement

The skinfold measurement is a method that is more convenient and fairly reliable with a caliper. Several skinfold sites should be used and the

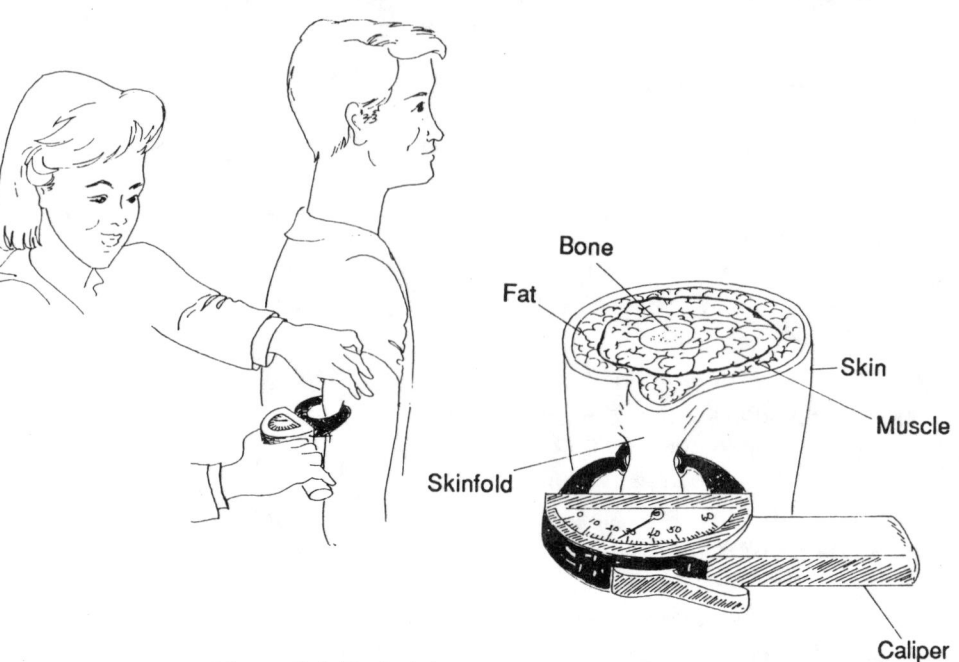

Figure 8-3. Technique for taking skinfold measurement.

measurement should be made by the same person and may vary slightly. The use of calipers should be learned by each person so measurements can be taken throughout one's life. Calipers ranging from twenty dollars to several hundred dollars are available for skinfold measurement.

Approximately 50% of the fat in the body is subcutaneous fat which is stored just beneath the skin or in skinfolds, and the remainder of fat is in the muscles and various organs (refer to Fig. 8.1). **Calipers** are used to measure the thickness of a fold of skin and the fat directly under the skin. Several skinfold measurements should be taken at specific body sites; the thickness of these skinfolds can be used to estimate total body fat. Most skinfold techniques have a standard error of about 3 to 3.5%.

Guidelines to Determine Skinfold Measurement

1. Practice this technique as much as possible. One of the greatest sources of error is not being able to locate and measure the skinfold site accurately.
2. Skinfold measurements should be made on the **right side** of the body. Refer to Fig. 8.4 for the skinfold sites to be measured. Use Lab 8.2, Skinfold Assessment, to record.
3. Measure only the fold of skin (with its subcutaneous fat) at the appropriate site. If there is difficulty in distinguishing fat from muscle,

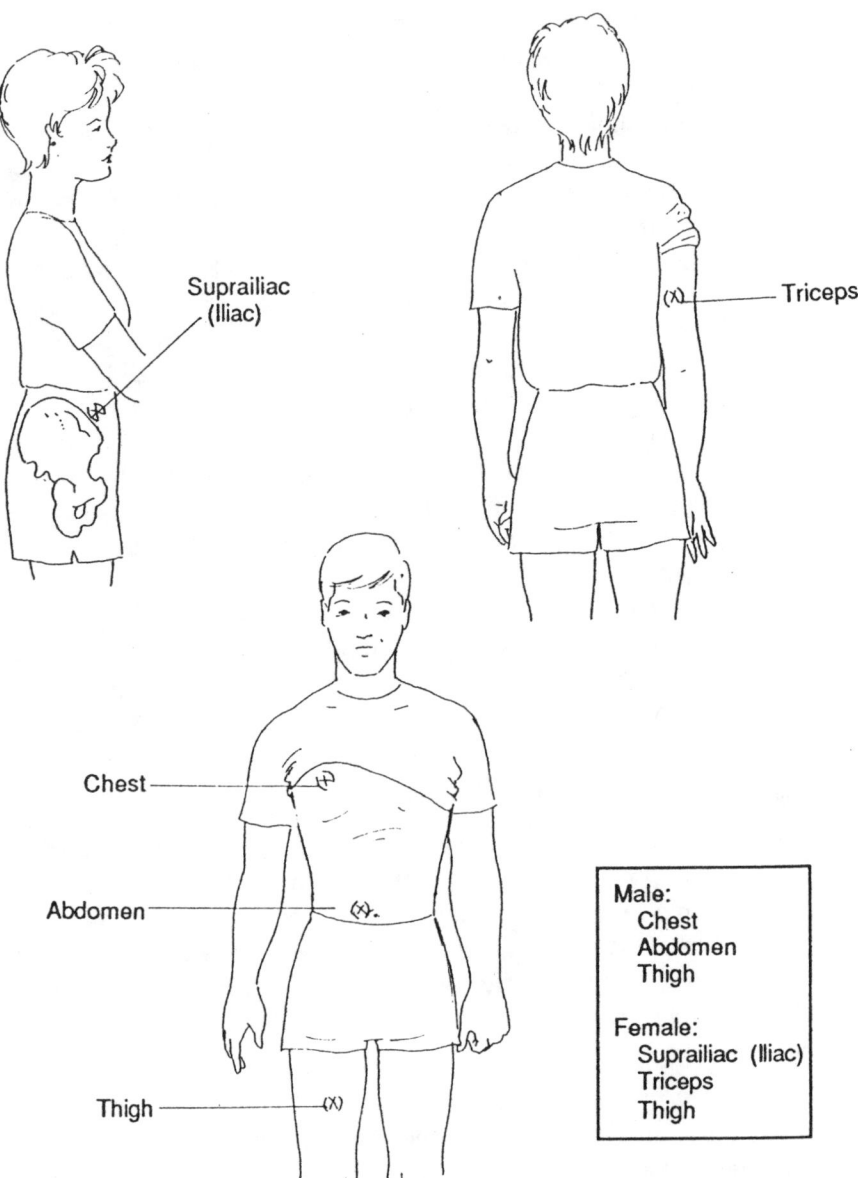

Figure 8-4. Skinfold Sites

have the subject contract and relax underlying muscle to aid in the identification of the subcutaneous fat.

4. The skinfold should be lifted up between the thumb and index finger. Since the thumb and index finger are used to "pinch" the skinfold, it may be necessary to trim the nails.

5. The caliper should be placed right next to the thumb and index finger (1 cm.; 1/4 to 1/2 inch away) and at a depth that is equal to the skinfold. The caliper as well as the thumb and index finger should be perpendicular to the fold of skin.

6. The skinfold reading should be taken with 2 to 3 seconds once the tension has been completely released in the caliper tips. Measurements are recorded in millimeters and can be recorded to the nearest 0.5 mm or 0.1 mm depending on the type of calipers used.

7. Make three skinfold measurements at each skinfold site. Use the average of the three values to determine measurement. If the readings vary by more than 3 mm, an additional reading should be taken. If it is still difficult to obtain consistent measurements, the average of the three most representative readings will be used for that particular skinfold site.

8. The subject's skin should be dry. Wet skin may be easier to grasp and this additional skin would increase the skinfold reading.

9. Obtain percent fat by adding together all three skinfold measurements and looking up the values on Tables 8.4 for men and 8.5 for women.

Circumferences (Body Girth)

These measurements are less accurate than the skinfold technique but better than the height-weight tables and should be used with other methods in monitoring body fatness. They can be easily done by the individual with a standard non-elastic tape measure. Measurements are usually done in inches, but can be done in millimeters. These measurements generally give a fair indication of whether the fat is increasing or decreasing.

Use the following procedure in making circumference measurements:

1. Women should measure their height (without shoes) and the circumference of hips at the widest point. Pull the tape so that it is snug and does not cause an indentation in the natural line of the skin.

2. Men should measure the circumference of the waist at the navel and their weight without shoes or clothes. The tape should be snug at the navel and should not cause an indentation in the natural line of the skin.

TABLE 8.4
PERCENTAGE OF BODY FAT - MEN
(Sum of Chest, Abdominal and Thigh Skinfolds)

Sum of Skinfolds (mm)	Age to the Last Year								
	Under 22	23 to 27	28 to 32	33 to 37	38 to 42	43 to 47	48 to 52	53 to 57	Over 57
8-10	1.3	1.8	2.3	2.9	3.4	3.9	4.5	5.0	5.5
11-13	2.2	2.8	3.3	3.9	4.4	4.9	5.5	6.0	6.5
14-16	3.2	3.8	4.3	4.8	5.4	5.9	6.4	7.0	7.5
17-19	4.2	4.7	5.3	5.8	6.3	6.9	7.4	8.0	8.5
20-22	5.1	5.7	6.2	6.8	7.3	7.9	8.4	8.9	9.5
23-25	6.1	6.6	7.2	7.7	8.3	8.8	9.4	9.9	10.5
26-28	7.0	7.6	8.1	8.7	9.2	9.8	10.3	10.9	11.4
29-31	8.0	8.5	9.1	9.6	10.2	10.7	11.3	11.8	12.4
32-34	8.9	9.4	10.0	10.5	11.1	11.6	12.2	12.8	13.3
35-37	9.8	10.4	10.9	11.5	12.0	12.6	13.1	13.7	14.3
38-40	10.7	11.3	11.8	12.4	12.9	13.5	14.1	14.6	15.2
41-43	11.6	12.2	12.7	13.3	13.8	14.4	15.0	15.5	16.1
44-46	12.5	13.1	13.6	14.2	14.7	15.3	15.9	16.4	17.0
47-49	13.4	13.9	14.5	15.1	15.6	16.2	16.8	17.3	17.9
50-52	14.3	14.8	15.4	15.9	16.5	17.1	17.6	18.2	18.8
53-55	15.1	15.7	16.2	16.8	17.4	17.9	18.5	18.1	19.7
56-58	16.0	16.5	17.1	17.7	18.2	18.8	19.4	20.0	20.5
59-61	16.9	17.4	17.9	18.5	19.1	19.7	20.2	20.8	21.4
62-64	17.6	18.2	18.8	19.4	19.9	20.5	21.1	21.7	22.2
65-67	18.5	19.0	19.6	20.2	20.8	21.3	21.9	22.5	23.1
68-70	19.3	19.9	20.4	21.0	21.6	22.2	22.7	23.3	23.9
71-73	20.1	20.7	21.2	21.8	22.4	23.0	23.6	24.1	24.7
74-76	20.9	21.5	22.0	22.6	23.2	23.8	24.4	25.0	25.5
77-79	21.7	22.2	22.8	23.4	24.0	24.6	25.2	25.8	26.3
80-82	22.4	23.0	23.6	24.2	24.8	25.4	25.9	26.5	27.1
83-85	23.2	23.8	24.4	25.0	25.5	26.1	28.7	27.3	27.9
86-88	24.0	24.5	25.1	25.7	26.3	26.9	27.5	28.1	28.7
89-91	24.7	25.3	25.9	25.5	27.1	27.6	28.2	28.8	29.4
92-94	25.4	26.0	26.6	27.2	27.8	28.4	29.0	29.6	30.2
92-97	26.1	26.7	27.3	27.9	28.5	29.1	29.7	30.3	30.9
98-100	26.9	27.4	28.0	28.6	29.2	29.8	30.4	31.0	31.6
101-103	27.5	28.1	28.7	29.3	29.9	30.5	31.1	31.7	32.3
104-106	28.2	28.8	29.4	30.0	30.6	31.2	31.8	32.4	33.0
107-109	28.9	29.5	30.1	30.7	31.3	31.9	32.5	33.1	33.7
110-112	29.6	30.2	30.8	31.4	32.0	32.6	33.2	33.8	34.4
113-115	30.2	30.8	31.4	32.0	32.6	33.2	33.8	34.5	35.1
116-118	30.9	31.5	32.1	32.7	33.3	33.9	34.5	35.1	35.7
119-121	31.5	32.1	32.7	33.3	33.9	34.5	35.1	35.7	36.4
122-124	32.1	32.7	33.3	33.9	34.5	35.1	35.8	36.4	37.0
125-127	32.7	33.3	33.9	34.5	35.1	35.8	36.4	37.0	37.6

Source: A.S. Jackson and M.L. Pollock, "Practical Assessment of Body Composition," *The Physician and Sportsmedicine* 13, No. 5, (May, 1985):86. Used by permission.

TABLE 8.5
PERCENTAGE OF BODY FAT - WOMEN
(Sum of Triceps, Iliac, and Thigh Skinfolds)

Sum of Skinfolds (mm)	Under 22	23 to 27	28 to 32	33 to 37	38 to 42	43 to 47	48 to 52	53 to 57	Over 57
8-10	1.3	1.8	2.3	2.9	3.4	3.9	4.5	5.0	5.5
11-13	2.2	2.8	3.3	3.9	4.4	4.9	5.5	6.0	6.5
14-16	3.2	3.8	4.3	4.8	5.4	5.9	6.4	7.0	7.5
17-19	4.2	4.7	5.3	5.8	6.3	6.9	7.4	8.0	8.5
20-22	5.1	5.7	6.2	6.8	7.3	7.9	8.4	8.9	9.5
23-25	6.1	6.6	7.2	7.7	8.3	8.8	9.4	9.9	10.5
26-28	7.0	7.6	8.1	8.7	9.2	9.8	10.3	10.9	11.4
29-31	8.0	8.5	9.1	9.6	10.2	10.7	11.3	11.8	12.4
32-34	8.9	9.4	10.0	10.5	11.1	11.6	12.2	12.8	13.3
35-37	9.8	10.4	10.9	11.5	12.0	12.6	13.1	13.7	14.3
38-40	10.7	11.3	11.8	12.4	12.9	13.5	14.1	14.6	15.2
41-43	11.6	12.2	12.7	13.3	13.8	14.4	15.0	15.5	16.1
44-46	12.5	13.1	13.6	14.2	14.7	15.3	15.9	16.4	17.0
47-49	13.4	13.9	14.5	15.1	15.6	16.2	16.8	17.3	17.9
50-52	14.3	14.8	15.4	15.9	16.5	17.1	17.6	18.2	18.8
53-55	15.1	15.7	16.2	16.8	17.4	17.9	18.5	18.1	19.7
56-58	16.0	16.5	17.1	17.7	18.2	18.8	19.4	20.0	20.5
59-61	16.9	17.4	17.9	18.5	19.1	19.7	20.2	20.8	21.4
62-64	17.6	18.2	18.8	19.4	19.9	20.5	21.1	21.7	22.2
65-67	18.5	19.0	19.6	20.2	20.8	21.3	21.9	22.5	23.1
68-70	19.3	19.9	20.4	21.0	21.6	22.2	22.7	23.3	23.9
71-73	20.1	20.7	21.2	21.8	22.4	23.0	23.6	24.1	24.7
74-76	20.9	21.5	22.0	22.6	23.2	23.8	24.4	25.0	25.5
77-79	21.7	22.2	22.8	23.4	24.0	24.6	25.2	25.8	26.3
80-82	22.4	23.0	23.6	24.2	24.8	25.4	25.9	26.5	27.1
83-85	23.2	23.8	24.4	25.0	25.5	26.1	28.7	27.3	27.9
86-88	24.0	24.5	25.1	25.7	26.3	26.9	27.5	28.1	28.7
89-91	24.7	25.3	25.9	25.5	27.1	27.6	28.2	28.8	29.4
92-94	25.4	26.0	26.6	27.2	27.8	28.4	29.0	29.6	30.2
92-97	26.1	26.7	27.3	27.9	28.5	29.1	29.7	30.3	30.9
98-100	26.9	27.4	28.0	28.6	29.2	29.8	30.4	31.0	31.6
101-103	27.5	28.1	28.7	29.3	29.9	30.5	31.1	31.7	32.3
104-106	28.2	28.8	29.4	30.0	30.6	31.2	31.8	32.4	33.0
107-109	28.9	29.5	30.1	30.7	31.3	31.9	32.5	33.1	33.7
110-112	29.6	30.2	30.8	31.4	32.0	32.6	33.2	33.8	34.4
113-115	30.2	30.8	31.4	32.0	32.6	33.2	33.8	34.5	35.1
116-118	30.9	31.5	32.1	32.7	33.3	33.9	34.5	35.1	35.7
119-121	31.5	32.1	32.7	33.3	33.9	34.5	35.1	35.7	36.4
122-124	32.1	32.7	33.3	33.9	34.5	35.1	35.8	36.4	37.0
125-127	32.7	33.3	33.9	34.5	35.1	35.8	36.4	37.0	37.6

Source: A.S. Jackson and M.L. Pollock, "Practical Assessment of Body Composition," *The Physician and Sportsmedicine* 13, No. 5, (May, 1985):86. Used by permission.

3. Use Fig. 8-5. Men: With a straight edge, connect body weight vs. waist girth. Women: Connect height vs. hip girth. The point at which the straight edge crosses the body fat line will indicate the amount of body fat.

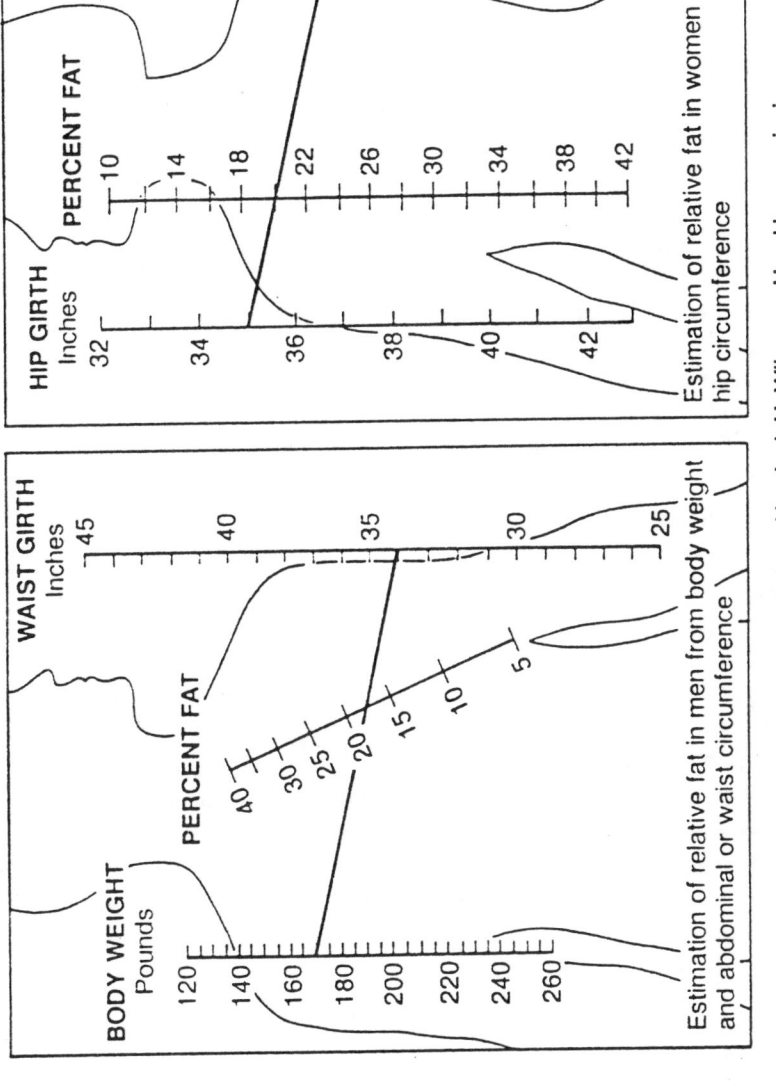

Nomograms developed by Jack H. Wilmore. Used by permission.

Figure 8-5. Nomogram for Estimating Percent Body Fat (Women: Height vs. Hip Girth; Men: Body Weight vs. Waist Girth)

Mirror

If still in doubt about being overweight, remove all clothing and take a long, hard look at the body in a full-length mirror. Appraise the body from various angles. Look for flab or excess fat. If still uncertain, jump up and down while looking at the body in the mirror; if it jiggles, begin that food plan and exercise program today!

WEIGHT LOSS

Scientists generally divide the body into four components — water, bone tissue, protein tissue and fat. For the purposes of weight loss, the body composition will be condensed into two components: body fat and lean body mass.

Body fat is the total amount of fat in the body which consists of both essential fat and storage fat. Essential fat is necessary in body structures such as the nerve tissue, bone marrow, heart, brain and cell membranes. Additional essential fat located in adult females is associated with the reproductive processes (breast tissue). Storage fat is a deposit of excess energy; the major storage site is the fat tissue cells just under the skin (subcutaneous fat). However, some fat is stored deep in the body. When the subcutaneous fat is separated by connective tissue into small compart-ments, it is known as cellulite which gives a dimpled look to the skin. **Cellulite is just plain fat.** Refer to Lab 8.5 to record results.

Lean body mass (fat-free mass) consists of those tissues other than body fat which includes primarily muscles, bones and other body organs such as the heart, brain, liver, and kidneys. Lean body mass is approxi-mately 70% water while adipose tissue (fat) is less than 10% water.

Body composition may be influenced by a number of factors such as age, sex, diet, exercise and genetics. As we get older the muscle mass may decrease, generally because of physical inactivity and the metabolism slows down. By the age of 70, the body needs about 15 percent fewer calories than it needed at the age of 20. There are small differences between boys and girls up to the age of puberty, but at this age the differences become much more. For procreation of the species, females generally deposit more fat tissue, while males develop more muscle tissue. Diet, such as water restrictions and starvation, can also affect the body composition over a short period but its main effects are seen over a longer period of time. Over-consumption will lead to increased body fat storage. **An aerobic exercise program such as walking, jogging, or running will help build muscle and reduce fat tissue.**

TABLE 8.6
RATINGS OF BODY FAT PERCENTAGE LEVELS

Rating	Males	Females
Essential fat	no less than 5%	no less than 10%
Lean	5-9%	10-14%
Good	10-14%	15-20%
Acceptable	15-19%	21-24%
Too fat	20-24%	25-29%
Obese	25 % or over	30 % or over

Note: Above ratings are approximate values. Individuals should strive for good or acceptable level.

Role of Metabolism

The increase in oxygen delivery to the exercising muscles which increases the body's burning mechanism is referred to as the **role of metabolism**. **Metabolism** is how the body utilizes its fuel to function, thus transforming foods into fuel. The body requires twice as much oxygen to burn one pound of fat as to burn one pound of carbohydrates. Therefore, the more capable the body is in utilizing oxygen, the more fat is burned. **Long, slow distance** (LSD), aerobic exercise of 45 minutes within target heart rate zone utilizes more oxygen, therefore utilizing fat. The best way to increase the metabolic furnace is by increasing the activity; therefore, increasing the metabolism increases the oxygen delivery to the exercising muscles.

Role of Exercise

Government organizations are encouraging physical activity in every person's daily life (refer to U. S. Dietary Guidelines, 1995). Research has documented that vigorous, sustained exercise in the presence of oxygen is necessary to utilize body fat. During aerobic exercise, the body utilizes a combination of carbohydrates and fats for fuel. In the first twenty minutes of exercise, the body utilizes more carbohydrates than fats. After twenty minutes, unless an individual has carbohydrate loaded, the ratio begins to change and more fat is utilized. As a person becomes fit, he/she is capable of utilizing more fat because trained muscles, in the presence of oxygen, utilize fat more efficiently. However, keep in mind that in order for a muscle to use fat as a source of energy, there must be carbohydrates present.

Many adults do not use walking, jogging, or running as an exercise for weight loss because their fitness level is low and they cannot sustain a moderate level of exercise intensity for a long period of time. However, the more exercise is done, the more the body will begin to adapt; therefore, the period of exercise can be longer. Physical exercise forces the body to expend energy (utilize calories) and the more intense the exercise, the more energy it requires. It also revs up the BMR [basal (**or resting**) metabolic rate] for hours afterward, which helps the fat-utilizing process.

Aerobic activities which use large muscle groups and which are performed in a continuous manner expend the greatest amount of calories.

TABLE 8.7

Activity	Calories Expended
Walking (.5 miles)	83
Fitness Walking (1.1 miles)	100
Jogging (1.5 miles)	160
Running (1.8 miles)	180
Cycling (2.4 miles)	102
Swimming (600 yards)	110
Aerobic Dancing	105

Walking is more economical than running; therefore, fewer calories are expended for a given distance of walking than running. If walking vigorously at a high speed (**fitness walking**), more energy is expended than jogging at the same speed. Walking is a very effective means to expend calories. Intensity and duration are very important in total energy expenditure; more exercise results in a greater total weekly caloric expenditure. **Approximately three to six times per week is sufficient to lose weight safely.** Refer to Appendix G for the Surgeon General's report on physical activity and health, including examples of moderate amounts of activity.

Exercise may help to keep resting metabolic rate up while dieting. It increases the number of calories used during exercise and keeps the metabolic rate elevated after the workout is completed. Even after the exercise session, the body continues to utilize energy (calories) at a faster pace for several hours. Aerobic exercises, which use the large muscle groups of the body, are continuous in motion, enjoyable, and include the **FITT formula** (previously discussed), expend the greatest amount of energy (calories).

Due to aging and weight loss, bones become brittle due to the loss of calcium. It is important to consume an adequate amount of calcium: a minimum of 1,200 mg per day for men and women 19 through 24 years old, and 800 mg/day for adults over 24. Post-menopausal women need additional calcium of 1,500 mg per day. **Peak bone mass does not occur**

until a person reaches 27 years of age. At some time after the peak is reached, calcium begins to be lost from the bones as a natural part of aging. This process can eventually lead to **osteoporosis** if too little calcium is "on reserve." Women can increase calcium intake by drinking more skim and/or low fat milk, eating more low-fat yogurt and other dairy products; green vegetables (broccoli and kale), salmon and sardines with the bones provide some calcium. Weight bearing exercise slows down bone loss. Refer to Chapter Seven, Nutrition, Mineral Section for additional information on osteoporosis.

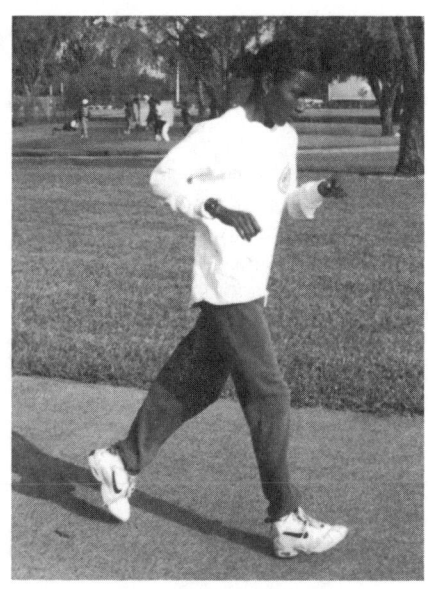

Exercise helps reduce stress and tension. Refer to Chapter Nine, Stress Management, for additional information. Exercise alters body composition in favor of lean tissue and it raises the metabolic rate as long as the body is conditioned. Lean muscle expends more calories than fat tissue. Exercise increases self-esteem and the psychological benefits of feeling and looking healthy are achieved. A person who diets without exercising loses both lean and fat tissue. If the person gains weight without exercising, the gain is mostly in the form of fat. Fat tissue expends fewer calories to maintain itself, so if the person eats the same amount of food as before, the person's weight will be higher than previously. This is known as the **"yo-yo syndrome"** of dieting. For permanent weight loss and fat reduction, it is important to remove weight safely and slowly. Losing weight too quickly may result in injury and/or illness; thus causing the person to have to discontinue the program.

Weight loss that occurs slowly and consistently is most likely to be effective. A weight loss rule of thumb is to lose no more than one to two pounds weekly. The American Heart Association recommends that no more than 30% of daily calories should come from fat (margarine, low-fat cheese, and lean meat). Of the remaining 70%, at least **58-60% should come from carbohydrates** (cereal, rice, potatoes, pasta, and vegetables), and **10-12% from protein** (lean meats, poultry, fish, beans). **To**

TABLE 8.8
INCREASING CALORIC EXPENDITURE BY PHYSICAL ACTIVITY

Remember to accumulate 30 minutes or more of moderate physical activity on most, preferably all, days of the week.
Examples of moderate physical activities for healthy U.S. adults walking briskly (3-4 miles per hour) conditioning or general calisthenics home care, general cleaning racquet sports such as table tennis mowing lawn, power mower golf—pulling cart or carrying clubs home repair, painting fishing, hand/casting jogging swimming (moderate effort) cycling, moderate speed (about 20 miles per hour) gardening canoeing leisurely (2.0-3.9 miles per hour) dancing
Source: Adapted from Pate, et al. *Journal of the American Medical Association, 1995, Vol. 273, p. 404.*

lose one pound of fat per week, the person should have a caloric deficit of no more than 500 calories a day (3500 calories a week) from one's normal diet and consume a minimum of 2200 calories a day for women and 2800 for men to maintain adequate nutrient status. For daily living, the National Research Council (1989) states that a person with no exercise should consume 2200 kcal per day for women and 2800 kcal per day for men to get the correct nutrients the body needs. The American Dietetic Association recommends a variety of foods containing 2000 to 3000 per day to provide adequate nutrients. Exercisers will require more calories per day than non-exercisers.

Spot Reduction

Research indicates that a person cannot lose fat in particular locations by using local isolated exercises in order to deplete local fat deposits. Fat cells release fat into the blood (not the muscle) and the fat is shared by all the muscles.

Spot-reducing exercises, such as sit-ups for the abdominal area or side bends to lose fat from the side of the waist, do not work. Fat cells shrink throughout the body as a result of reduced caloric intake. A balanced exercise program will tone muscles in those spots by developing and strengthening muscle tissue under the stored body fat.

Fad Diets

Food is a companion for some people that will not "talk back." It is an addiction. There are diet books on the best-seller list which could be very dangerous because these diets are nutritionally unbalanced. They may emphasize one food or food group and the elimination of others. Staying on these for a long time could jeopardize the individual's health. Kidney stones, fatigue, nausea, irregular heart beats, dizziness, and muscle loss may be some of the side effects.

Diets that claim quick weight loss, **"burn fat"** or **"burn away"** excess pounds often send dieters into a cycle of quick weight loss, then rebound weight gain when normal eating is resumed. It is not advisable to go on a crash or fad diet for a week or more. There is evidence that cycles of weight loss and gain (**yo-yo dieting**) can make the person even fatter by slowing metabolism and making it easier to gain. Ninety to ninety-five percent of dieters put the weight back on plus additional weight in a short time. A lasting weight loss cannot happen overnight; it is a lifetime endeavor. Jane Brody, author of *Jane Brody's Nutrition Book* (1987), states, "Every fad diet is nutritionally unbalanced in one way or another, and some are downright dangerous, even if followed by healthy people for a relatively short time."

Fad diets are "scams." They differ from the basic rule: eat each day less calories, exercise more, and do it forever. Go on a healthy food plan; stay with a regular exercise program; and lose pounds safely and permanently.

Fasting, Liquid, and Low Calorie Diets

According to *Running Research News* (July/August, 1986), a twenty-four hour fast decreases endurance capacity at competitive exercise intensities. Fasting confuses the body and it burns up the wrong tissue. **Fasting** causes approximately 2/3 loss from lean body tissue or muscle and 1/3 loss from fatty tissue. When nutrients are very low, the body maintains blood glucose level by converting the available amino acids in the tissue of muscle to glucose. Fasting can precipitate gout and severe depression as well as cause sudden death due to heart rhythm abnormalities.

Low calorie and/or liquid diets may cause rapid weight loss but may be dangerously short of certain nutrients. **Women must eat a minimum of 2200 calories per day and men 2800 calories to get sufficient nutrients.** Anything below this amount is semi-starvation. Very low calorie diets may be justified if the individual is fifty pounds overweight and have health problems associated with obesity, such as heart disease. On a low calorie diet, the body develops a lower metabolic rate, therefore requiring less nutrients. Ninety-five percent of the people gain the weight back on a low calorie liquid diet. These diets may cause a low-grade damage to the organs of the heart, liver and kidneys. **Close medical supervision is advisable when using these diets.**

High protein/low carbohydrate diets are known for delivering dramatic weight loss in the first few weeks. Low carbohydrate diets may cause kidney disorder, loss of muscle tissue, fatigue, and dizziness. These diets work by starving the body of its normal fuel. Most of the weight loss is water. The body must break down stored sugar and protein (process that releases water). Once off the diet, the body replaces water and the weight is quickly regained. High protein diets may cause excessive fluid loss or deterioration of muscle tissue and cause the body to lose calcium and bone.

Weight Reducing Drugs and Diet Aids

Drugs should never be taken unless prescribed by a physician for the treatment of specific health problems such as congestive heart failure or high blood pressure. Drugs and drug combinations can be dangerous and sometimes fatal.

Diet aids (weight pills, candy, gum, etc.) are a dieter's dream. These pills dehydrate the body. Some pills may help control the appetite (give a feeling of fullness) as long as they being taken but may have serious side effects. Amphetamines and diuretics are two common diet pills. They are highly addictive and have adverse reactions on the heart and central nervous system. Amphetamines involve the thyroid gland, cause nervousness and speed up the metabolism, thus making the individual "hyper." Stronger doses are required as the body becomes tolerant. **Diuretics or "water pills" cause rapid water loss (dehydration), not fat loss; once the pills are stopped, the water and pounds return.** Dehydration could interfere with proper function of the muscles and may disrupt the body's salt balance, causing heart rhythm abnormalities.

Gums, candies depend on benzocaine (mild topical anesthetic) which curbs the appetite and numbs the tongue (taste buds), therefore reducing the sense of taste.

Laxatives should not be used to lose weight. They also eliminate water from the body, not fat, by increasing the water content of the stool. Laxatives interfere with the absorption of essential vitamins, minerals and potassium (needed for muscle contraction). Laxatives may also cause permanent crippling of bowel muscle function which may lead to constipation.

Fiber pills are intended to be taken with water and fill the stomach before meals, thus giving a fullness feeling. The pills will not work unless fewer calories are eaten than normal and are not recommended for long term weight loss. Drinking water before meals may be more helpful than taking fiber pills and is less expensive. Diet pills may be dangerous, causing high blood pressure, headaches, nausea, excess sweating, or even blood clotting in the brain to sensitive people. Diet aids do not contribute to permanent weight loss and are not recommended.

Prescription Appetite Suppressants

In 1997 the FDA banned Redux and Pondimin (combined with phentermine and called fen-phen), two of the most popular diet drugs in the United States. Strong evidence was present that these drugs could seriously damage heart valves and even cause death. Phentermine remains as a prescription drug but is being scrutinized for possible side effects.

These drugs worked by increasing the level of the brain chemical serotonin, which curbs hunger and makes those who take the drugs feel full. They were to be prescribed along with an exercise program and proper diet.

Passive Exercise and Weight Reducing Gimmicks

Gimmick approaches promising rapid weight loss remain popular. Beware of reducing salons and health clubs that promote diet plans or food supplements and gimmicks. It is advisable to have a complete physical examination by a physician before joining a reducing salon. Studies indicate that repeated losing and regaining of extra pounds is more damaging to physical health than remaining overweight. Therefore, it is important to find a food plan and an exercise program for a lifetime and forget the gimmicks, diets, and crash programs. Most of these devices are of little value. Gimmicks such as rubber suits, steam baths, vibrators (tables, pillows, belts), massage, body wraps, and motor driven cycles/rowing machines are not necessary for a successful weight management program.

Rubber suits cause sweating, not weight loss. The suit raises body heat and core temperature can rise during exercise to a dangerous level. Air (the most effective means of cooling the body) does not contact the skin and sweat is not eliminated. The weight loss is due to loss of body fluid which causes changes in water metabolism and in kidney and circulatory functions.

Steam baths and saunas remove body fluids. Rapid and excessive fluid loss is potentially dangerous because it can cause severe dehydration and chemical imbalance. Drinking water immediately after a sweat session results in an immediate return to normal weight.

Vibrators (tables, pillows, belts) result in minimum caloric expenditure and do not cause weight loss. They are potentially dangerous to pregnant women, and may aggravate back problems.

Massage burns very few calories. It is relaxing and may improve circulation but will not reduce weight.

Body wraps (wrapping the body in bandages soaked in a "special formula") may alter the body circumference but the body will regain its original size within a short time. This practice could be dangerous.

Motor-driven cycles and rowing machines are devices which do the work for a person and may help maintain flexibility and increase circulation. They are not as effective as the body doing the work. The harder a person works during exercise, the greater the benefits derived.

There is no easy, fast method or a device to lose body fat. A combination of eating fewer calories, exercising more, and doing it forever is the safest way to have a healthy body. Oprah Winfrey is an example of a person who went on a quick fix and found it did not work. Soon she realized that a sensible diet and a good exercise program was the best plan.

Behavior Modification

A person must set realistic goals (women, 1/2-1 lb.; men, 1-2 lbs. weight loss per week) and must be motivated to lose weight for the program to be successful. An individual must take the responsibility for his/her life. Recent studies show that adults who watch three or more hours of television per day are twice as likely to be obese as those who watch television for one hour. Behavior modification changes the behaviors of the individual of underexercising and overeating. When a behavior of eating less calories and expending more calories through exercise is met, the outcome is successful.

Guidelines for Weight Loss Behavior Modification

1. **Keep a record or diary of present eating behaviors in order to measure future progress.** Be aware of these behaviors daily.
2. **Eliminate the behaviors that prompt eating inappropriately such as watching television, talking on the telephone, eating in different locations.** Eat at regular meal times and in designated areas (kitchen or dining room).
3. **Keep a variety of nutritious foods available and encourage family members to eat these foods as well.** Eat small portions, exercise more and keep active.
4. **Eat slowly.** Alter eating response. Slow down (pause for two to three minutes), put down utensils, swallow before reloading the fork.
5. **Have others near when eating and ask them to be supportive and provide encouragement.**
6. **Measure and weigh foods.** Regularly updating records of food intake, exercise, and weight change. Plan rewards (new outfit, movie).

7. **Track your progress with a tape measure, not the scale.** As you exercise and burn off fat, you're gaining lean muscle and getting slimmer and stronger. Scales cannot differentiate between lean muscle mass and fat, and may not show any loss in pounds, since muscle is denser than fat and weighs more. So measure inches, not pounds, when you chart your progress.

Guidelines for a Safe Weight Loss Program

1. The program should be a nutritionally adequate food plan and medically safe. Commit to healthy eating—starting today!
2. Consume a minimum of **eight glasses of water daily** and keep the stomach full. Limit beverages (caffeine, colas, alcohol).
3. **Do not skip meals,** eat only at scheduled times and places, and eat bulky foods (lettuce, celery, carrots, fruits) as snacks between meals. Eat three meals each day from the Food Guide Pyramid. Eating smaller portions of five to six meals a day has been shown to result in more weight loss than the standard three meals a day for some individuals. Avoid snacks after the evening meal.
4. **Breakfast is essential** because it launches the metabolism into "go." **To lose weight, consume about 25 percent of the daily calories at breakfast, 50 percent at lunch (before 1:00 P.M.., with only 25 percent at the evening meal.** Eat the most food when you are the most active. Eat meals slowly (20-30 minutes), chew each mouthful of food ten plus times, put the utensil down between each mouthful. It takes the appetite control center about 20 minutes to receive the message that you have eaten enough. Say "No thanks" when someone offers you food.
5. **Avoid stimulants, diuretics, dehydration techniques (saunas, steam baths), laxatives and pills.**
6. **Eat lots of complex carbohydrates such as fruits, vegetables, bread and pasta.** Count calories daily and do not exceed the daily target. The body needs approximately 2200-2800 calories daily. A simple method which may be used to determine the minimum amount of calories to be consumed in a weight loss program is to multiply the body weight by 10 (or add a zero to body weight). For example, a 140 lb. person should try a 1400 Kcal diet (140 x 10 = 1400) as the daily intake guide. Smaller individuals may need less calories (1000-1200); however, lean body mass and metabolic rate are determinants. Losing 1/2 -1 pound per week is advisable to keep the weight off— more than 2 pounds, you lose water and muscle. **Carbohydrate foods should consist of 58-60%; proteins, 10-12%; and fats, 30% (preferably 20-25%) and less of the daily calories of the diet.**

7. **Do not eat while watching television.** Eat at regular mealtimes and in designated areas such as the dining room or kitchen.
8. **Learn from failure.** You are only human. Decide how you can be successful in the future.
9. **Avoid fats**, especially ice cream, cookies, candy and soft drinks. After 8-12 weeks you should lose your taste for fatty foods. Avoid fat substitutes and use less refined foods.
10. **Leave the table** as soon as you finish eating.
11. **Make a list and only buy what's on it**. Shop for groceries when you are not hungry and get rid of high calorie "treats."
12. **Plan activities when you are most likely to snack.**
13. **Maintain a regular exercise program** (expends calories and tones body). Weight loss should be gradual. Walking after a meal will expend fat while it is still in the bloodstream and before it reaches the fat storage.

Guideline for Determining Body Fat Loss

To lose 1 pound of fat

$$\frac{3500 \text{ calories}}{7 \text{ days per week}} = 500 \text{ calories a day less than maintenance number.}$$

To lose 2 pounds of fat

$$3500 \text{ calories} \times 2 = \frac{7000 \text{ calories}}{7 \text{ days per week}} = 1,000 \text{ calories a day less than maintenance number.}$$

Note: **Always eat 2200-2800 calories per day.** A daily food plan of less than 1,200 calories per day may be deficient in nutrients the body needs for growth, repair and energy necessary to perform daily activities. Consult a physician if eating less calories. A safe weight loss (1/2 to 1 pound per week for women and 1-2 pounds per week for men) can be accomplished by eating less and exercising more. Refer to Lab 8.1.

WEIGHT MAINTENANCE

Weight maintenance (**staying the same weight**) is remaining at the same composition of fat to the amount of lean that is carried in the body. To remain at this constant weight, energy must be in balance; for example: "energy in" (eating) is equal to the "energy out" (expenditure, exercise). To remain at the same weight, one must intake (eat) the amount of calories expended (burned up) each day. During the process of aging the metabo-

Shoes

Why run? → prevent injury
→ comfort (better exer)

- nylon/mesh uppers (cooler)
- good brand
- where to buy - try out
- kinds: motion control
  - stability
  - cushioned
  - (lightweight training)
  → pronation/supination

- Clothing
- cold-weather; don't overdress
- warm weather - minimal
- Chafing/rubbing
- no weights

- heat cramp
- heat exhaus → stop
  - shade
  - heat stroke water
- H₂O 8oz/15min

Safety

- pairs
- headphones (volume → look!)
- toward traffic
- 911/call boxes/Sports Med

Mechanics

- posture - tall, but relaxed
- arms @ 90° angle (jogging: hands can be a little lower
- hands (fingers together, thumb on finger)
- arms don't cross midline
- stride: knee in front of ankle (90°)
- heel - toe
- breath: naturally w/ rhythm

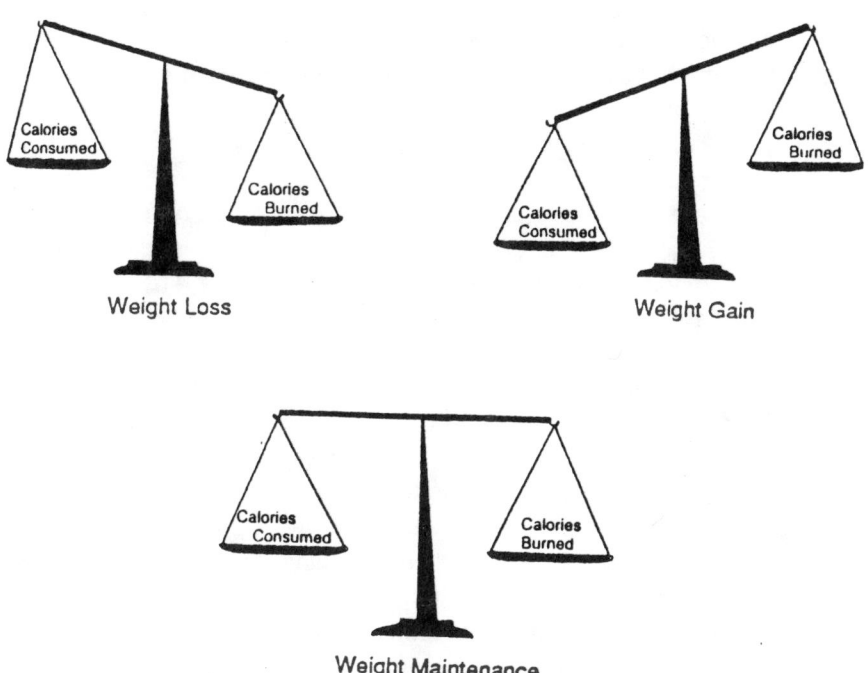

Weight Loss

Weight Gain

Weight Maintenance

lism slows down and the individual may be less active. One must select a variety of nutritious foods (food plan) and eat less calories as one ages.

Guideline for Determining Weight Maintenance

1. Record present weight, in pounds: _____
2. Record number, value of the
   type of lifestyle: _____
   14 calories per lb — sedentary
   15 calories per lb — relatively active
   16 calories per lb — very active
   20 calories per lb — vigorous activity (athlete)
3. Multiply 1 times 2: _____

Result: Individual's weight maintenance number, or the calories needed to eat each day to maintain current weight. Refer to Lab 8.1 to record results.

WEIGHT GAIN

Less than ten percent of the population may have difficulty gaining body weight. These individuals may have the desire to increase their lean body weight (not fat) in order to improve performance, appearance, body image, and self concept.

In order to increase lean body weight, adequate rest and sleep, increased caloric intake, and a safe weight training program should be effective. The increased body weight should be lean body mass and not body fat. If an individual consumes more calories than are used, whether the calories are from carbohydrates, proteins, or fat, weight will be gained. The food plan must be higher in calories, obtaining adequate amounts of dietary protein, and still be nutritious, while the exercise program should be designed to increase muscle mass.

Approximately 14 grams of protein per day above normal protein requirements is suggested in increasing muscle tissue. This protein can be obtained in small amounts of food such as two ounces of meat, fish, cheese, or poultry or two glasses of milk. Gaining about one pound per week is a safe approach after acquiring basic strength through a month of weight training. Weight training is recommended as a means to gain lean body weight, muscle mass and strength. However, some aerobic exercise is necessary for good health. Increased food intake (calories) should compensate for depleting calories aerobically.

To add one pound of body muscle, the caloric requirement is 2,500 calories (this includes approximately 600 calories for the muscle and the extra energy needed for exercise to develop the muscle). The daily caloric excess, over the maintenance number above is 360 calories. Refer to Lab 8.1 to record results.

Guideline for Determining Lean Weight Gain

1 pound of muscle gain:

$$\frac{2500 \text{ calories equivalent of 1 pound of muscle}}{7 \text{ days in a week}} = 360 \text{ daily excess calories to eat, over maintenance number.}$$

CHAPTER SUMMARY

Obesity in our society is a serious medical problem which contributes to a variety of diseases and disorders and leads to premature death. However, obesity is reversible. A nutritious food plan and aerobic exercises for lifetime are appropriate in changing an individual's weight. Treatment programs may be successful on a short-term basis, most of the weight loss is regained by the majority of the people. A diet is no longer viewed as a temporary aid in weight loss but as a permanent lifetime commitment in eating behaviors to ensure adequate weight management. For permanent weight management, continue the same program each day throughout life, rather than following off and on patterns.

Exercise gimmicks are expensive, time consuming and do not work. **There is no such thing as "effortless exercise."** Weight reducing drugs and diet pills are dangerous. Weight loss must be permanent to be successful; therefore, it is a lifetime decision.

To lose or gain weight, there must be an imbalance of energy. To lose fat, expenditure has to be greater (a loss of 500 cals./day/1 lb. of fat loss); and to gain lean, the intake has to be a greater number (adding 360 cals./day/lb of muscle gain). For weight maintenance, (balance must be met) caloric input (eating) must be equal to caloric output (daily activity).

During the behavior modification process, it is imperative to be aware of past negative behaviors and try to avoid these situations. As soon as Americans realize that they can't starve it off, sleep it off, or melt it off and replace those patterns with living one day at a time, setting and achieving one goal at a time, they will keep off extra weight and fat. Weight control is a learned behavior. Eat less, exercise more, and do it for a lifetime. "If you think you can or you think you cannot, you are *always* right." *— Henry Ford, American Industrialist (1863 - 1947).*

CHAPTER NINE

Stress Management

WHAT IS STRESS?

Dr. Hans Selye, "the father of stress research," defines stress as "the nonspecific response of the human organism to any demand that is placed upon it." The term **"nonspecific"** indicates that the body will react in a similar fashion, regardless of the nature of the event that led to the stress response. In essence, stress is any condition that forces a person to change or adjust to any situation that is new, frightening, threatening, or exciting. Individuals are constantly subjected to strain or pressure (stress) throughout their lives. Any kind of change can be stressful. Stress is caused by both major and minor life events. Stress is caused by major life changes such as marriage, death of a loved one or a new job, but minor daily hassles cause stress too. The pressures of daily life, like waiting in line when in a hurry, add up and eventually cause as much stress as major life changes. The body must learn to adjust to the stress or tension of major and minor life events.

The way in which an individual reacts to stress has been defined by Dr. Selye as either **"eustress or distress."** **Eustress**, or **positive stress**, is mentally or physically stimulating, such as a job promotion, getting a degree, and pay increase. **Distress**, or **negative stress**, is feeling over-whelmed, unable to relax, exhausted, isolated, depressed or anxious. Distress can be harmful or unpleasant, therefore deteriorating health and performance, such as the loss of a spouse, job or promotion. The individual's reaction, not the situation, determines whether the stress is eustress (positive) or distress (negative).

Awareness of the stress or tension will help in coping with it. Stress is a normal part of living. Everyone has to deal with responsibilities, goals, pressures, and/or negative situations. Daily hassles, events (a death in the family), or individuals (authoritarian boss), are unavoidable. One must give oneself positive messages or "self talk," and maintain a positive attitude in dealing with these situations. Remember that patience is man's greatest virtue. It is often said that if "we can manage our stress, we can manage our lives." A positive attitude can help one get through daily chaos and is one of the characteristics of good mental health. Positive people tend to fare better than negative people. Looking on the bright side of life may help one enjoy life more fully and manage the stress in one's life. Being positive will make one feel better, look better, stay independent and active and more relaxed around people. Attitude is contagious. Think about it: Is your's worth catching?

The effects of stress are cumulative unless positive coping techniques are employed. Approximately 50 to 70 percent of all illnesses are either caused or made more serious by stress. For this reason, learning about stress and stress management is an important part of being healthy.

Several ailments have such a strong relationship to stress that they have been called "stress diseases." These include: bowel problems, stomach ulcers, lower back pain, high blood pressure, cholesterol concentration, colitis, migraine headaches, diabetes, and heart disease. Managing stress helps reduce the risk of these **"stress diseases."** In addition, one is less likely to become dependent on prescription drugs and alcohol. Pills that advertise themselves as **"stress vitamins,"** are not the best choice. Lack of sufficient vitamins and minerals in the daily diet may indicate a need to take a vitamin-mineral supplement that supplies a balanced assortment of nutrients, not in "megadoses" but in amounts properly needed daily.

Because stress disrupts the immune system, managing stress may even help prevent certain kinds of cancer. Stress does deplete the body's nutrient reserves; it drains protein from muscle and lean tissue, vitamins and minerals from every cell of the body, and calcium from the skeleton. Most people cannot eat during a stressful situation, nor can they digest food because the stress response suppresses the digestive activity in favor of muscular activity. Going without food depletes the reserves of the body's nutrients. Nutrition and exercise go hand-in-hand to build up stress defenses.

MANAGING STRESS

Stress management is defined as a way of dealing with stress. Managing stress well involves two strategies:
1. One for sailing along, when moment-to-moment adjustments can keep the person on course.
2. Stormy situations. A person who maintains a strong program of personal health during ordinary times is best able to withstand crises when they occur.

The following three factors will be discussed in helping to manage stress in life:

1. Recognize the signs and symptoms of stress.
2. Identify and remove the stressor. Admit there is a problem.
3. Cope with stress using stress management techniques.

RECOGNIZING SIGNS AND SYMPTOMS OF STRESS

A tense person is often fatigued or has a persistent tired feeling. Dr. Kenneth Cooper suggests checking the heart rate early in the morning and then rechecking it later in the day. A normal increase would be about 10 beats; however, if the heart rate is increasing 20-30 beats per minute, this suggests a manifestation of stress.

Another method is checking hand temperature. In normal conditions, the hand temperature should be about the same temperature as the neck. If the hands are cooler, this could be an indication of stress.

Hiding stress does not resolve it. Ignoring and denying stress increases its negative effects. A vital step in effective stress management is to recognize symptoms of stress.

Early Symptoms of Stress	Advanced Symptoms of Stress
Constipation	Tightness/Pain in chest
Biting nails	Rapid heart rate
Nausea	Loss of sex drive
Poor concentration	Temper explosions
Fatigue	Low grade infection
Muscular aches	Eating too much
Grinding teeth	Insomnia
Stuttering	Depression
Finger/Toe tapping	Drinking excessively
Increased sweating	Nightmares
Frustration	High blood pressure
Anger	Impotence
Dizziness	Stomach pain
Dry mouth	Hives/skin rash or acne

Fortunately, all of these signs do not occur at one time. Stress varies from person to person and from day to day within the same individual. Also different signs of stress may be noticed by various people on the same individual. Refer to Lab 9.1, Symptoms of Stress, to record results.

IDENTIFYING OR REMOVING THE STRESSOR

The first technique in any stress management program is to attempt to identify and remove the stressor (cause of stress). Most people either do not want to accept that they are under too much stress or

WHAT IS YOUR CURRENT LEVEL OF STRESS?

STRESSO

Answer the following questions by checking the appropriate ( ) with an **X**.

YES	NO	AT TIMES		
( )	( )	( )	1.	Do you frequently drum your fingers on a table or desk top?
( )	( )	( )	2.	When thinking do you frequently pull a lock of hair, your ear, or scratch your scalp?
( )	( )	( )	3.	Do you curl up your toes when sitting?
( )	( )	( )	4.	Do you grip a pencil so tight your fingers become numb?
( )	( )	( )	5.	Do you frequently clasp or unclasp your hands, or twist objects in your hands?
( )	( )	( )	6.	Do you frequently grind your teeth while awake or asleep?
( )	( )	( )	7.	Does your posture and movement appear stiff?
( )	( )	( )	8.	Do you frequently twist your ring, cross or uncross your legs, or wrap your feet around each other?
( )	( )	( )	9.	Do you worry a lot or have tension headaches?
( )	( )	( )	10.	Are you frequently tired, angry, or frustrated?
( )	( )	( )	11.	Are you frequently constipated?
( )	( )	( )	12.	Do you have trouble sleeping?

SCORING: After checking each question give yourself a +1 for every NO answer; a -1 for every YES answer; and a -1/2 for every AT TIMES answer.

+

8-12	"Far Out Man or Lady"
5-7	Loose
3-4	Above Average Looseness
1-2	Average Looseness

–

8-12	"Like a Clock Spring"
5-7	Highly Stressed
3-4	Above Average Stress
1-2	Average Stress

"Stresso" was developed by Dr. Clancy Moore and is reprinted from Stokes, Moore, Moore, and Schultz, *Fitness: The New Wave, Third Edition.* Winston-Salem, NC: Hunter Textbooks, Inc. 1992.

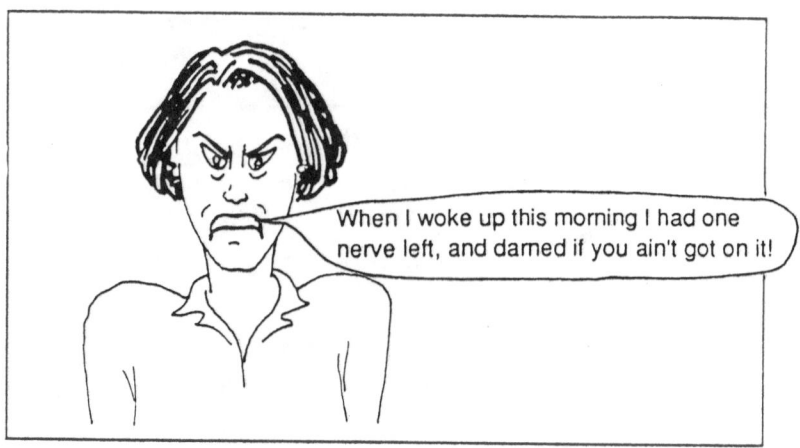

they fail to recognize the signs and symptoms of their stress. In some situations, removing the stressor may be impossible. For example, the first year on the job, death of a close friend or family member, intolerable supervisor, etc., are situations in which little can be done to eliminate the stressor. However, stress can still be handled by learning how to cope with the situation. A cardiologist has stated, **"Rule 1 is don't sweat the small stuff; and Rule 2 is it's all small stuff and if you can't fight it and you can't flee — go with the flow."** (American Heart Association, 1984) However, stress can still be managed through the use of adequate relaxation techniques.

STRESS MANAGEMENT TECHNIQUES

There are numerous stress management techniques which may help reduce stress. These techniques may be used to prevent stress from accumulating if practiced regularly. They can also be used for temporary relief of stress when signs of stress are evident. Some individuals may find techniques which may work for them, such as reading a favorite book, cross stitching, playing a game, and/or walking or jogging. However, for those who don't already have a healthy way of reducing stress, the following techniques will be discussed: **breathing exercises, visualization, meditation, progressive relaxation, massage and acupuncture, balanced diet, rest and sleep, aerobic exercise, expressing feelings, outside interests, time alone, affirmations and imaging, reframing thoughts, humor, and support systems and professional assistance.**

When performing nonexercise relaxation techniques, assume a comfortable position, either sitting or lying on the back (pillow under knees), feet separated, toes pointing outward, palms open, and eyes closed. In a quiet, pleasant and well-ventilated room each exercise should be repeated eight to ten times whenever feeling tense. Continue the exercise for 15-20 minutes. When finished, sit quietly for several minutes, and open eyes when ready.

Breathing Exercises

Probably the simplest way to induce a state of relaxation is through **breathing exercises**. Such methods have been used for centuries in India and the Orient as a means of developing better mental, physical and emotional stamina. Breathing exercises can be learned in a few minutes and should be used regularly to quiet the body's natural reactions to stress. These exercises are performed one at a time and not all of them together at a time.

Breathing exercises should concentrate on a slow, deep inhalation followed by a slow, deep exhalation. The person concentrates on "breathing away" the tension and inhaling fresh oxygen to the entire body. Some examples of breathing exercises are:

1. **Inhale slowly and deeply through the nose.** Once reaching a full inhalation, hold that position for about 3 seconds and concentrate, "My body is very calm and relaxed." Exhale slowly. The words "peace," "calm," "one," etc., may also be used while concentrating.

2. **Inhale slowly and mentally count from one to five.** Exhale gradually and mentally count down from five to one.

3. **Breathe faster on the count of ten, then slower the lower the number.**

4. **In abdominal breathing place one hand on the abdomen and the other hand on the chest.** Slowly breathe in and out so that the hand on the abdomen rises when inhaling and falls when exhaling. The hand on the chest should not move much.

5. **Sit in an upright position or stand straight up.** Breathe through the nose and gradually fill up the lungs from the bottom up. Hold the breath for several seconds. Now exhale slowly by allowing complete relaxation of the chest and abdomen.

6. **Combine breathing and stretching.** Stretch arms overhead toward the ceiling when inhaling deeply. Exhale slowly as the arms are lowered to the side.

Visualization

Do a little mental housecleaning to clear away the mental clutter during stressful situations. Imagine a peaceful scene you'd like to be in and "go" there; or imagine that you're floating or drifting in the clouds. Visualize how one may cope with the stressor or how one may relax when the stressor is present. Repeat the exercise for 5 to 15 minutes. Refer to Lab 9.2, Relaxation Techniques.

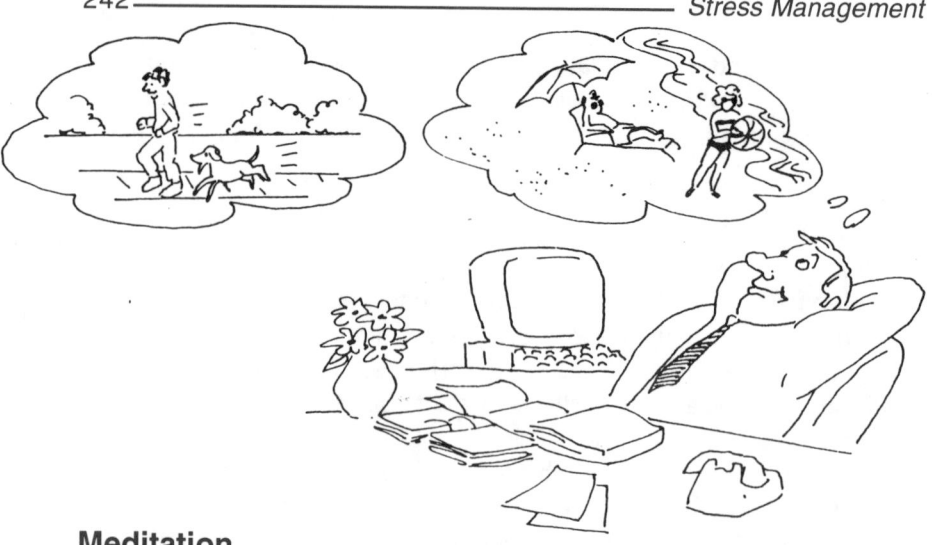

Meditation

Meditation is mental exercise which affects body processes. Gaining control of attention is the purpose of meditation. Meditation involves choosing to focus on something repetitive (word or phrase) or something unchanging (an object or spot on the wall).

To feel calm, close eyes and focus or think of a peaceful word or phrase. Use words or phrases which produce comfort. Repeatedly say it from 5 to 15 minutes. Meditation is one of the most popular relaxing techniques because it can be learned easily and quickly.

Progressive Relaxation

Progressive relaxation is a technique developed by Edmund Jacobson (1938) which helps individuals recognize and release tension by progressively contracting and relaxing the muscles. Relaxation techniques may be learned from an individual, therapist, books and tapes. Proper conditions are important for learning and practicing relaxation. A quiet room and comfortable furniture that completely supports the body such as a sofa, recliner, bed, or carpeted floor in a dimly lit room is recommended. Clothing should be loose and comfortable.

Sit or lie in a way that allows a feeling of relaxation without tensing any muscles to hold the position. A pillow placed under the knees may be helpful if stretched out on the floor. Eyes should be closed. Contract or tense the muscles to become familiar with the feeling of contraction and tension. Individuals with a heart condition, high blood pressure or stroke may only want a mild contraction of the muscles. The contraction period should last 5 to 10 seconds, slowly release the tension, going completely limp for about 30 seconds. While relaxing, concentrate on the feeling of

The suggested technique is as follows:

1. Toes	7. Stomach	13. Shoulders
2. Feet	8. Back	14. Neck
3. Ankles	9. Chest	15. Mouth
4. Calf	10. Hands	16. Forehead, nose and eyes
5. Thighs	11. Forearms	17. Top of head
6. Buttocks	12. Upper arms	

When performing non-exercise relaxation techniques, assume a comfortable position, either sitting or standing. With eyes closed, perform the relaxation techniques.

1. Contract the fist—ball up the hand, until you feel tension (muscular) and discomfort.

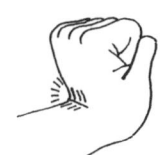

2. Relax the fist, allowing the sensation of muscular reaction to occur.

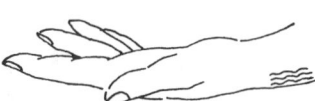

3. Lift shoulders up until you feel tension and discomfort in the back.

4. Relax shoulders and feel muscles relax in neck and upper back.

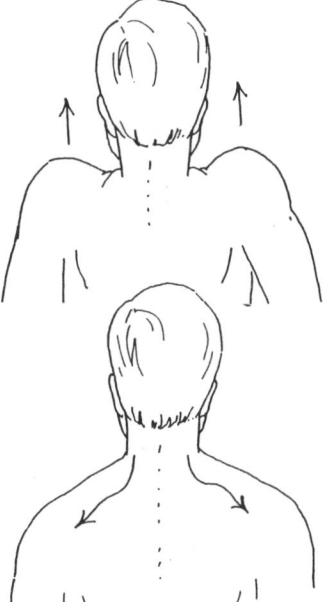

decreasing tension. All major muscles should be relaxed until the entire body becomes relaxed. As one becomes familiar with the tension and relaxation sensations in the muscles, the relaxation session can be shortened.

Practice the technique each day in 15 to 20 minute sessions. Select a time of day when not rushed; do not hurry relaxation. Performing a few exercises is better than none at all but the completion of the entire sequence yields the best results. Refer to Laboratory 9.2, Relaxation Techniques.

Massage and Acupressure

Several forms of massage for relaxing exist, but acupressure (pressing down on points of the body where muscle tension often occurs) is a popular form. Various objects can be used but the hands are recommended to employ pressure. Several techniques such as gliding, kneading, and caressing are used. A simple massage of the various muscles of the body can be done by most individuals. Use caution and seek professional assistance when pressing down hard on the vertebrae, neck and lower back.

A Balanced Diet

The body receives nutrients from food which provide the fuel it needs to combat the effects of stress in daily activities. Proper foods include those high in fiber, low in fat, and with abundant vitamins and minerals. Individuals under chronic stress should increase protein intake with the leanest sources of protein: poultry, fish, lean cuts of beef and low-fat or skim dairy products. A diet high in complex carbohydrates should consist of the most calories in one's daily food plan. A well-balanced diet based on the Food Guide Pyramid is essential for stress management.

Rest and Sleep

Adequate rest and sleep are necessary to avoid tiredness and fatigue. When the body is deprived of rest and sleep, mental, physical and emotional processes will deteriorate.

There is no consensus about how much sleep is needed, but approximately 6 to 8 hours of restful sleep per night would probably be sufficient. A person's rate of growth influences the need for sleep. Young individuals who are growing rapidly and older individuals whose recuperative powers are less efficient often require more sleep. Being rested and relaxed is an important step against stress.

Aerobic Exercise

Exercise can be stressful to a person but it may also be an effective means of reducing stress and aid muscle tension release. Individuals participating in regular aerobic activities may experience improvement in their outlook on life. Research shows that regular exercise decreases many stress disorders and shortens the recovery time of emotional trauma in many individuals.

It is recognized that the cardiovascular system seems to be most seriously affected by stress; therefore, it is necessary to have a strong cardiorespiratory system in order to cope with stress sufficiently. Good cardiorespiratory endurance and resting heart rate have been shown to decrease blood pressure for some individuals. Both the blood pressure and heart rate rise in a stressful activity; therefore it is important to decrease the negative effects of stress.

Physical activity is one of the simplest means to control stress. According to Dr. Selye, **physical fitness serves as a sort of "inoculation against stress."** A report from the National Institute of Mental Health notes that "present clinical and experimental evidence overwhelmingly supports the view that a single bout of vigorous exercise can reduce levels of anxiety in both normal and clinically anxious individuals."

One theory is that exercise frees the mind from the stressor contributing to anxiety. The better the fitness level, the better one can withstand the tension of everyday life situations. Another theory suggests that exercise decreases muscular tension and induces a state of muscular relaxation. In addition, one theory suggests that the feeling of achievement to do something for one's self is a stress resolver.

Drugs, alcoholic beverages, painkillers, or tranquilizers do not provide a long-term solution to reducing stress and may also produce stress. Some individuals may need additional help from biofeedback (utilizes machines to monitor certain processes of the body). Stretching, brisk walking, jogging and/or running may aid in reduction of muscle tension. In addition, a change in activity, a massage, sauna, hot bath or shower may alleviate tension and anxiety in most individuals.

For extensive coverage of these and other methods of stress reduction, the following books are highly recommended: *Guide to Stress Reduction* by L. John Mason, *Controlling Stress and Tension* by D. Girdano and G. Everly; *Progressive Relaxation* by Dr. Edmund Jacobson; *The Relaxation Response* by Dr. Herbert Benson.

Expressing Feelings

It is important to deal with situations as they occur instead of keeping them inside. When feelings are not expressed and are kept within, anger results, which may get out of control. Also, ulcers can be avoided when situations are handled in a timely manner.

Outside Interests

Everyone should become involved in additional activities other than the work or home routine. A hobby may be helpful to totally remove oneself from stressful situations found in everyday life. Hobbies allow concentration on something entirely different. Choose a hobby that will allow mind and body to relax and escape the presence of the normal everyday world. An exercise regimen consisting of walking, jogging or running may be an excellent hobby.

Time Alone

Some time of each day should be spent doing activities that are enjoyed, a time to pamper oneself. Take approximately 15 to 30 minutes each day and consider it "your time" for quiet and peace. Closing the eyes, quietly meditating, resting the head or placing the feet on a chair may help to eliminate fatigue so that one can face the stress and clear the thinking in order to distinguish between that which is "worth fighting about" and items less important. This may be a time for reading a 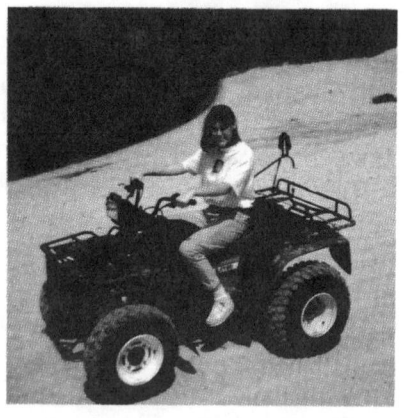 favorite book, listening to music, walking or jogging in the park, exercising, or just enjoying peace and quiet. It does not matter what is done with that special time—what matters is that one can relax, unwind and enjoy those special moments.

Affirmations and Imaging

Positive coping messages or affirmations can help to manage stress. Affirmations are methods of self talk used to replace negative thoughts with positive thoughts, thus improving self-esteem.

In addition to using positive messages, imaging plays an important role in stress management. Imaging is imagining being successful at an endeavor. Imagine participation in a 5K Run. A self-talk suggestion is "I am going to complete the race; I have prepared for this race as much as possible." Use imaging ability to visualize crossing the finish line. Relax and visualize everything under control. This is an example of using affirmation and imaging skills in combination with physically preparing for success.

Reframing Thoughts

Reframing suggests changing the way of looking at something, learning to be an optimist instead of a pessimist. When under stress, what a person thinks often helps to change the impact stress has on the body. Use positive phrases and descriptions to describe yourself or situations. Avoid negative words such as should have, ought to, never, don't; instead use positive terms such as good, success, and accepted.

Humor

Don't worry, be happy! Find the humorous side of everyday life situations. Laughter is a natural stress reliever. It is impossible to be angry or depressed when laughing. Laughter sources can be found in books, friends, pets, family members, comedy shows, television, an simply people-watching. Spend time with upbeat people who have a good sense of humor and who stimulate laughter and feelings of self-worth. Your outlook on life will improve with a daily dose of laughter.

Support Systems

Everyone needs someone on whom to depend in times of a major or minor need. Support systems can come from friends, church, family, school events, or clubs or organizations. Each one needs someone to share both good and bad times and positive and negative experiences. It is helpful to use support systems when experiencing stressful events.

Professional Assistance

It's a sign of strength to seek assistance when needed. Take advantage of a psychiatrist, psychologist, social worker, local hospital or health care facility, community mental health services, a doctor, clergy, or family counselor. **Empathy** — the understanding one receives from talking with a trusted, supportive friend or spouse — quickly cures most psychological injuries and releases the stress. **It isn't necessary to be alone with problems.**

STRESS MANAGEMENT GUIDELINES

The following ideas suggest ways to cope with stress.

1. **Total daily relaxation (20 minutes)** listening to music, napping, meditating, day dreaming, etc. Make a commitment and do it.
2. **Join community education classes** and learn a new activity.
3. Take a walk (park, beach, shopping mall); enjoy nature.
4. **Pamper yourself.** Take a warm bath, shower or dip in the whirlpool.

5. **Control weight.** Avoid foods high in fat, salts and sugars.

6. Take a **ten minute break** for every four hours of work.

7. **Say "no" to overburdening yourself** with too many commitments. Delegate responsibility. Rank priorities in order so that the most important items get done.

8. **Communicate feelings** effectively (I feel angry, sad, upset, etc.). Think positive. Believe in yourself.

9. **Socialize with friends** (one night per week).

10. **Plan in advance** by making weekly and monthly projections.

11. **Organize work.** Take one activity at a time. Decide which is most important, do it, and cross off items as completed. Don't build more tasks into your day than you can complete.

12. **Don't worry, be happy.** Take action and solve problems. Don't put it off until tomorrow.

13. **Make adjustments**, be flexible and make the best of all situations. Don't live by the clock. Get on with life.

14. **Take time for yourself.** A two weeks vacation, recreational activities, rest and play. Try something you always wanted to do but never made time for previously.

15. **Choose relaxation activities** that will allow you to forget everything except what you are doing.

16. Before going to bed, **spend a few minutes clearing your mind** of the day's events. When you go to bed relaxed, you will sleep better.

17. **Laugh, express humor, love and like yourself.** Do something completely spontaneous for a change and don't feel guilty afterward.

Unpleasant stress to the body can be minimized by keeping it well-nourished, relaxed, rested and strong. Controlling and managing stress **EARNS** healthier lifestyles and habits for all individuals. "**EARNS**" stands for: **E**xercise **A**erobically, **R**elaxation, **N**utrition and **S**leep

---

PRESCRIPTION FOR A "WELLNESS" LIFESTYLE

• Exercise	• Pursue activities	• Good health habits
• A balanced diet	• Continue to learn	• Contribute to others
• Stay in charge	• Develop a support system	• Keep a sense of humor

CHAPTER SUMMARY

Stress affects people differently and people react to stress in different ways. Recognizing shortcomings and how to adjust and to cope with stressful ways of life will depend mostly on the individual. Various diseases and health problems, such as hypertension, stroke, ulcers, coronary heart disease, allergies, tension headaches and cancer, can be traced to stress. It does not matter which stress management technique is used, as long as it works to alleviate stress. Physical coping techniques of reducing stress include aerobic exercise, breathing exercises, visualization, meditation, massage, acupressure, expressing feelings, developing outside interests, spending time alone, affirmation and imaging, humor, support systems, diet, rest, sleep, and progressive relaxation. Experimenting with different techniques and finding which one works best is important. Talking with a trusted individual can often help one find a solution to problems. Learning to take time out from busy schedules and enjoying the pleasures which life brings should be a priority of each individual. **By taking charge of one's life, one can take charge of one's health.**

APPENDIXES

A. References and Suggested Readings.....252

B. Muscles of the Body 260

C. Chapter Evaluations 262

D. Laboratories 281

E. Shoe and Foot Types 331

F. Additional Nutrition Information 333

G. A Report of the Surgeon General:
Physical Activity and Health...................337

APPENDIX A
REFERENCES AND SUGGESTED READINGS

American Cancer Society. 1994. *Cancer Facts and Figures.* Atlanta, ACS.

American College of Sports Medicine. 1983. "Proper and Improper Weight Loss Programs." *Medicine and Science in Sports and Exercise,* 15: IX.

American College of Sports Medicine. 1995. *Guidelines for Exercise Testing and Prescription.* Fifth Edition. Baltimore: Williams & Wilkins.

American Dietetic Association. 1987. Position of the American Dietetic Association: Nutrition Physical Fitness and Athletic Performance for Adults. *Journal of American Dietetic Association,* 87: 933-939.

American Heart Association. 1992. *Heart Facts.*

American Heart Association. 1995. *Lifestyles of the Trim and Healthy.* Dallas: American Heart Association.

American Heart Association (Greater Long Beach Chapter). 1984. "Stress—Bona Fide A.H.A. Risk Factor." *Heart Lines Issue* (February). 41:1.

American Running and Fitness Association: News release. 1995. "Drink Up . . . Your Performance Depends on It."

Anderson, B. 1989. "The Flex Factor." *Runner's World.* 24(2): 38-41.

Anderson, B. 1989. "Eight Minutes to Stretch." *Women's Sports and Fitness.* 11(8):18

Anderson, B. 1989. *Stretching.* Bolinas, CA: Shelter Publishing, Inc.

Anderson, D. 1994. "Autumn Excitement." *Runner's World.* 29(9):34

Anderson, D. 1994. "On the Threshold." *Runner's World.* 29(7):38.

Anderson, K. 1989. "Push It." *Runner's World,* 24 (8): 40-44.

Anderson, O. 1998. "The Best Workout You Can Do." *Runner's World.* 33(3): 34.

Anderson, O. 1997. "Hill, Yes!" *Runner's World.* 32(4): 42.

Anderson, O. 1989. "Raising Your Carbo Consciousness."*Women's Sports and Fitness,* 11(8): 18.

Applegate, L. 1998. "Eight Simple Ways to Boost Your Energy." *Runner's World* 33(3): 26.

Applegate, L. 1996. "Burning Desire."*Runner's World* 31(1): 22-23.

Applegate, L. 1996. "Fluid News You Can Use." *Runner's World* 31(7):26.

Applegate, L. 1989. "Eat, Drink and Be Faster." *Runner's World.* 24(5): 30.

ARAPCS Newsletter. 1990. "More on Beta Carotene." XI (2): 8.

Armstrong, R. B. 1984. "Mechanisms of Exercise-induced Delayed Onset Muscular Soreness: A Brief Review." *Medicine and Science in Sports and Exercise.* 16: 529.

Averbuch, G. 1984. *The Woman Runner.* New York: Cornerstone Library.

Barahona, M. 1996. "The Protein Problem." *Weight Watchersd* 29(3):22.

Beanm, A. and Will-Weber, W. 1995. "Kicking Butt," *Runner's World* 30(1): 32

Bell, A. 1990. "Miracle at Your Fingertips." *The Walking Magazine,* 5(1): 47-49.

Benson, H. 1985. *Beyond the Relaxation Response.* New York: Berkley Publishers.

Benson, H. 1975. *The Relaxation Response.* New York: William Morrow and Company.

Benson, R. 1988. Videotape:*In Training with Coach Benson.* Atlanta: Florida Runners Camp.

Benson, R. 1994. *Precision Running With Your Polar Electronic Heart Rate Monitor.* Port Washington, NY: Polar CIC Inc.

Berger, B. G., Friedmann, E. and Eaton, M. 1988. "Comparison of Jogging, the Relaxation Response, and Group Interaction for Stress Reduction." *Journal of Sport and Exercise Psychology,* 10: 431-447.

Blair, S. Horton, E. et al. 1996. "Physical Activity, Nutrition, and Chronic Disease." *Medicine and Science in Sports and Exercise* 28(3): 335-349.

Bloom, M. 1990. "Cross Training: Testing the Waters." *Runner's World* 25(5):46-54.

Branner. T. 1993. *The Safe Exercise Handbook,* Second Ed. Dubuque, IA: Kendall/Hunt.

Brenner, J. 1987. "Help Yourself to Happy Feet."*Women's Sports and Fitness.* 11(7): 58.

References, continued

Brody, J. 1987. *Jane Brody's Nutrition Book.* New York: W. W. Norton Company.
Brownell, K. D. 1989. "The Ups and Downs of Yo-Yo Dieting. *Reebock Instructor News.* 3(1):3.
Brunick, T. and Wischnia, B. 1994. "Spring Buyer's Guide." *Runner's World.* 24(10): 49-70.
Brzycki, M. 1996. "Q & A on Steroid Use." *Coach and Athletic Director* 65(9): 75-81.
Burfoot, A. 1994. "Formula for Success." *Runner's World.* 29(10): 90-91
Burton, B. T. et al. 1985. "Health Implications of Obesity: NIH Consensus Development Conference. *International Journal of Obesity.* 9: 155.

Cahill, D. M. 1990. "The Fat Experiment." *The Walking Magazine.* 5(1): 29-35.
Cahill, K. M. 1989. "Muscles, the Great Protectors." *The Walking Magazine.* 4(3): 27-33.
Cantor, R. 1989. "Give Yourself Proper Support."*Runner's World.* 24(7): 50-54.
Castleman, M. 1996. Nature's Cures. Emmaus, PA: Rodale Press.
Cawood, F. 1995. *High Blood Pressure Lowered Naturally.* Peachtree City, PA: FC & A Publishing.
Chasnov, M. 1989. "The Ice Is Right." *Runner's World.* 24(7): 34.
Christie, C. "Shoes: Buy by Feel." *The Walking Magazine.* 5(2): 24-27.
Coleman, E. 1996. "How Many Calories Do You Really Need?" *Runner's World* 31(6): 29.
Colfer, G. R. and Chevrette, J. M. 1980. *Running for Fun and Fitness.* Dubuque, IA: Kendall-Hunt Publishing Company.
Cooper, K. H. 1982. *The Aerobics Program for Total Well-being: Exercise, Diet, Emotional Balance.* New York: Bantam.
Cooper, K. H. 1994. *Antioxidant Revolution.* Nashville, TN: Thomas Nelson.
Corbin, C. B. and Lindsey, R. 1994. *Concepts of Physical Fitness with Laboratories.* 8th Ed. Dubuque, IA: Wm. C. Brown.
Corbin, C. B. and Pangrazi, R. P. 1996. "How Much Physical Activity Is Enough?" *Journal of Health, Physical Education, Recreation and Dance* 67(4): 33-37.
Costill, D. L. 1986. *Inside Running: Basics of Sports Physiology.* Indianapolis: Benchmark Press, Inc.
Coyle, E. 1995. Fat Metabolism During Exercise." *Sports Science Exchange* 8(6):1.
Cross Training. 1986. Editors of *Runner's World.* Emmaus, PA: Rodale Press, Inc.

Daniels, J. 1990. "Cruise Control." *Runner's World.* 25(6): 75-82.
Daniels, J. 1994. "The 2-2 T-20: A Great Way to Carry Out Your Lactate-Threshold Workouts." *Running Research.* 10(2): 7-8.
Daniels, J., Fitts, R., and Sheehan, G. 1978. *Conditioning for Distance Running.* New York: John Wiley & Sons.
Davis, K. 1989. "Pregnant and Fit." *Women's Sports and Fitness.* 11(5): 31-43.
Delhagen, K. 1989. "Swimming vs. Running." *Women's Sports and Fitness.* 24(9): 20.
Delhagen, K. 1989. "The Runner's Companion."*Women's Sports and Fitness.* 11(7):31-43.
Delliger, B., Newnham, B., and Morgan, W. 1978. *The Running Experience.* Chicago: Contemporary Books, Inc.
Dintiman, G. B., Davis, R. G., Pennington, J. C., and Stone, S. F. 1989. *Discovering Lifetime Fitness: Concepts of Exercise and Weight Control.* 2nd ed. St. Paul, MN: West.
Dintiman, G. B. and Ward, R. D. 1988. *Sport Speed.* Champaign, IL: Leisure Press.
Drum, T. 1993. *'Fraid Nots.* Pompano Beach, FL: Tom Drum, Inc.
Durkin, J. F. 1990. "If the Shoe Fits." *Runner's World.* 25(4): 46-48.
Durkin, J. F. 1989. "Stress Fractures." *Runner's World.* 24(10): 28.

Edwards, S. 1993. *The Heart Rate Monitor Book.* Port Washington, NY: Polar CIC Inc.
Ellis, J. 1989. "Heavy Duty." *Runner's World.* 24(10): 50-54.
Ellis. J. 1989. "Between a Sock and a Hard Place." *Runner's World.* 24(8): 28.

Fenton, M. 1994. "Pieces of Resistance." *Walking.* 9(5): 28-32.
Fisher, A. G. and Allsen, P. E. 1980. *Jogging.* Dubuque, IA: Wm. C. Brown.
Fixx, J. F. 1977. *The Complete Book of Running.* New York: Random House.
Floyd, P. A., Mimms, S. & Yelding-Howard. 1998. *Personal Health: Perspectives and Lifestyles.* Englewood, CO: Morton Publishing Company

References, continued

Floyd, P. et al. 1993. *Wellness: A Lifetime Commitment.* Winston-Salem, NC: Hunter Textbooks Inc.
Food and Nutrition Board, National Academy of Sciences-National Research Council. 1980. *Recommended Dietary Allowances.* Washington, D.C.: U.S. Government Printing Office.

Galloway, J. G. 1997. "Galloway on Training." *Runner's World.* 32(3):38.
Galloway, J. G. 1996. *Marathon!* Atlanta: Philippides Publications.
Galloway, J. G. 1984. *Galloway's Book on Running.* Bolinas, CA: Shelter Publications.
Girandola, R. N. 1988. *Running for Lifetime Fitness: A Scientific and Personal Guide.* Englewood Cliffs, NJ: Prentice-Hall.
Greenberg, J. S. 1990. *Stress Management.* 3rd. ed. Dubuque, IA: Wm. C. Brown.
Greenleaf, J. E. 1983. "Drinking and Water Balance During Exercise and Heat Acclimation. *Journal of Applied Physiology: Respiratory, Environmental and Exercise Physiology.* 54: 414-419.
Guilland, J. et al. 1989. "Vitamin Status of Young Athletes Including the Effects of Supple-mentation. *Medicine and Science in Sports and Exercise.* 21: 441.

Hafen, B. Q. and Hoeger, W. W. K. 1994. *Wellness: Guidelines for a Healthy Lifestyle.* Englewood, CO: Morton.
Hales, D. 1994. *An Invitation to Health,* 6th ed. Redwood City, CA: Benjamin/Cummings.
Haskell, W., Scala, J., and Whitman, J. 1982. "Use of Nutritional Supplements by Athletes. *Nutrition and Athletic Performance.* Palo Alto, CA: Bull Publishing. 106-155.
Henderson, J. 1988. *Total Fitness: Training for Life.* Dubuque, IA: Wm. C. Brown.
Henderson, J. 1985. *Running for Fitness, for Sport, and for Life.* Dubuque, IA: Wm. C. Brown.
Higdon, H. 1994. "The Single Best." *Runner's World.* 29(6):81-89.
Higdon, H. 1993. Marathon: The Ultimate Training and Racing Guide. Emmaus, PA: Rodale Press.
Hoeger, W. W. K. 1994. *Lifetime Physical Fitness and Wellness: A Personalized Program.* 3rd ed. Englewood, CO: Morton.
Human Nutrition Information Service. 1992. *Food Guide Pyramid.* Hyattsville, MD: U. S. Department of Agriculture.

Jacobson, E. 1938. *Progressive Relaxation.* 2nd ed. Chicago: Chicago Press.
Jacobson, E. 1970. *You Must Relax.* New York: McGraw-Hill.

Kardong, D. 1987. "The Games Runners Play." *Runner's World.* 22(8): 61-67.
Kasperek, G. J. and Snider, R. D. 1987. "Effect of Exercise Intensity and Starvation on Activation of Branched-chain Keto Acid Dehydrogenase by Exercise. *American Journal of Physiology.* 252: E33-E37, as cited by Lemon, 1987.
Kellett, J. 1986. "Acute Soft Tissue Injuries—A Review of the Literature." *Medicine and Science in Sports and Exercise.* 18: 489.
Kevles, B. 1989. "When You Haven't Got Time for the Pain." *Women's Sports and Fitness.* 11(6):12.
Kipp, D. "Stress and Nutrition." *Contemporary Nutrition.* 7(9): 7.
Kleiner, S. M. 1995. "The Role of Meat in an Athlete's Diet." *Sports Science Exchange* 8(5): 1-2.
Koplan, J. P., Discovick, D. S., and Goldbaum, G. M. 1985. "The Risks of Exercise: A Public View of Injuries and Hazards. " *Public Health Reports.* 100 and 180.
Kramer, M. and Wells, C. 1995. "Does Physical Activity Reduce Risk of Estrogen-dependent Cancer in Women?" *Medicine and Science in Sports and Exercise* 28(3): 332-334.
Kravitz. L. 1990. "Getting in Step." *Women's Sports and Fitness.* 2(3): 18.
Kuehls, D. 1995. "All Gain, No Pain." *Runner's World.* 30(5): 50-55
Kuehls, D. 1995. "Long May You Run." *Runner's World.* 30(8): 46-51.
Lamb, D. R. 1984. *Physiology of Exercise.* New York: Macmillan.
Laskau, H. 1987. Videotape: *The Health Walking Technique.* Action East.

References, continued

Lewis, J. 1981. *Nutrition Notes. Dietary Guidelines.* Bowling Green, OH: Bowling Green State University.

Liebman, B. 1989. *Nutrition Action Health Letter.* 16(2). 5-6.

Lindsey, R. and Corbin, C. 1989. "Questionable Exercises—Some Safe Alternatives. *Journal of Physical Education, Recreation, and Dance.* 60(8): 26-32.

Lindsey, R., Jones, B. J., and Whitley, A. V. 1989. *Fitness for the Health of It.* Dubuque, IA: Wm. C. Brown.

Lombardi, V. P. 1989. *Beginning Weight Training.* Dubuque, IA: Wm. C. Brown.

Madsen, M.1989. "Things That Go Bump in Your Foot." *Women's Sports and Fitness.* 11(7): 14-16.

Makalous, S .L., Arauj, M. A., and Thomas, T. R. 1988. "Energy Expenditure During Walking with Hand Weights." *The Physician and Sportsmedicine.* 16(4): 139-48.

Malley, S. 1989. "Diet Daze." *Runner's World.* 24(10): 86-93.

Mannherz, R. E. 1989. "Stress Injuries of the Extensor Mechanism." *Sports Medicine Update.* 4(3): 7-8.

Masseo, S., Shier, N. and Lindeman, A. 1996. "Nutritional Supplements: An Update for Coaches and Athletes." *The Physical Educator* 53(1): 34-42.

McCarthy, P. 1989. "How Much Protein Do Athletes Really Need?" *Physician and Sportsmedicine.* 17: 170.

McGlynn, G. 1990. *Dynamics of Fitness: A Practical Approach.* 2nd ed. Dubuque, IA: Wm. C. Brown.

McGuire, R. 1989. "The Ankle: A Classy Joint." *Women's Sports and Fitness.* 11(8): 52-55.

Melograno, V. J., and Klinzing, J. E. 1988. *An Orientation to Total Fitness.* 4th ed. Dubuque, IA: Kendall/Hunt.

Menninger, R. W. 1978. "Coping With Life's Strains. *U. S. News and World Report.* 5:80.

Miller, G. 1990. "Stepping Up to Fitness." *Reebok Instructor News.* 3(2): 7.

Montoye, H. J., Christian, J. L., Nagle, F. J., and Levin, S. M. 1988. *Living Fit.* Menlo Park, CA: Benjamin/Cummings.

Morgan, W. P. and Goldston, S. 1987. *Exercise and Mental Health.* New York: Hemisphere Publishing Corporation.

Morgan, W. 1984. *Coping with Mental Stress: The Potential and Limits of Exercise Intervention. (Final Report).* Bethesda: National Institute of Mental Health.

National Institutes of Health. 1995. "Eat 5 Fruits and Vegetables a Day." National Cancer Institute.

Newsweek. 1989. "Vitamins: New RDAs." Nov. 6: 84.

Nieman, D. C. 1993. *Fitness and Your Health.* Palo Alto, CA: Bull.

Nieman, D. C. 1989. "Exercise and the Mind." *Women's Sports and Fitness.* 22(7): 54-57.

Nieman, D. C. 1989. "Exercise: How Much Is Enough? How Much Is Too Much?" *Women's Sports and Fitness.* 22(5): 31-34.

Noakes, Tim. 1991. *The Lore of Running.* Champaign, IL: Leisure Press.

Norris, W. A. and Fanning, W. L. 1989. *Concepts and Strategies for a Lifetime of Fitness.* Winston-Salem, NC: Hunter Textbooks Inc.

Nutrition Action Newsletter. 1991. "Taking Supplements Seriously," 18(8), 1-8.

Obarzanek, E., Velletri, P. 1996. "Dietary Protein and Blood Pressure. *Journal of American Medical Association* 275(20), 1598-1602.

O'Shea, M. 1995. "Parade's Guide to Better Fitness." *Parade.* July 2, 1995: 12-13.

Osler, T. 1978. *Serious Runner's Handbook.* Mountain View, CA: Anderson/World, Inc.

Pangrazi, Robert P., Corbin, C., and Welk, G. J. "Physical Activity for Children and Youth." *JOHPERD* 67:4, 38-43.

Pengelly, S. 1995. "Breathing-Part I." *The Pursuit of Excellence.* 3(1): 1-2.

Pengelly, S. 1995. "Breathing-Part II." *The Pursuit of Excellence.* 3(2): 1-2.

Pollock, M. L., Wilmore, J. H., and Fox III, S. M. 1984. *Exercise in Health and Disease.* Philadelphia: Sanders.

256

References, continued

Prevention 1994. "Train Your Body to Trim Your Tummy," 46(5), 51-53.
Prevention 1994. "How to Lose 10 Stubborn Pounds." 46(6), 58-60.
Prevention 1996. "Fill Up, Slim Down," 48(3), 98-103.
Prevention 1996. "Burn Fat—Faster." 48(6), 96-100.
Prevention 1996. "Low-fat Heaven," 48(2), 65-72.
Prevention 1996. "Make Exercise Automatic." 48(1), 73-78.

Rapaport, J. 1996. "Running on Empty," *Women's Sports and Fitness,* May/June, 93-94.
Reader's Digest. 1994. "Dump that Diet." May, 123-125.
Reebock Instructor News. 1990. "Risky Exercises." 3(2): 6.
Reebock Instructor News. 1990. "Reebock Presents 'Step Training.'" 3: 5.
Reebock Walk Instructor's Manual. 1988. Canton, MA: Reebok International Ltd.
Reid, J. G. and Thomson, J. M. 1985. *Exercise Prescription for Fitness.* Englewood Cliffs, NJ: Prentice-Hall.
Reynolds, W. and Anderson, O. 1994. "Specific Strength." *Runner's World* 29(12): 50-57.
Rhea, D. Jamber, E., and Wiginton, K. 1996. "Preventing Eating Disorders in Female Athletes." *Journal of Physical Education, Recreation and Dance* 67(4):66-68.
Rhein, S. and Hoffman, C. J. 1995. "Fueling the Human Machine for Optimal Performance." *Coach and Athletic Director* 65(5), 66-69.
Rogers, E. 1988. "If You Eat Less, Will You Live Longer?" *Women's Sports and Fitness.* 10(2): 26.
Rodgers, B. and Welch, P. 1991. *Masters Running and Racing.* Emmaus, PA: Rodale Press.
Rosato, F. D. 1990 *Fitness and Wellness.* 2nd ed. St. Paul, MN: West.
Rosato, F. D. 1988. *Jogging for Health and Fitness.* 2nd ed. Englewood, CO: Morton.
Rudow, M. 1975. *Race Walking.* Mountain View, CA: World Publications.
Running and FitNews. 1991. "Cross Training with In-Line Skates." 9(12):1.
Running and FitNews. 1992. "In the Long Run." 10(8): 4,5
Running and FitNews. 1992. "New Ways to Use Carbohydrate Supplements." 10(2): 3.
Running and FitNews. 1991. "Running During Pregnancy." 9(7): 1-4.
Running and FitNews . 1994. "Backward Running and Walking." 12(6):1.
Running and FitNews. 1994. "Iron Stores." 29(5): 3-4.
Running and FitNews . 1995. "Don't Measure It, Just Do It!" 13(7): 1.
Running and FitNews . 1993. "Exercise Improves Quality of Life: In Sickness and in Health." 11(10):1.
Running and FitNews . 1994. "Breathing Workouts." 12(6): 4-5.
Running and FitNews . 1994. "Endurance: Always Top Priority. 12(8): 2.
Running and FitNews . 1994. "Fine Tuning Your Running Before Races." 12(9): 1.
Running Injury-free. 1986. Editors of *Runner's World.* Emmaus, PA: Rodale Press.
Running Research News. 1991. "After the Things Those Runners Said." 7(5): 5-7.
Running Research News. 1985. "Caring for Muscles Before and After Exercise." 1(1): 3.
Running Research News. 1986. "Cycling vs. Running." 2 (1): 4.
Running Research News. 1985. "Dehydration and Water Intoxication: A Delicate Balance?" 1(2): 6.
Running Research News. 1987. "Detraining: Losing Fitness a Slow Process." 3(5): 1-2.
Running Research News. 1991. "Don't Put Your Running Recovery on Ice." 7(5): 5-7.
Running Research News. 1986. "Eating or Fasting Before a Run: Which Is Better?" 2(1): 2-3.
Running Research News. 1985. "Endurance and Strength Training: Compatible?" 1(1):1-2.
Running Research News. 1986. "Effective Warm-Ups." 2 (3): 2-3.
Running Research News. 1992. "German Runners Find Right Dose of Threshold Running." 8(4): 1-3.
Running Research News. 1992. "Hill Leaping 'Bounces Away Need for Lots of Oxygen, Leads to More Efficient Running in Recent Swedish Research." 8(2): 1-4.
Running Research News. 1987. "How Well Does the Wet Vest Work?" 3(3): 5.
Running Research News. 1988. "Improving Your Running Economy: A Neglected Aspect of Training." 4(4) 1, 3-4.
Running Research News. 1987. "In Search of the Optimal Interval Workout: Which Expert Should You Believe?" 3(2): 1-3.

References, continued

Running Research News. 1987. "Intense Running a Mood Lifter." 3(6): 4-5.

Running Research News. 1986. "Interval Length, Frequency, and Training Duration. 2 (2): 2-3.

Running Research News. 1985. "Intervals: How Fast and How Long? The '80 and 90' Rules." 1(3): 1-2.

Running Research News. 1990. "Keeping Cramps from Crimping Your Running: Experts Offer Their Advice.: 6(2): 1-7.

Running Research News. 1985. "Mental Strategies for Runners." 1(2): 1-2.

Running Research News. 1991. "Methods of Producing Peak Performance: Can You Peak for More Than a Week?" 7(2) 1-5.

Running Research News. 1985. "Muscle Stretching: What Are Its Benefits?" 1(3): 6.

Running Research News. 1986. "Relief Intervals: Jog, Don't Walk." 2(4): 2-3.

Running Research News. 1989. "Running Economy Remains Elusive to Even the Most Earnest Experts. 5(5): 1, 3-5.

Running Research News. 1986. "Should You Run Before Stretching?" 2(6): 3.

Running Research News. 1988. "Sports Drink Upheaval at Recent ACSM Meeting: For Long Runs, Water Is No Longer the Drink of Champions: Previously Shunned Salt May Be an Important Ingredient in Sports Beverages." 4(4): 1-3.

Running Research News. 1991. "Sports Drink Update: Beginning with Bolus Better Than Slurping Small Samples." 7(4): 1-4.

Running Research News. 1992. "A Stitch in Time Can Ruin a Race; Become a 'Left-Footed Exhaler' to Reduce Your Risk." 8(3): 8-10.

Running Research News. 1986. "Techniques of Muscle Stretching." 2(1): 7-8.

Running Research News. 1989. "The Carbohydrate Story: Quick Replacement Is Not Good Enough—You Also Need the Right Amount." 5(1): 1-2.

Running Research News. 1988. "Unique Training Strategy Reduces Muscle Soreness." 4(1): 3-4.

Running Research News. 1987. "Weight Training: Can It Benefit Your Long-distance Running?" 3(1): 1, 3-4.

Running Research News. 1985. "What to Drink Before and During a Run." 1(2): 3-4.

Running Research News. `992. "Antioxidants to the Rescue," 28(10: 30-32.

Running Research News. 1990. "Shoe Buyer's Guide—Glossary." 25(4): 44.

Running Research News. 1995. "Two-Week Cycle Plus Ten-Day Taper Leads to Huge Gains in Anaerobic Capacity." 11(1): 9-10.

Running Research News. 1995. "It's Now Official: Strength Training Can Improve Your Running Economy." 11(4): 8-10.

Running Research News. 1994. "Three Are Enough! A Trio of Strength Training Exercises Will Improve Your Stride Length and Frequency." 10(1): 1-6.

Running Research News. 1994. "More Evidence That Runners Can Pedal Their Way to Faster Race Times." 10(5): 10.

Running Research News. 1994. "Forget About Pre-Marathon Coffee Consumption: Caffeine Improves Your Interval Workouts." 10(5): 8.

Running Research News. 1994. "The 2-2 T-20: A Great Way to Carry Out Your Lactate-Threshold Workouts." 10(2): 7-8.

Running Research News. 1994. "The 10K Corner: Tips on Training for 10K Races." 10(2): 9.

Running Research News. 1994. "Top Researchers Use Carolina Cruisin' to Find Tapering Heaven." 10(3): 1-3.

Running Research News. 1995. "What About the Dehydration Question." 11(1): 11-12.

Sacks, M. H. and Sachs, M. L. 1981. *Psychology of Running.* Champaign, IL: Human Kinetics Publishing, Inc.

Sargent, R. and Trexler, M. L. 1989. "Nutrition for Exercise."*Fitness Management.* 5: 21.

Schmidt, S. B. 1989. "Reform Food Labels Now!" *Nutrition Action.* 16(2): 8-9.

Seiger, L. H. and Hesson, J. 1990. *Walking for Fitness.* Dubuque, IA: Wm. C. Brown.

Selye, H. 1974. *Stress Without Distress.* Philadelphia: J. B. Lippincott.

Selye, H. 1978. *The Stress of Life.* New York: McGraw-Hill.

Sharkey, B. J. 1979. *Physiology of Fitness.* Champaign, IL: Human Kinetics.

References, continued

Sheehan, G. 1989. "Viewpoint: Heat Success." *Runner's World.* 24(7): 16.
Sheehan, G. 1988. "Dial 'C' for Comfort." *Runner's World.* 23(12): 14.
Shorter, F. 1987. "Beyond Running: An Olympic Gold Medalist Has Learned the Value of Cross-Training." *Runner's World.* 22(6): 24-30.
Simon, H. B. 1989. "Should You Walk With Weights?" *Walking Magazine.* 4 5): 62-64.
Simopoulos, A. P. 1989. "Nutrition and Fitness." *Journal of the American Medical Association.* 261: 2862.
Slavin, J. L. et al. 1988. "Amino Acid Supplements: Beneficial or Risky?" *Physician and Sportsmedicine* 16: 221.
Smith, T. 1994. "The Key Is Carbohydrate for the Marathon, Too." *Running and Fit News.* 12(7): 4-5.
Smith, T. 1995. "Hit the Hills." *Running and Fit News* 13(1): 4-5.
Stanford, B. 1989. "Caffeine and Athletes." *Physician and Sportsmedicine.* 17: 193.
Stokes, R., Moore, A. C., Moore, C., and Shultz, S. 1992. *Fitness: The New Wave.* 3rd ed. Winston-Salem: Hunter Textbooks Inc.
Surgeon General's Report on Physical Activity and Health, July 11, 1996.
Sweetgall, R., Rippe, J. and Katch, F. 1985. *Rockport's Fitness Walking.* New York: Putnam.

The Complete Runner. 1974. Editors of *Runner's World.* New York: Avon.
The Rockport Guide to Fitness Walking. 1989. Marlboro, MA: Rodale Press, Inc.
Thompson, T. 1989. "Be Injury-Free: Eliminate the Terrible Ten." *Women's Sports and Fitness.* 11(4): 24-25.
Timmermans, H. and Martin, M. 1987. "Top Ten Potentially Dangerous Exercises." *Journal of Physical Education, Recreation, and Dance.* 58(8): 29-31.
Training Smart. 1986. Editors of *Runner's World.* Emmaus, PA: Rodale Press, Inc.
Tucker, L. A. and Friedman, G. M. 1989. "Television Viewing and Obesity in Adult Males." *American Journal of Public Health.* 79:516.
Tufts University Diet and Nutrition Letter. 1990. "New RDAs Call for More Calcium, Less Sodium." 7(11): 1-2.

Ullyot, J. L. 1980. *Running Free.* New York: G. P. Putnam's Sons.
Ullyot, J. L. 1976. *Women's Running.* Mountain View, CA: World Publications.
U. S. Department of Health and Human Services. 1995. *Nutriton and Your Health:Dietary Guidelines for Americans,* 4th ed.
University of California, Berkeley Wellness Letter. 1994. "Antioxidants: Never Too Late. 10(8): 2.
University of California, Berkeley Wellness Letter. 1994. "The Latest on Caffeine and Pregnancy." 10(6): 2.
University of California, Berkeley Wellness Letter. 1992. "Better Walking Workouts." 8(12): 4,5.
University of California, Berkeley Wellness Letter. 1990. "Relief: Exercise Injuries, Part II. 6(8): 4-5.
University of California, Berkeley Wellness Letter. 1990. "Should You Give Up on Oats? . . . Should You Give Up on Coffee?" 6(7): 2-3.
University of California, Berkeley Wellness Letter. 1990. "Where to Get an Accurate Cholesterol Test." 6(6): 2.
University of California, Berkeley Wellness Letter. 1990. "Exercise Without Injury." 6(6): 4-5.
University of California, Berkeley Wellness Letter. 1990. "Fresh Fish Findings." 6(6): 6-7.
University of California, Berkeley Wellness Letter. 1990. "Is McDonald's 'Poisoning' America?" 3.
University of California, Berkeley Wellness Letter. 1990. "Muscle Cramps: S-T-R-E-T-C-H Spells Relief." 6(4): 6.
University of California, Berkeley Wellness Letter. 1990. "Muscle Cramps: Don't Lose Sleep Over Calf Cramps. 6(4): 6.

References, continued

University of California, Berkeley Wellness Letter. 1994. "Udder Confusion." 10(8): 1-2.
University of California, Berkeley Wellness Letter. 1994. "Ask the Experts." 10(6): 8.
University of California, Berkeley Wellness Letter. 1996. "Should You Be Eating More Protein or Less?" 12(9):4.
University of California, Berkeley Wellness Letter. 1996. "Olestra: Just Say No." 12(5): 1.
University of California, Berkeley Wellness Letter. 1996. "The Push-up: Still the Best." 12 (9): 6.
University of California, Berkeley Wellness Letter. 1996. "Make 'Folacin' a Household Word. 12(8): 1.
University of California, Berkeley Wellness Letter. 1996. "Just Do It." 12(6): 8.
University of California, Berkeley Wellness Letter. 1996. "Antioxidants: The Key to Good Health." 12(7): 1-2.
University of California, Berkeley Wellness Letter. 1996. "Beata Carotene Pills: Should You Take Them?" 12(7): 1.
University of California, Berkeley Wellness Letter. 1989. "Winter—A Great Time for Exercise." 6(3): 6.
University of California, Berkeley Wellness Letter. 1989. "Ask the Experts." 6(3): 8.
University of California, Berkeley Wellness Letter. 1989. "Are We Too Concerned About Cholesterol?" 6(2): 4-5.
Uram, P. 1980. *The Complete Stretching Book.* Mountain View, CA: Anderson World, Inc.

Voy, R. O. 1986. "Water Soluble Vitamins Not Safe in Megadoses." *Physician and Sportsmedicine.* 14: 52.

Walk Leader Manual. 1989. Marlboro, MA: The Rockport Walking Institute.
Walsh, J. 1996. "Are You Going to Swallow That?" *Women's Sp[orts and Fitness,* September, 75-76.
Wasserman, Y. 1996. "Nutrients to the Max." *Weight Watchers* 29(4): 20.
Weight Watchers. 1994. "Are You Too Good?" 27(2), 23-26.
Whitney, E. N., Hamilton, E., and Rolfes, S. R. 1990. *Understanding Nutrition.* 5th Ed. St. Paul: West.
Whitney, E. N. and Sizer, F. S. 1989. *Essential Life Choices.* St. Paul: West.
Wiita, B., Stanbaugh, I., and Buch, J. 1995. "Nutrition Knowledge and Eating Practices of Young Female Athletes." *Journal of Physical Education, Recreation and Dance* 66(3): 36-41.
Williams, M. H. 1990. *Lifetime Fitness and Wellness: A Personal Choice.* 2nd Ed. Dubuque, IA: Wm. C. Brown.
Williams, M. H. 1988. *Nutrition for Fitness and Sport.* 2nd ed. Dubuque, IA: Wm. C. Brown.
Williams, M. 1985. *Lifetime Physical Fitness: A Personal Choice.* Dubuque, IA: Wm. C. Brown.
Williams, M. H. 1983. "Vitamin Supplementation and Physical Performance," in *Report of the Ross Symposium on Nutrient Utilization During Exercise.* E. L. Fox, ed. Columbus, OH: Ross Laboratories, pp. 26-30.
Williams, M. 1974. *Drugs and Athletic Performance.* Springfield, IL: Charles C. Thomas.
Willix, R. and Anderson, M. 1990. "Cross Training in Athletics. What Is It? How It Can Help Your Running." *East Coast Runner.* 1(1): 17.
Wilson, B. 1990. "Choosing Shoes—What to Look For at the Running Store. *Florida Sports.* 4(1): 30-31.
Wischina B. & Brunick, T. 1997. "Choosing The Right Shoe." 32(4):52.

Yanker, G. 1983. *The Complete Book of Exercise Walking.* Chicago: Contemporary.
Yoshimura. H. and coauthors. 1980. "Anaemia During Hard Physical Training (Sports Anaemia) and Its Causal Mechanism with Special Reference to Protein Nutrition." *World Review of Nutrition and Dietetics.* 35. 1-86.

APPENDIX B
MUSCLES OF THE BODY

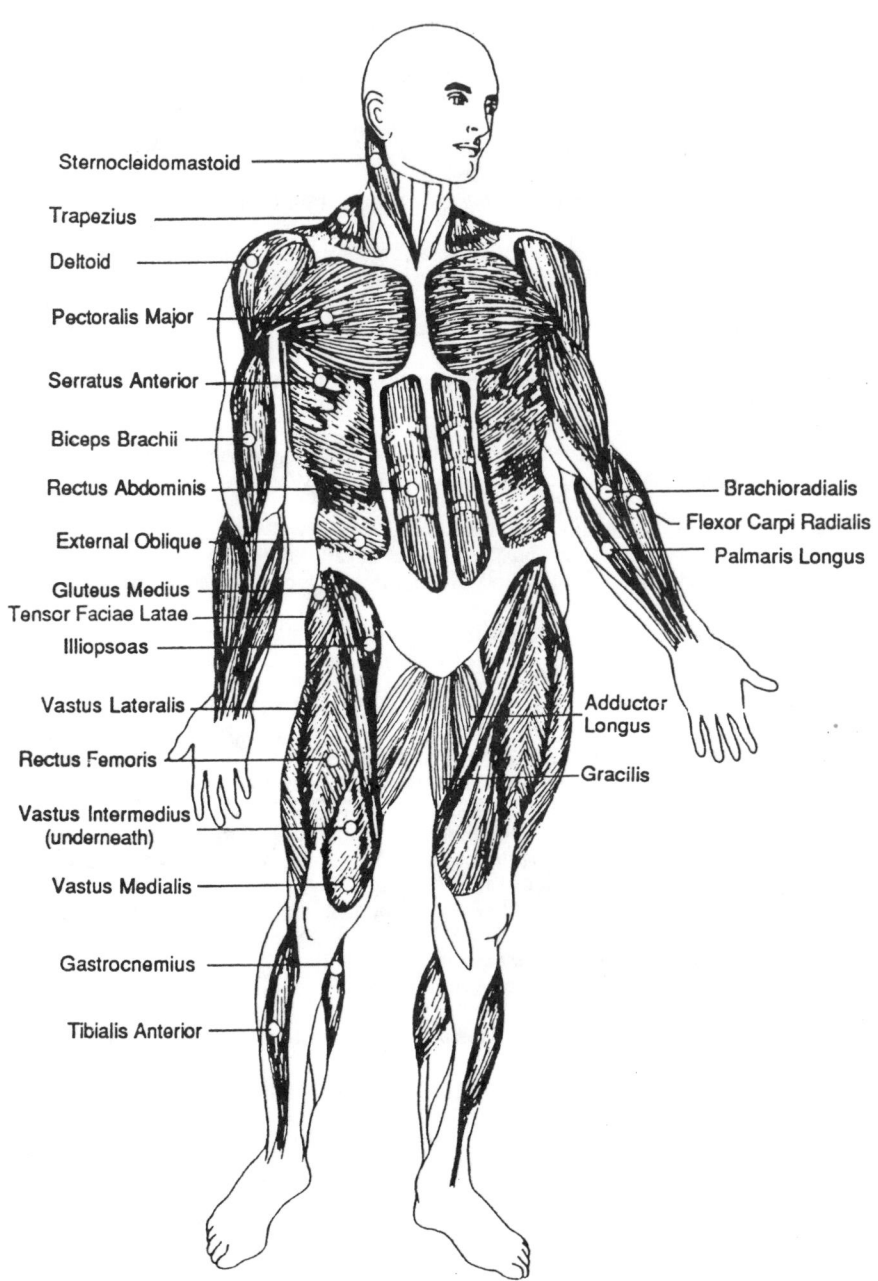

Sternocleidomastoid

Trapezius

Deltoid

Pectoralis Major

Serratus Anterior

Biceps Brachii

Rectus Abdominis

External Oblique

Gluteus Medius
Tensor Faciae Latae

Illiopsoas

Vastus Lateralis

Rectus Femoris

Vastus Intermedius
(underneath)

Vastus Medialis

Gastrocnemius

Tibialis Anterior

Brachioradialis

Flexor Carpi Radialis

Palmaris Longus

Adductor
Longus

Gracilis

APPENDIX B
MUSCLES OF THE BODY

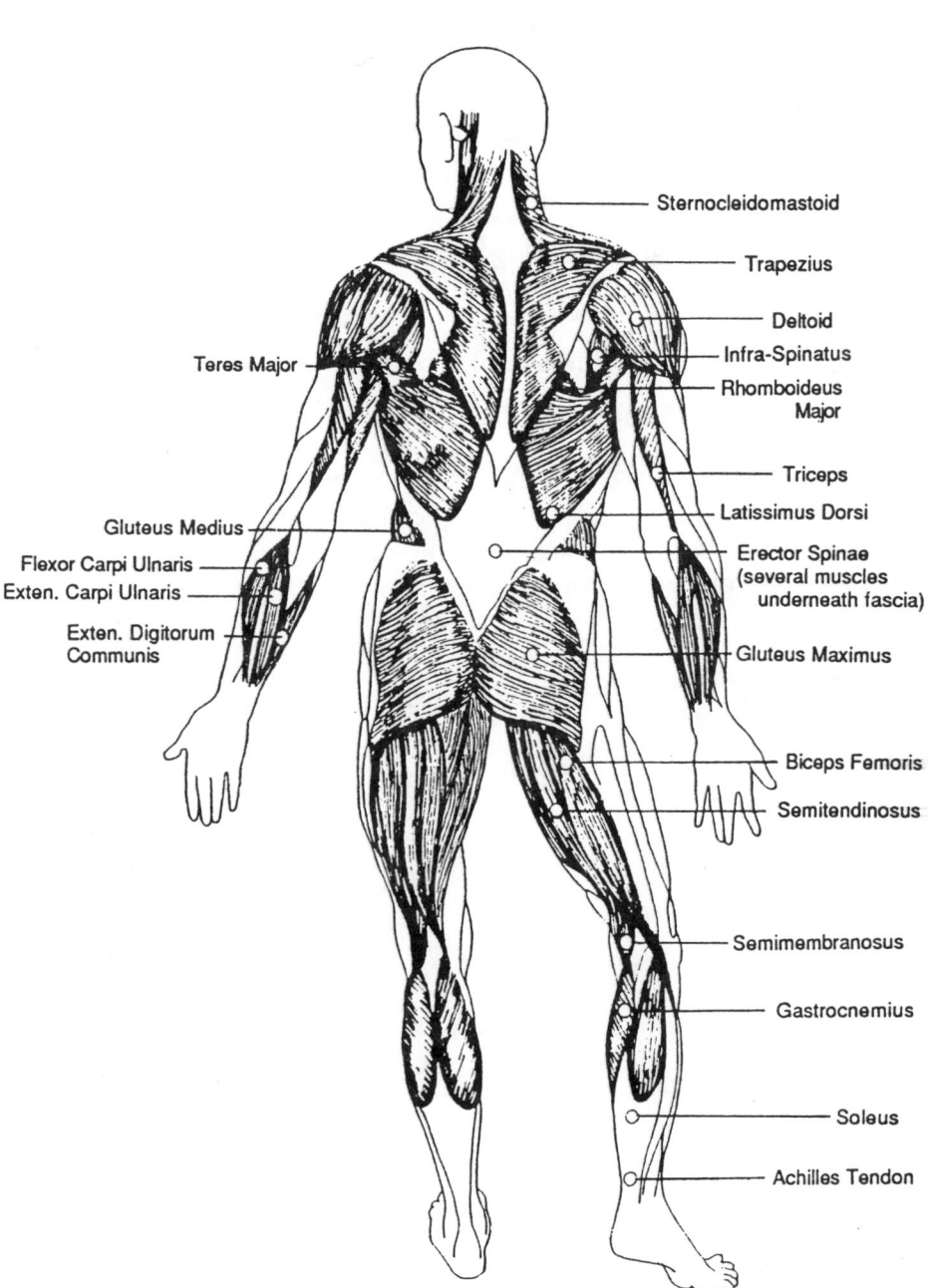

Sternocleidomastoid

Trapezius

Deltoid

Infra-Spinatus

Rhomboideus Major

Teres Major

Triceps

Latissimus Dorsi

Gluteus Medius

Erector Spinae (several muscles underneath fascia)

Flexor Carpi Ulnaris

Exten. Carpi Ulnaris

Exten. Digitorum Communis

Gluteus Maximus

Biceps Femoris

Semitendinosus

Semimembranosus

Gastrocnemius

Soleus

Achilles Tendon

APPENDIX C
CHAPTER EVALUATIONS

1. Lifetime Fitness Through Walking,
    Jogging, and Running 263

2. Preparation 265

3. Training Principles 267

4. Training Programs 269

5. Fitness Enhancing Programs 271

6. Common Injuries: Prevention and Care 273

7. Nutrition 275

8. Weight Management 277

9. Stress Management 279

CHAPTER ONE EVALUATION
Lifetime Fitness Through Walking, Jogging and Running

Name _____ Section _____ Date _____

1. Define and explain the five health-related components of fitness.

2. Define wellness.

3. List the components of wellness.

CHAPTER TWO EVALUATION

Preparation

Name _____ Section _____ Date _____

1. Do I need a physical examination before I begin an exercise program? Explain.

2. What type of clothing should be worn when exercising in warm, cold, and wet weather?

3. What type of shoes should be worn when exercising?

4. Why are sauna or rubber suits dangerous during walking, jogging, or running?

5. Are hand and wrist weights necessary? Explain.

6. Explain anabolic steroids and what happens to the body when using steroids.

7. What precautions must be taken when exercising in hot and humid conditions?

8. What precautions must be taken when exercising in cold weather?

CHAPTER THREE EVALUATION
Training Principles

Name _____ Section _____ Date _____

1. What does good standing posture contribute to walking, jogging, or running mechanics?

2. Describe arm position, lean of body, stride, foot plant, and foot pushoff for walking, jogging, or running (whichever activity you have adopted). Be sure to indicate the activity described.

3. Explain the difference between aerobic and anaerobic activities.

4. List 5 physiological benefits from walking, jogging, and running.

5. What contribution do walking, jogging, and running have on muscular response and which type of muscle fibers are most suited to endurance?

6. What motivational techniques are used by walkers, joggers, and runners?

7. What psychological benefits will be derived from walking, jogging, and running?

8. Explain what the initials FITT represent for the exercise prescription guidelines.

9. Explain what the initials FITT represent for the lifetime activity recommendations.

10. What is the purpose of determining the target heart zone and how is that information used during a walking, jogging, and running workout following the exercise prescription guidelines?

11. How long should an aerobic workout last when following the lifetime activity recommendations?

12. Why is the type of exercise important?

13. What is the purpose of overloading and how should it be applied in a walking, jogging, or running program?

14. What happens when an exerciser experiences retrogression?

CHAPTER FOUR EVALUATION
Training Programs

Name _____ Section _____ Date _____

1. What is the value and purpose of testing prior to beginning a walking, jogging, and running programs?

2. What is the benefit of following a program developed by a walking, jogging, and running authority?

3. When planning a walking, jogging, and running program what precautions should be taken to prevent risk of injury?

4. What procedures should be followed prior to adding speedwork to your training program and during your speed workout?

5. Give one example of a speed workout.

6. What suggestions are advocated regarding the inclusion of a long distance workout in your training program?

7. Cite precautions for women walkers, joggers, and runners during pregnancy.

8. From reading this chapter, what warm-up and cool-down procedures have you established?

9. Explain your plan for drinking and eating prior to, during and after a race or workout.

10. Comment on the effects of heat on your workout or race pace.

CHAPTER FIVE EVALUATION
Fitness Enhancing Programs

Name _____ Section _____ Date _____

1. Define flexibility.

2. Which type of flexibility exercising is recommended and how is the technique performed?

3. What are the benefits from improved strength?

4. What happens to muscle fibers as a result of strength training?

5. Name and describe the type of strength exercising that is most popular.

6. How many sets and repetitions are recommended before increasing weight in a weight training program?

7. For weight training, describe the breathing and time involved in exerting a force and also in the relaxation or weight lowering phase.

8. What benefits do plyometric exercises provide?

9. Which alternate aerobic activity do you prefer to substitute in your walking, jogging, or running program?

10. How would you perform that alternate aerobic activity and for what length of time, distance, or intensity?

CHAPTER SIX EVALUATION

Common Injuries: Prevention and Care

Name _____ Section _____ Date _____

1. Explain the difference between an acute and overuse injury.

2. List six guidelines which should be used to prevent common injuries.

3. What causes muscle soreness?

4. Define shin splints and describe the recommended treatment for shin splints.

5. What causes a side stitch while walking, jogging, or running?

6. What causes muscle cramps and what do you do about cramps?

7. What is the standard treatment for most injuries regarding walking, jogging, or running? Explain.

8. When should heat be applied to an injury?

CHAPTER SEVEN EVALUATION
Nutrition

Name _____ Section _____ Date _____

1. Explain the difference between a calorie and a kilocalorie (kcal).

2. Does cooking affect the amount of calories contained in food? Explain.

3. List and explain the purpose of the six major nutrients required by the human body. What are the suggested percentages of the three energy nutrients?

4. Explain the difference between saturated, monunsaturated, and polyunsaturated fats.

5. Define atherosclerosis.

6. What is HDL and why is it good?

7. What is osteoporosis and how can it be prevented?

8. Do women who exercise have special needs? Explain.

9. Are caffeine and alcohol detrimental to good health? Explain.

10. What are the problems associated with fast foods?

11. Explain the difference between iron-deficiency anemia and sports anemia.

12. List several instances in which vitamin and mineral supplements may be necessary.

13. Do athletes or individuals who train for long periods of time need a special diet? Explain.

14. What is listed on the label of a food item?

15. Calculate the percentage of fat in this lunch meat: Fat—10g., Calories—100, Sodium—220 mg., Protein—5g.

16. List and explain the seven dietary guidelines for Americans.

CHAPTER EIGHT EVALUATION
Weight Management

Name _____ Section _____ Date _____

1. Explain the term "food plan."

2. Name and explain four theories of obesity.

3. Explain anorexia nervosa, bulimia, amenorrhea, and anorexia athletica.

4. What is the most effective exercise for losing weight?

5. What is spot reduction?

6. Are rubberized or plastic suits and steam baths an effective way to lose weight? Explain.

7. What is the difference between cellulite, adipose tissue and fat?

8. Are mechanical vibrators, figure-wraps, whirlpool/steam and massages useful in losing weight? Explain.

9. Are health clubs, salons, and/or spas necessary? Why?

10. Why are high protein/low carbohydrate diets not recommended for weight reduction?

CHAPTER NINE EVALUATION
Stress Management

Name _____ Section _____ Date _____

1. Define stress.

2. Explain the difference between eustress and distress.

3. When is stress most likely to occur?

4. What is the singularly most important deterrent to stress?

5. List several symptoms of stress in a person's life.

6. How can daily hassles be avoided?

7. Name and explain several of the physical coping techniques for managing stress.

APPENDIX D
LABORATORIES

1.1 Health-related Components of Fitness 283

2.1 Foot Evaluation 285

2.2 Shoe Selection 287

3.1 Walking Mechanical Analysis 289

3.2 Racewalking Mechanical Analysis 291

3.3 Jogging/Running Mechanical Analysis 293

3.4 Target Heart Rate Zone 295

4.1 Risko 297

4.2 Walking/Jogging/Running Schedule/Goals 301

4.3 Weekly Walking/Jogging/Running Log 303

5.1 Strength Workout and Progress Chart 305

7.1 Dietary Habits Evaluation 307

7.2 Daily Nutritional Evaluation 309

7.3 Calories Per Day Formulas 315

7.4 Food Guide Pyramid 317

8.1 Estimation of Ideal Body Weight.............................. 319

8.2 Skinfold Assessment.. 321

8.3 Circumference Measurements/Weight Loss 323

8.4 Weight Control Progress Chart................................. 325

9.1 A Stress Level Checklist 327

9.2 Relaxation Techniques 329

Laboratory 1.1
Health-Related Components of Fitness

Name ——————————————————— Section ——— Date ———

Using the example below, identify each of the health-related components of fitness.

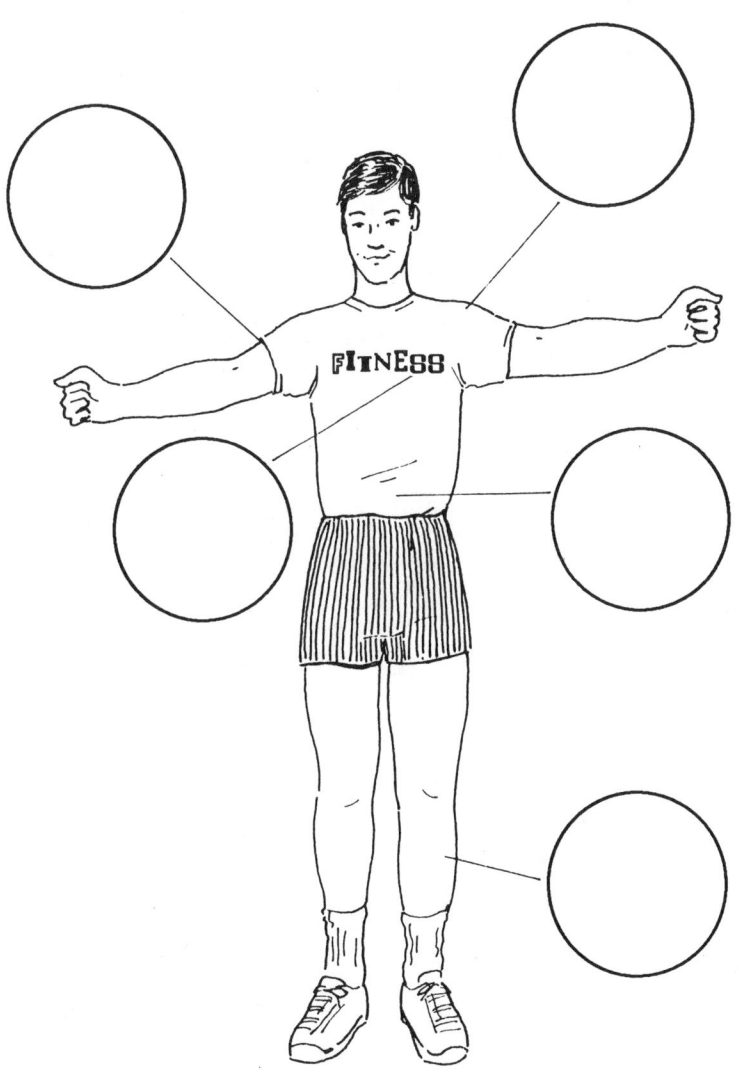

Laboratory 2.1:   Foot Evaluation

Name _____   Section _____   Date_____

	Right	Left
Blisters	_____	_____
Bunions	_____	_____
Corns	_____	_____
Calluses	_____	_____
Deformed toes	_____	_____
Dry skin	_____	_____
Low longitudinal arch	_____	_____
Low metatarsal arch	_____	_____
Nails (ingrown)	_____	_____
Overpronation	_____	_____
Oversupination	_____	_____
Toeing in	_____	_____
Toeing out	_____	_____
Others	_____	_____

Key: A — Good (no problem)
       B — Slight problem
       C — Moderate problem
       D — Needs attention immediately

Comments:

_____

_____

_____

_____

Laboratory 2.2: Shoe Selection

Name _____ Section _____ Date _____

Purpose:
1. To assist in determining individual shoe needs.
2. To become familiar with a variety of walking and/or jogging/running shoes when selecting a quality shoe.

Results:
1. What are your individual needs in the selection of walking/jogging or running shoes?

   1. Foot shape and size: _____

   _____

   2. Foot structure characteristics (degree of pronation or no pronation):

   _____

   _____

   3. Body weight: _____

   _____

   4. Present level of physical activity: _____

   _____

   5. Primary workout: _____

   _____

   6. Mode of exercise (walking, jogging, or running): _____

   _____

2. Visit the library and review the annual shoe issue of *Runner's World* magazine. Select a number of shoe brands that rate high in areas you feel are important to meet your individual needs.

3. Visit a local walking or running shoe store and try on several shoe brands/styles before making your final shoe selection.

Conclusions:

1. Briefly discuss the six important characteristics to look for when selecting a quality shoe.

    1. shape _____

              _____

    2. construction _____

              _____

    3. midsole _____

              _____

    4. outsole _____

              _____

    5. weight _____

              _____

    6. sizes _____

              _____

2. What brand and style will best meet your individual needs? Why?

_____

_____

_____

_____

_____

_____

_____

_____

_____

_____

_____

Laboratory 3.1: Walking Mechanical Analysis

Name _____ Section _____ Date _____

Directions: Use this checklist to analyze body positioning and mechanics.

AREA OF FOCUS	GOOD	NEEDS CORRECTION	
Head	Forward	Down	Up
	_____	_____	_____
Shoulders	Relaxed	Tight	
	_____	_____	
Arms	Bent 90°	Bent 90°+	Hanging Down
	_____	_____	_____
Armswing	Forward and back (Does not cross midline of body)	Across mid-line of body	Out to side away from body
	_____	_____	_____
Slight lean of body	Forward from ankle	Forward from waist	Straight or backward
	_____	_____	_____
Stride	Normal (Knee slightly bent and above foot as plant)	Overextended (Foot beyond knee as foot plants)	Underextended (Short steps Almost shuffle)
	_____	_____	_____

(Continued on Back)

Checklist, continued

AREA OF FOCUS	GOOD	NEEDS CORRECTION	
Body Movement	Forward	Up and down (bounce)	
	_____	_____	
Foot Plant	Heel first Foot 40° to surface	Flat foot	
	_____	_____	
	Straight	Turned in	Turned out
	_____	_____	_____
Push Off	Big toe	2-5 toes	Flat-footed
	_____	_____	_____

Laboratory 3.2: Racewalking Mechanical Analysis

Name _____ Section _____ Date _____

Directions: Use this checklist to analyze body positioning and mechanics.

AREA OF FOCUS	GOOD	NEEDS CORRECTION	
Head	Forward	Down	Up
	_____	_____	_____
Shoulders	Relaxed	Tight	
	_____	_____	
Arms	Bent 90°	Bent 90°+	Hanging Down
	_____	_____	_____
Armswing	Forward and back (Does not cross midline of body)	Across mid-line of body	Out to side away from body
	_____	_____	_____
Slight lean of body	Forward from ankle	Forward from waist	Straight or backward
	_____	_____	_____
Stride	Normal (Knee slightly bent and above foot as plant)	Overextended (Foot beyond knee as foot plants)	Underextended (Short steps Almost shuffle)
	_____	_____	_____

(Continued on Back)

Checklist, continued

AREA OF FOCUS	GOOD	NEEDS CORRECTION	
Body Movement	Forward	Up and down (bounce)	
	_____	_____	
Foot Plant	Heel first Foot 90° angle to shin	Flat foot	
	_____	_____	
	Straight	Turned in	Turned out
	_____	_____	_____
Support Leg	Straight when under body	Bent (creeping) when under body	
	_____	_____	
Push Off	2-5 Toes	Big Toe	Flat-footed
	_____	_____	_____
Hip Action	Relaxed/Smooth	Tight/Restricted	
	_____	_____	

Laboratory 3.3: Jogging/Running Mechanical Analysis

Name _____ Section _____ Date _____

Directions: Use this checklist to analyze body positioning and mechanics.

AREA OF FOCUS	GOOD	NEEDS CORRECTION	
Head	Forward	Down	Up
	_____	_____	_____
Shoulders	Relaxed	Tight	
	_____	_____	
Arms	Bent 90°	Bent 90°+	Hanging Down
	_____	_____	_____
Armswing	Forward and back (Does not cross midline of body)	Across mid-line of body	Out to side away from body
	_____	_____	_____

Note: Runners swing higher and faster than joggers.

Slight lean of body	Forward from ankle	Forward from waist	Straight or backward
	_____	_____	_____
Stride	Normal (Knee slightly bent and above foot as plant)	Overextended (Foot beyond knee as foot plants)	Underextended (Short steps Almost shuffle)
	_____	_____	_____

Note: Runners have a longer stride.

(Continued on Back)

294

Checklist, continued

AREA OF FOCUS	GOOD	NEEDS CORRECTION	
Body Movement	Forward	Up and down (bounce)	
	_____	_____	
Foot Plant	Heel first	Toes first	Flat foot
	_____	_____	_____
	Straight	Turned in	Turned out
	_____	_____	_____
Push Off	Big Toe	2-5 Toes	Flat-footed
	_____	_____	_____

Laboratory 3.4: Target Heart Zone

Name _____ Section _____ Date _____

Determine your target heat zone for aerobic exercise for your selected range by using the procedure below. During an aerobic workout, the exerciser should attempt to keep the heart rate within his/her target heart zone.

First, find your Resting Heart Rate (RHR) by taking your pulse for one minute after waking from a night's sleep or a nap without the assistance of an alarm and without getting up from the prone position. Next, find your Maximum Heart Rate (MHR) by subtracting your age from 220. Then, apply the formula below to determine the upper and lower limits of your training heart zone.

UPPER LIMIT = (MHR – RHR) x upper %

Example (70-85% range)

MHR	_____	200
– RHR	_____	– 75
=	_____	125
x .85	x_____%	x .85
=	_____	106
+ RHR	+_____	+ 75
UPPER LIMIT =	_____	181

LOWER LIMIT = (MHR – RHR) x lower %

MHR	_____	200
– RHR	_____	– 75
=	_____	125
x .70	x_____%	x .70
=	_____	87
+ RHR	+_____	+ 75
LOWER LIMIT =	_____	162

Laboratory 4.1: Risko

Name _____ Section _____ Date _____

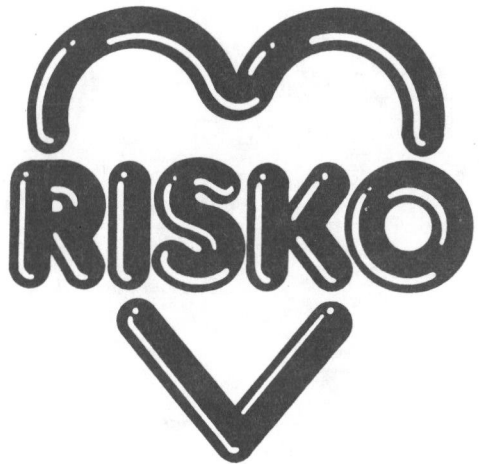

A HEART HAZARD APPRAISAL

Reprinted by permission of

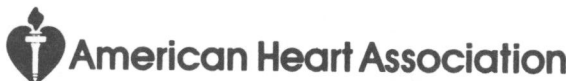 **American Heart Association**

* The RISKO heart hazard appraisal is an indicator of risk for adults who do not currently show evidence of heart disease. However, if you already have heart disease, it is very important that you work with your doctor in reducing your risk.
* The original concept of RISKO was developed by the Michigan Heart Association.
* It has been further developed by the American Heart Association with the assistance of Drs. John and Sonja McKinlay in Boston. It is based on the Framingham, Stanford, and Chicago heart disease studies. The format of RISKO was tested and refined by Dr. Robert M. Chamberlain and Dr. Armin Weinberg of the National Heart Center at the Baylor College of Medicine in Houston.

* RISKO scores are based upon four of the most important modifiable factors which contribute to the development of heart disease. These factors include your weight, blood pressure, blood cholesterol level, and use of tobacco. If you are a woman, your score will also take into account your use of estrogen.
* The RISKO score you obtain measures your risk of developing heart disease in the next several years, provided that you currently show no evidence of such disease.
* The RISKO heart hazard appraisal is not a substitute for a thorough physical examination and assessment by your physician. Rather, it will help you learn more about your risk of developing heart disease and will indicate ways in which you can reduce this risk.

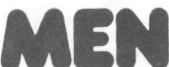

MEN

Find the column for your age group. Everyone starts with a score of 10 points. Work down the page *adding* points to your score or *subtracting* points from your score.

		54 OR YOUNGER	55 OR OLDER

1.WEIGHT

STARTING SCORE **10**   STARTING SCORE **10**

Locate your weight category in the table below If you are in

	54 OR YOUNGER	55 OR OLDER
weight category A	SUBTRACT 2	SUBTRACT 2
weight category B	SUBTRACT 1	ADD 0
weight category C	ADD 1	ADD 1
weight category D	ADD 2	ADD 3
	EQUALS ☐	EQUALS ☐

2.SYSTOLIC BLOOD PRESSURE

Use the first or higher number from your most recent blood pressure measurement If you do not know your blood pressure, estimate it by using the letter for your weight category If your blood pressure is

		54 OR YOUNGER	55 OR OLDER
A	119 or less	SUBTRACT 1	SUBTRACT 5
B	between 120 and 139	ADD 0	SUBTRACT 2
C	between 140 and 159	ADD 0	ADD 1
D	160 or greater	ADD 1	ADD 4
		EQUALS ☐	EQUALS ☐

3.BLOOD CHOLESTEROL LEVEL

Use the number from your most recent blood cholesterol test. If you do not know your blood cholesterol, estimate it by using the letter for your weight category. If your blood cholesterol is

		54 OR YOUNGER	55 OR OLDER
A	199 or less	SUBTRACT 2	SUBTRACT 1
B	between 200 and 224	SUBTRACT 1	SUBTRACT 1
C	between 225 and 249	ADD 0	ADD 0
D	250 or higher	ADD 1	ADD 0
		EQUALS ☐	EQUALS ☐

4.CIGARETTE SMOKING

If you

(If you smoke a pipe but not cigarettes, use the same score adjustment as those cigarette smokers who smoke less than a pack a day.)

	54 OR YOUNGER	55 OR OLDER
do not smoke	SUBTRACT 1	SUBTRACT 2
smoke less than a pack a day	ADD 0	SUBTRACT 1
smoke a pack a day	ADD 1	ADD 0
smoke more than a pack a day	ADD 2	ADD 3
	FINAL SCORE EQUALS ☐	FINAL SCORE EQUALS ☐

WEIGHT TABLE FOR MEN	YOUR HEIGHT FT IN	WEIGHT CATEGORY (lbs)				
		A	**B**	**C**	**D**	
Look for your height (without shoes) in the far left column and then read across to find the category into which your weight (in indoor clothing) would fall	5 1	up to 123	124-148	149-173	174 plus	Because both blood pressure and blood cholesterol are related to these risk factors for each weight category is printed at the bottom of the table
	5 2	up to 126	127-152	153-178	179 plus	
	5 3	up to 129	130-156	157-182	183 plus	
	5 4	up to 132	133-160	161-186	187 plus	weight, an estimate of
	5 5	up to 135	136-163	164-190	191 plus	
	5 6	up to 139	140-168	169-196	197 plus	
	5 7	up to 144	145-174	175-203	204 plus	
	5 8	up to 148	149-179	180-209	210 plus	
	5 9	up to 152	153-184	185-214	215 plus	
	5 10	up to 157	158-190	191-221	222 plus	
	5 11	up to 161	162-194	195-227	228 plus	
	6 0	up to 165	166-199	200-232	233 plus	
	6 1	up to 170	171-205	206-239	240 plus	
	6 2	up to 175	176-211	212-246	247 plus	
	6 3	up to 180	181-217	218-253	254 plus	
	6 4	up to 185	186-223	224-260	261 plus	
	6 5	up to 190	191-229	230-267	268 plus	
	6 6	up to 195	196-235	236-274	275 plus	
ESTIMATE OF SYSTOLIC BLOOD PRESSURE		119 or less	120-139	140-159	160 +	
ESTIMATE OF BLOOD CHOLESTEROL		199 or less	200-224	225-249	250 +	

WOMEN

Find the column for your age group. Everyone starts with a score of 10 points. Work down the page *adding* points to your score or *subtracting* points from your score.

	54 OR YOUNGER	55 OR OLDER

1. WEIGHT

Locate your weight category in the table below. If you are in

	STARTING SCORE [10]	STARTING SCORE [10]
weight category A	SUBTRACT 2	SUBTRACT 2
weight category B	SUBTRACT 1	SUBTRACT 1
weight category C	ADD 0	ADD 0
weight category D	ADD 2	ADD 1
	EQUALS [ ]	EQUALS [ ]

2. SYSTOLIC BLOOD PRESSURE

Use the 'first' or 'higher' number from your most recent blood pressure measurement. If you do not know your blood pressure, estimate it by using the letter for your weight category. If your blood pressure is

A	119 or less	SUBTRACT 2	SUBTRACT 3
B	between 120 and 139	SUBTRACT 1	ADD 0
C	between 140 and 159	ADD 0	ADD 3
D	160 or greater	ADD 1	ADD 6
		EQUALS [ ]	EQUALS [ ]

3. BLOOD CHOLESTEROL LEVEL

Use the number from your most recent blood cholesterol test. If you do not know your blood cholesterol, estimate it by using the letter for your weight category. If your blood cholesterol is

A	199 or less	SUBTRACT 1	SUBTRACT 3
B	between 200 and 224	ADD 0	SUBTRACT 1
C	between 225 and 249	ADD 0	ADD 1
D	250 or higher	ADD 1	ADD 3
		EQUALS [ ]	EQUALS [ ]

4. CIGARETTE SMOKING

If you

do not smoke	SUBTRACT 1	SUBTRACT 2
smoke less than a pack a day	ADD 0	SUBTRACT 1
smoke a pack a day	ADD 1	ADD 1
smoke more than a pack a day	ADD 2	ADD 4
	EQUALS [ ]	EQUALS [ ]

5. ESTROGEN USE

Birth control pills and hormone drugs contain estrogen. A few examples are 'Premarin 'Ogan 'Menstranol 'Provera 'Evex 'Menest 'Estinyl 'Meurium

- Have you ever taken estrogen for five or more years in a row?
- Are you age 35 years or older and are now taking estrogen?

No to both questions	ADD 0	ADD 0
Yes to one or both questions	ADD 1	ADD 3

	FINAL SCORE EQUALS [ ]	FINAL SCORE EQUALS [ ]

WEIGHT TABLE FOR WOMEN
Look for your height (without shoes) in the far left column and then read across to find the category into which your weight (in indoor clothing) would fall

YOUR HEIGHT FT IN	WEIGHT CATEGORY (lbs)			
	A	B	C	D
4 8	up to 101	102-122	123-143	144 plus
4 9	up to 103	104-125	126-146	147 plus
4 10	up to 106	107-128	129-150	151 plus
4 11	up to 109	110-132	133-154	155 plus
5 0	up to 112	113-136	137-158	159 plus
5 1	up to 115	116-139	140-162	163 plus
5 2	up to 119	120-144	145-168	169 plus
5 3	up to 122	123-148	149-172	173 plus
5 4	up to 127	128-154	155-179	180 plus
5 5	up to 131	132-158	159-185	186 plus
5 6	up to 135	136-163	164-190	191 plus
5 7	up to 139	140-168	169-196	197 plus
5 8	up to 143	144-173	174-202	203 plus
5 9	up to 147	148-178	179-207	208 plus
5 10	up to 151	152-182	183-213	214 plus
5 11	up to 155	156-187	188-218	219 plus
6 0	up to 159	160-191	192-224	225 plus
6 1	up to 163	164-196	197-229	230 plus
ESTIMATE OF SYSTOLIC BLOOD PRESSURE	119 or less	120-139	140-159	160 +
ESTIMATE OF BLOOD CHOLESTEROL	199 or less	200-224	225-249	250 +

Because both blood pressure and blood cholesterol are related to weight, an estimate of these risk factors for each weight category is printed at the bottom of the table

WHAT YOUR SCORE MEANS

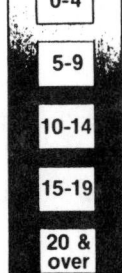

0-4
You have one of the lowest risks of Heart Disease for your age and sex.

5-9
You have a low to moderate risk of Heart Disease for your age and sex but there is some room for improvement.

10-14
You have a moderate to high risk of Heart Disease for your age and sex, with considerable room for improvement on some factors.

15-19
You have a high risk of developing Heart Disease for your age and sex with a great deal of room for improvement on all factors.

20 & over
You have a very high risk of developing Heart Disease for your age and sex and should take immediate action on all risk factors.

WARNING
- If you have diabetes, gout or a family history of heart disease, your actual risk will be greater than indicated by this appraisal.
- If you do not know your current blood pressure or blood cholesterol level, you should visit your physician or health center to have them measured. Then figure your score again for a more accurate determination of your risk.
- If you are overweight, have high blood pressure or high blood cholesterol, or smoke cigarettes, your long-term risk of heart disease is increased even if your risk in the next several years is low.

HOW TO REDUCE YOUR RISK

- Try to quit smoking permanently. There are many programs available.
- Have your blood pressure checked regularly, preferably every twelve months after age 40. If your blood pressure is high, see your physician. Remember blood pressure medicine is only effective if taken regularly.
- Consider your daily exercise (or lack of it). A half hour of brisk walking, swimming or other enjoyable activity should not be difficult to fit into your day.
- Give some serious thought to your diet. If you are overweight, or eat a lot of foods high in saturated fat or cholesterol (whole milk, cheese, eggs, butter, fatty foods, fried foods) then changes should be made in your diet. Look for the American Heart Association Cookbook at your local bookstore.
- Visit or write your local Heart Association for further information and copies of free pamphlets on many related subjects including:
  - Reducing your risk of heart attack.
  - Controlling high blood pressure.
  - Eating to keep your heart healthy.
  - How to stop smoking.
  - Exercising for good health.

SOME WORDS OF CAUTION

- If you have diabetes, gout, or a family history of heart disease, your real risk of developing heart disease will be greater than indicated by your RISKO score. If your score is high and you have one or more of these additional problems, you should give particular attention to reducing your risk.
- If you are a woman under 45 years or a man under 35 years of age, your RISKO score represents an upper limit on your real risk of developing heart disease. In this case your real risk is probably lower than indicated by your score.
- If you are a woman whose use of estrogen has contributed to a high RISKO score, you may want to consult your physician. Do not automatically discontinue your prescription.
- Using your weight category to estimate your systolic blood pressure or your blood cholesterol level makes your RISKO score less accurate.
  - Your score will tend to overestimate your risk if your actual values on these two important factors are average for someone of your height and weight.
  - Your score will underestimate your risk if your actual blood pressure or cholesterol level is above average for someone of your height or weight.

Laboratory 4.2:
Walking/Jogging/Running Schedule/Goals

Name _____ Section _____ Date _____

1. Fill in dates for the month.
2. Decide on the number of workout days per week.
3. Circle the date for each workout day.
4. Write in time or distance goal for each day.
    a. Start at current exercise times or distances

    or

    b. Based upon the exercise level determined by the aerobic test results, check suggested starting times or distances in the sample programs provided in Chapter 4.
5. Alternate hard and easy days or alternate exercise and rest days.
6. Increase no more than 10% weekly.
7. Schedule workouts of over 12 miles on alternate weeks.

CALENDAR

_____
Month

Month

Month

Laboratory 4.3: Weekly Walking/Jogging/Running Log

Name _____ Dates for Week _____

Day	Workout Goal	Workout Distance	Workout Time	Mid Workout Pulse	Post Workout Pulse	Workout Location	Weather Conditions	Comments
Monday								
Tuesday								
Wednesday								
Thursday								
Friday								
Saturday								
Sunday								

Total Weekly Mileage or Workout Time: _____

Name _____ Dates for Week _____

Day	Workout Goal	Workout Distance	Workout Time	Mid Workout Pulse	Post Workout Pulse	Workout Location	Weather Conditions	Comments
Monday								
Tuesday								
Wednesday								
Thursday								
Friday								
Saturday								
Sunday								

Total Weekly Mileage or Workout Time: _____

Lab 5.1. Strength Workout and Progress Chart

Name _____ Section _____ Date _____

S = Sets   R = Repetitions   D = Dosage (Example: Weight)

DATES:	EXERCISE																			

DATES:		S	R	D	S	R	D	S	R	D	S	R	D	S	R	D	S	R	D	S	R	D	S	R	D
EXERCISE																									

Laboratory 7.1: Dietary Habits Evaluation

Name _____ Section _____ Date _____

Circle Yes or No for the responses below. Add the number of yes scores and refer to the Dietary Habits Chart on the back of this page for your Dietary Habits Evaluation Rating.

Yes No 1. Do you eat a variety of foods daily?

Yes No 2. Do you eat breakfast daily?

Yes No 3. Do you eat lunch daily?

Yes No 4. Do you eat dinner 6:00 PM or before?

Yes No 5. Do you limit your snacks?

Yes No 6. Are your snacks nutritious?

Yes No 7. Do you drink 8-10 glasses of water daily?

Yes No 8. Do you eat from the Food Guide Pyramid daily?

Yes No 9. Do you eat less than one teaspoon of salt daily?

Yes No 10. Do you consume an adequate amount of vitamins in your diet without a supplement?

Yes No 11. Do you consume an adequate amount of minerals in your diet without a supplement?

Yes No 12. Does your diet contain 55-60% carbohydrates?

Yes No 13. Are less than 10% of the carbohydrates eaten, simple carbohydrates?

Yes No 14. Does your diet contain a high concentration of fiber daily?

Yes No 15. Does your diet contain 10-12% protein?

Yes No 16. Does your diet contain 20-25% fat?

Yes No 17. Do you limit the amount of saturated fat in your diet?

Yes No 18. Do you limit the amount of cholesterol in your diet?

Yes No 19. Do you limit your intake of caffeine to acceptable levels?

Yes No 20. Do you limit your intake of alcohol?

Total Yes Responses: _____

Dietary Habits Evaluation Rating Chart
(Circle your rating)

Score	Rating
19-20	Very Good
17-18	Good
15-16	Fair
11-14	Poor
10 or less	Very Poor

Laboratory 7.2:   Daily Nutritional Evaluation

Name _____ Section _____ Date _____

1. Using the "Daily Food and Calorie Inventory" on the following pages,
    list all fluids and food consumed over a three-day period. This should
    be representative of your daily dietary habits. After recording all food
    consumed, complete the following questions.

    A. Determine your average carbohydrate intake.   _____ Kcals

    B. Determine your average protein intake.   _____ Kcals

    C. Determine your average fat intake.   _____ Kcals

    D. Determine your total average daily calories
        consumed.   _____ Kcals

    E. What % of your daily intake (D) is carbohydrates? _____ %

    F. What % of your daily intake (D) is proteins?   _____ %

    G. What % of your daily intake (D) is fats?   _____ %

2. How does your diet compare with the recommended amount
    described below?

Recommended Intake	Actual Intake
Carbohydrates = 55-60%	_____
Proteins = 10-12%	_____
Fats = < 30%	_____

3. List three suggestions that you are willing to practice to improve your
    daily nutritional standards.

    1. _____

    2. _____

    3. _____

DAILY FOOD CALORIE INVENTORY
DAY 1

BREAKFAST

Food	Amount	Calories	Carbo.	Protein	Fat
Totals					

LUNCH

Food	Amount	Calories	Carbo.	Protein	Fat
Totals					

DINNER

Food	Amount	Calories	Carbo.	Protein	Fat
Totals					

SNACKS

Food	Amount	Calories	Carbo.	Protein	Fat
Totals					

Total Number of Calories (Day 1) = _____

Laboratory 7.2: Daily Nutritional Evaluation, cont'd

Name _____ Section _____ Date _____

DAILY FOOD CALORIE INVENTORY
DAY 2

BREAKFAST

Food	Amount	Calories	Carbo.	Protein	Fat
Totals					

LUNCH

Food	Amount	Calories	Carbo.	Protein	Fat
Totals					

DINNER

Food	Amount	Calories	Carbo.	Protein	Fat
Totals					

SNACKS

Food	Amount	Calories	Carbo.	Protein	Fat
Totals					

Total Number of Calories (Day 2) = _____

DAILY FOOD CALORIE INVENTORY
DAY 3

BREAKFAST

Food	Amount	Calories	Carbo.	Protein	Fat
Totals					

LUNCH

Food	Amount	Calories	Carbo.	Protein	Fat
Totals					

DINNER

Food	Amount	Calories	Carbo.	Protein	Fat
Totals					

SNACKS

Food	Amount	Calories	Carbo.	Protein	Fat
Totals					

Total Number of Calories (Day 3) = _____

Laboratory 7.2: Daily Nutritional Evaluation, cont'd

Name _____ Section _____ Date _____

1. Total Calories for Each Meal

	DAY 1	DAY 2	DAY 3
Breakfast			
Lunch			
Dinner			
Snacks			
TOTALS			

2. Totals for Three Days
    A. Calories = _____
    B. Grams of Carbohydrates = _____
    C. Grams of Protein = _____
    D. Grams of Fats = _____

3. Average Per Day
    A. Calories = _____
    B. Grams of Carbohydrates = _____
    C. Grams of Protein = _____
    D. Grams of Fats = _____

4. Average Calories Per Day Per Nutrient
    A. Multiply average grams of carbohydrates per day by 4 = _____
    B. Multiply average grams of protein by 4 = _____
    C. Multiply average grams of fat by 9 = _____

5. Percentage of Calories from Each Nutrient
    A. Divide average calories per day from carbohydrates by average total calories per day.
      Calories from Carbohydrates ÷ Total Calories = _____

    B. Divide average calories per day from protein by average total calories per day.
      Calories from Protein ÷ Total Calories = _____

    C. Divide average calories per day from fat by average total calories per day.
      Calories from Fat ÷ Total Calories = _____

Laboratory 7.3. Calories Per Day Formulas

Name_____ Section_____ Date_____

Carbohydrates

Your total calories per day = ——————

Multiplied by 58 or 60 = —————— carbohydrate calories per day

Divided by 4 (1 gram of   grams of total carbohy-
carbohydrate has 4 calories) =—————— drates allowable per day

Proteins

Your total calories per day = ——————

Multiplied by .10 or .12 = ————— protein calories per day

Divided by 4 (1 gram of   grams of total protein
protein has 4 calories) = ————— allowable per day

Fats

Your total calories per day = —————

Multiplied by .25 or .30 = ————— fat calories per day

Divided by 9 (1 gram of   grams of total fat
fat has 9 calories) = ————— allowable per day

Laboratory 7.4
Food Guide Pyramid: A Guide to Daily Food Choices

Name_____Section _____ Date_____

Fill in the blanks to describe the food groups included in the Food Guide Pyramid and the number of servings recommended for each group.

_____ , _____ , & _____
Use _____

_____ , _____ ,   _____ , _____ ,
& _____ Group   _____ , _____ ,
_____ Servings   _____ & _____ Group
                                        _____ Servings

_____ Group   _____ Group
_____ Servings   _____ Servings

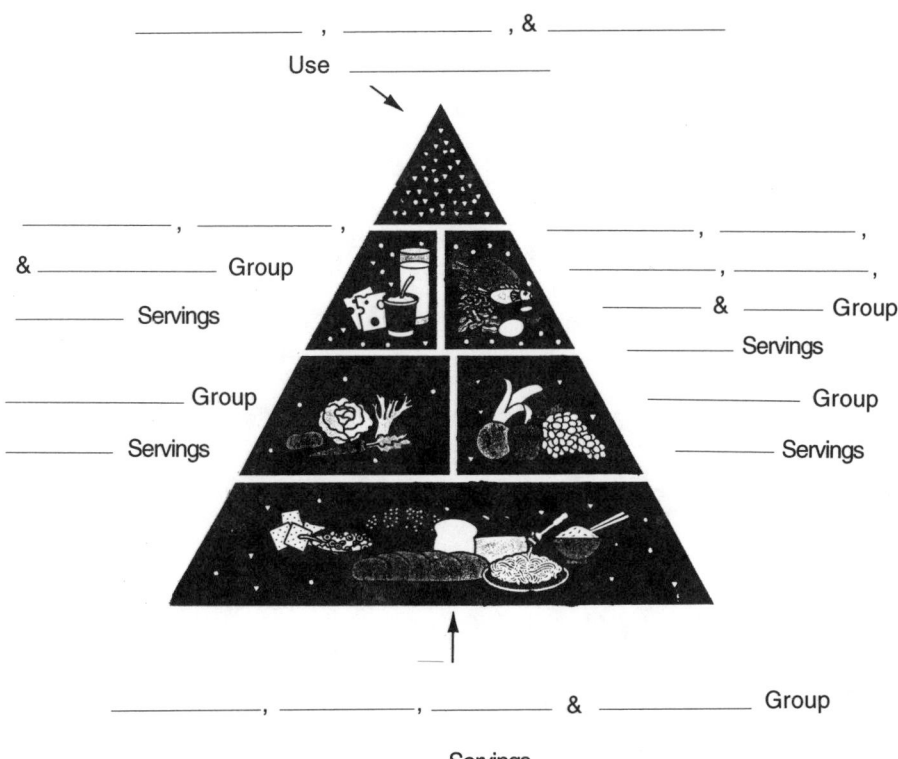

_____ , _____ , _____ & _____ Group
_____ Servings

Laboratory 8.1: Estimation of Ideal Body Weight

Name _____ Section _____ Date_____

Men: 106 pounds for the first five feet   = _____

        +06 pounds for each additional inch   = _____

        + or - 10% to account for individual differences   = _____
                    (small or large frame)

Women: 100 pounds for the first five feet   = _____

        +05 pounds for each additional inch   = _____

        + or - 10% to account for individual differences   = _____
                    (small or large frame)

        Modifications for African Americans:
        Men: 110 lbs. for the first 5 feet of height
        Women: 104 lbs. for the first 5 feet of height.

Weight Loss

To lose 1 pound of fat, subtract 500 calories a day, less maintenance number (3,500 calories ÷ 7 days in a week = 500 calories).

To lose 2 pounds of fat, subtract 1000 calories a day, less maintenance number (3,500 calories x 2 = (7000 calories ÷ 7 days in a week = 1000 calories).

Maintain Current Weight

1. Record present weight in pounds: = _____

2. Record number value of the lifestyle   = _____
                  x 14 (sedentary)
                  x 15 (relatively active)
                  x 16 (very active)
                  x 20 (vigorous activity)

3. Multiply 1 times 2:   = _____

Weight Gain

To gain lean weight, add 360 calories over maintenance intake number (2,500 calories equivalent of 1 pound of muscle ÷ 7 days in a week = 360 daily excess calories over maintenance number of calories).

Laboratory 8.2:   Skinfold Assessment

Name _____ Section _____ Date_____

Following the guidelines for skinfold measurements in Chapter 8, record results below.

	Current	**Goal**	**Results**
Weight:	_____	_____	_____

Skinfold   Measurements:

Women

Triceps	_____	_____	_____
Suprailiac	_____	_____	_____
Thigh	_____	_____	_____
Sum of above	_____	_____	_____
% Body Fat	_____	_____	_____

Men

Chest	_____	_____	_____
Abdomen	_____	_____	_____
Thigh	_____	_____	_____
Sum of above	_____	_____	_____
% Body Fat	_____	_____	_____

Comments:

_____

_____

_____

Laboratory 8.3: Circumference Measurements/Weight Loss

Name _____ Section _____ Date _____

Directions: Following the instructions in Chapter 8, record results below.

Men

Weight _____ lbs.

Waist Circumference _____ in.

Percentage of Body Fat _____

Rating _____

Women

Height _____ in.

Hip Circumference _____ in.

Percentage of Body Fat _____

Rating _____

(Measure to nearest 1/8")

	Current	Goal	Results
Weight	_____	_____	_____
Bust/Chest	_____	_____	_____
Waist	_____	_____	_____
Hips	_____	_____	_____
Thigh	_____	_____	_____
Calf	_____	_____	_____
Upper Arm	_____	_____	_____
Fat %	_____	_____	_____

Comments:

_____

_____

_____

_____

Laboratory 8.4: Weight Control Progress Chart

Name _____ Section _____ Date _____

Age _____   Sex   _____

Resting Heart Rate   (RHR)   _____

Resting Blood Pressure   (RBP)   _____

Present Weight _____

Pounds to be lost _____

Target Weight _____

Exercise Heart Rate Training Zone:

_____ (minimum) to _____ (maximum)

Exercise(s) _____

_____

_____

_____

_____

Progress Chart

Week	RHR	RBP	Exercise	Time/ Distance	Caloric Intake	Weight
1						
2						
3						
4						
5						
6						
7						
8						
9						
10						
11						
12						
13						
14						
15						
16						

Laboratory 9.1: A Stress Level Checklist

Name_____Section _____ Date_____

Stress may affect you in many adverse ways. Learn how to recognize the symptoms in order to rechannel your energy. Take steps to identify and alleviate your stress if you have any of the warning signs listed below. Check those symptoms which apply to you.

____ Acne - rash - hives

Back or shoulder/neck pain
____ (muscular pain)

____ Breathlessness

____ Poor concentration

____ Diarrhea

____ Dry mouth

____ Fatigue - elevated heart rate

____ Finger/toe tapping

____ Grinding teeth

____ Headaches

Hostility or losing temper
____ more often

____ Insomnia

____ Impotence

____ Increase or loss in appetite

____ Low-grade infection

____ Nausea - vomiting

____ Nightmares

____ Restlessness

____ Stomach pain

____ Tiredness

Feeling consistently
____ disappointed

Anger or feeling out of
____ control

____ Biting nails

____ Crying

____ Depression

____ Dizziness

Excessive habits—
smoking, eating, alcohol
____ consumption

____ Fear - panic - anxiety

____ Frustration

Hands shake or tremble/
____ cold, clammy hands

____ High blood pressure

Increased perspiration
____ (sweating)

____ Unusual irritability

____ Jumpy - nervous tics

____ Loss of sex drive

Muscular aches or
____ spasms

____ Nervous laughter

____ Pacing

Speech problems -
____ stuttering

____ Tightness or pain in chest

Tendency to blame
____ mistakes on others

Feel short-changed about
____ life

Laboratory 9.2: Relaxation Techniques

Name _____ Section _____ Date _____

Goal: To practice the conscious release of muscular tension (relaxation).
Equipment Needed: Towels, pillows, or comfortable chair.

Procedure:

1. To determine your stress level, mark (x) each of the early and advanced symptoms of stress which apply to you in Chapter 9. (Refer to Lab 9.1.)

2. Practice the breathing exercises described in Chapter 9.

   A. What was your category of tenseness? _____

   B. Did this technique help you release muscular tension? _____

3. Practice the visualization and/or meditation techniques described in Chapter 9.

   A. What was your category of tenseness? _____

   B. Did this technique help you release muscular tension? _____

4. Practice the progressive relaxation technique as described in Chapter 9.

   A. What was your category of tenseness? _____

   B. Did this technique help you release muscular tension? _____

5. Practice using affirmations and Imaging described in Chapter 9.
   A. What was your category of tenseness? _____

   B. Did this technique help you release muscular tension? _____

APPENDIX E
SHOE AND FOOT TYPES

CHOOSING THE RIGHT SHOE

Motion-Control Shoes

Motion-control shoes are the most control-oriented and rigid running shoe. Designed to limit overpronation (or slow the rate at which a runner overpronates), motion-control shoes are generally heavy and very durable. Features included are medial post (for pronation control), a polyurethane midsole (for midsole durability) and a carbon-rubber outsole (for outsole durability). Many are built on a straight last, which offers stability and maximum medial support.

These shoes are suggested if you are an overpronator who needs control features and places a premium on durability; or you wear orthotics and want a firm midsole and deep heel counter; or you are a heavy runner who needs extra durability and control. Motion-control shoes are often recommended for runners who have flat feet.

Stability Shoes

Stability shoes offer a good blend of cushioning, medial support and durability. To provide stability, these shoes often have a medial post or two-density midsole. They are usually built on a semi-curved last. These shoes are suggested if you are a midweight runner who doesn't have any severe motion-control problems and wants a shoe with some medial support and good durability. Stability shoes are often good for runners with normal arches.

Cushioned Shoes

Cushioned shoes generally have the softest (or most cushioned) midsoles and the least medial support. They are usually built on a semi-curved or curved last to encourage foot motion, which is helpful for underpronators (who have rigid, immobile feet). These shoes are suggested if you are an efficient runner who doesn't overpronate and doesn't need any extra medial support. Runners with high arches often do best in cushioned shoes.

Lightweight Training Shoes

Lightweight training shoes are lighter versions of standard trainers. Usually built on a semi-curved or curved last, lightweight trainers are for fast-paced training or racing. Some lightweight trainers are relatively stable; others are not. These shoes are suggested if you are a quick, efficient runner who wants a light second shoe for fast-pacing training; or you want a racing shoe, but want more support and cushioning than you'd get from one of the pure, superlight racers.

DETERMINE YOUR FOOT TYPE

The Normal Foot

Normal feet have a normal-sized arch and leave an imprint that has a flare but shows the forefoot and heel connected by a wide band.

A normal foot lands on the outside of the heel, then rolls inward (pronates) slightly to absorb shock. Runners with a normal foot and normal weight are usually considered biomechanically efficient and don't require motion-control shoes. Best shoe is a semi-curved and stability shoes with moderate control features such as a two-density midsole.

The Flat Foot

Flat feet have a low arch and leave a nearly complete imprint. The imprint looks like the whole sole of the foot. This imprint usually indicates an overpronated foot that strikes on the outside of the heel and rolls inward (pronates) excessively. Over time, this may cause many different kinds of overuse injuries. The best choice is a straight or semi-curved shoe. Best shoes include motion-control or stability shoes with firm midsoles and control features that reduce the degree of pronation. Stay away from highly cushioned, curved-lasted shoes that lack stability and control.

The High-Arched Foot

High-arched feet leave an imprint showing a very narrow band connecting the forefoot and heel. A curved, high-arched foot is generally termed a supinated or underpronated foot (the terms are synonymous). This type of foot usually doesn't pronate enough, so it is not an effective shock absorber. The best choice is a curved shoe. Cushioned shoes with plenty of flexibility to encourage foot motion are recommended. Stay away from motion-control or stability shoes, which reduce foot mobility.

APPENDIX F
ADDITIONAL NUTRITION INFORMATION

TIPS TO CUT FAT FROM YOUR DIET

- Eat less fried food.
- Go easy on adding fats, such as butter or margarine on toast and mayonnaise on sandwiches.
- Drink fortified skim milk, and choose dairy products (such as cheese) made from skim or low-fat milk.
- Eat meatless main dishes at least several times a week.
- Eat more fish and skinless poultry; bake, broil or stew it.
- Eat no more than 4 to 6 ounces of lean meat, poultry and fish a day and no more than 1 to 3 teaspoons of oils/fats daily. Keep meat portions to the size of a deck of cards.
- Limit fatty meats, such as corned beef, sausage, hotdogs, luncheon meats, spareribs, regular ground beef and heavily marbled meat.
- Eat red meat only a few times a week. Choose lean cuts, such as loin, round, rump or flank. Trim all visible fat before you cook, and cook the meat so the fat can drain away from it.
- Use meat for flavoring, as in chili, rather than as a main dish.
- Remove skin from chicken and turkey before you cook it.
- Cook stews, soups and gravies a day ahead; refrigerate and lift off congealed fat.
- Bake, broil, roast, steam, stir-fry or stew foods instead of frying them.
- Eat no more than four egg yolks a week, including the ones you use in cooking.
- Eat in moderation. Know when to stop. Make changes gradually.
- Learn to read food labels. Fat grams are listed on most food labels.
- Use the 3 gram rule. Read labels and look for more foods that have 3 grams or fewer of fat for every 100 calories.
- Practice fat balancing. When you eat high-fat foods, select low-fat foods to balance out the meal, or try eating high-fat foods in smaller portions or less frequently.

FAT CONTENT OF VARIOUS CHEESES

Type of Cheese	% Calories from Fat
"Diet" or "Light"	25–50
Ricotta (part skim)	52
Mozzarella (part skim)	56
Parmesan	59
Provolone	66
Swiss	66
Ricotta (whole milk)	67
Mozzarella (regular)	68
Brie	74
Cheddar	74
American	75
Cream cheese	90

COMBINATIONS FOR COMPLETE PROTEIN

- Legumes + nuts/seeds = complete protein
- Nuts/seeds + green vegetables = complete protein
- Green vegetables + grains = complete protein
- Grains + legumes = complete protein

Incomplete protein – yield complete protein

- Beans + rice
- Peanut butter sandwich
- Tofu + rice + green vegetables

Charts on this and the preceding page reprinted from *Personal Health: Perspectives and Lifestyles*, ©1998 by Morton Publishing Company.

APPENDIX G
PHYSICAL ACTIVITY AND HEALTH:
A Report of the Surgeon General

A NEW VIEW OF PHYSICAL ACTIVITY
This report brings together, for the first time, what has been learned about physical activity and health from decades of research. Among its major findings:
- People who are usually inactive can improve their health and well-being by becoming even moderately active on a regular basis.
- Physical activity need not be strenuous to achieve health benefits.
- Greater health benefits can be achieved by increasing the amount (duration, frequency, or intensity) of physical activity.

THE BENEFITS OF REGULAR PHYSICAL ACTIVITY
Regular physical activity that is performed on most days of the week reduces the risk of developing or dying from some of the leading causes of illness and death in the United States. Regular physical activity improves health in the following ways:
- Reduces the risk of dying prematurely.
- Reduces the risk of dying from heart disease.
- Reduces the risk of developing diabetes.
- Reduces the risk of developing high blood pressure.
- Helps reduce blood pressure in people who already have high blood pressure.
- Reduces the risk of developing colon cancer.
- Reduces feelings of depression and anxiety.
- Helps control weight.
- Helps build and maintain healthy bones, muscles and joints.
- Helps older adults become stronger and better able to move about without falling.
- Promotes psychological well-being.

A MAJOR PUBLIC HEALTH CONCERN
Given the numerous health benefits of physical activity, the hazards of being inactive are clear. Physical inactivity is a serious, nationwide problem. Its scope poses a public health challenge for reducing the national burden of unnecessary illness and premature death.

WHAT IS A MODERATE AMOUNT OF PHYSICAL ACTIVITY?

As the examples listed in the box show, a moderate amount of physical activity* can be achieved in a number of ways. People can select activities that they enjoy and that fit into their daily lives. Because amount of activity is a function of duration, intensity and frequency, the same amount of activity can be obtained in longer sessions of moderately intense activities (such as brisk walking) as in shorter sessions of more strenuous activities (such as running):[†]

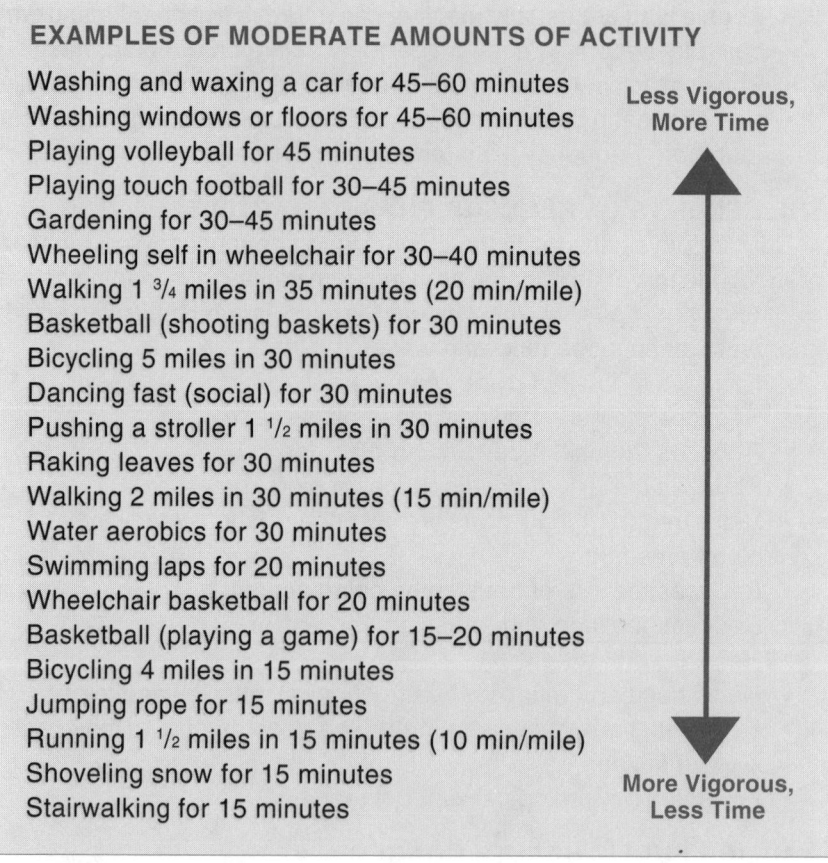

EXAMPLES OF MODERATE AMOUNTS OF ACTIVITY

Washing and waxing a car for 45–60 minutes
Washing windows or floors for 45–60 minutes
Playing volleyball for 45 minutes
Playing touch football for 30–45 minutes
Gardening for 30–45 minutes
Wheeling self in wheelchair for 30–40 minutes
Walking 1 ¾ miles in 35 minutes (20 min/mile)
Basketball (shooting baskets) for 30 minutes
Bicycling 5 miles in 30 minutes
Dancing fast (social) for 30 minutes
Pushing a stroller 1 ½ miles in 30 minutes
Raking leaves for 30 minutes
Walking 2 miles in 30 minutes (15 min/mile)
Water aerobics for 30 minutes
Swimming laps for 20 minutes
Wheelchair basketball for 20 minutes
Basketball (playing a game) for 15–20 minutes
Bicycling 4 miles in 15 minutes
Jumping rope for 15 minutes
Running 1 ½ miles in 15 minutes (10 min/mile)
Shoveling snow for 15 minutes
Stairwalking for 15 minutes

Less Vigorous, More Time

More Vigorous, Less Time

---

* A moderate amount of physical activity is roughly equivalent to physical activity that uses approximately 150 Calories (kcal) of energy per day, or 1,000 Calories per week.

† Some activities can be performed at various intensities; the suggested durations correspond to expected intensity of effort.

PRECAUTIONS FOR A HEALTHY START

To avoid soreness and injury, individuals contemplating an increase in physical activity should start out slowly and gradually build up to the desired amount to give the body time to adjust. People with chronic health problems, such as heart disease, diabetes, or obesity, or who are at high risk for these problems should first consult a physican before beginning a new program of physical activity. Also, men over age 40 and women over age 50 who plan to begin a new vigorous physical activity program should consult a physician first to be sure they do not have heart disease or other health problems.

STATUS OF THE NATION—A NEED FOR CHANGE

Adults

- More than 60 percent of adults do not achieve the recommended amount of regular physical activity. In fact, 25 percent of all adults are not active at all.
- Inactivity increases with age and is more common among women than men and among those with lower income and less education than among those with higher income or education.

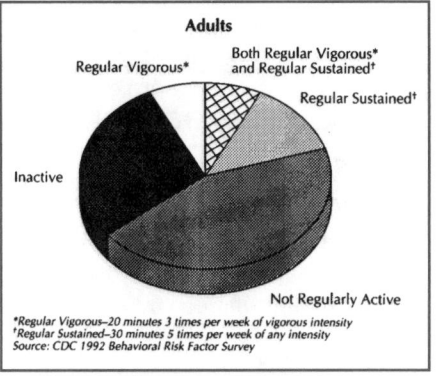

*Regular Vigorous–20 minutes 3 times per week of vigorous intensity
†Regular Sustained–30 minutes 5 times per week of any intensity
Source: CDC 1992 Behavioral Risk Factor Survey

Adolescents and Young Adults

- Nearly half of young people aged 12–21 are not vigorously active on a regular basis.
- Physical activity declines dramatically with age during adolescence.

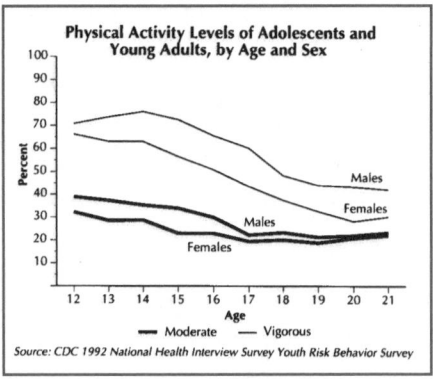

Source: CDC 1992 National Health Interview Survey Youth Risk Behavior Survey

- Female adolescents are much less physically active than male adolescents.

High School Students

- In high school, enrollment in daily physical education classes dropped from 42 percent in 1991 to 25 percent to 1995.
- Only 19 percent of all high school students are physically active for 20 minutes or more in physical education classes every day during the school week.

IDEAS FOR IMPROVEMENT

This report identifies promising ways to help people include more physical activity in their daily lives.

- Well-designed programs in schools to increase physical activity in physical education classes have been shown to be effective.
- Carefully planned counseling by health care providers and worksite activity programs can increase individuals' physical activity levels.
- Promising approaches being tried in some communities around the nation include opening school buildings and shopping malls for walking before or after regular hours, as well as building bicycle and walking paths separated from automobile traffic. Revising building codes to require accessible stairwells is another idea that has been suggested.

SPECIAL MESSAGES FOR SPECIAL POPULATIONS

Older Adults

No one is too old to enjoy the benefits of regular physical activity. Of special interest to older adults is evidence that muscle-strengthening exercises can reduce the risk of falling and fracturing bones and can improve the ability to live independently.

Parents

Parents can help their children maintain a physically active lifestyle by providing encouragement and opportunities for physical activity. Family events can include opportunities for everyone in the family to be active.

Teenagers

Regular physical activity improves strength, builds lean muscle, and decreases body fat. It can build stronger bones to last a lifetime.

Dieters

Regular physical activity burns Calories and preserves lean muscle mass. It is a key component of any weight loss effort and is important for controlling weight.

People with High Blood Pressure

Regular physical activity helps lower blood pressure.

People Feeling Anxious, Depressed or Moody

Regular physical activity improves mood, helps relieve depression, and increases feelings of well-being.

People with Arthritis

Regular physical activity can help control joint swelling and pain. Physical activity of the type and amount recommended for health has not been shown to cause arthritis.

People with Disabilities

Regular physical activity can help people with chronic, disabling conditions improve their stamina and muscle strength and can improve psychological well-being and quality of life by increasing the ability to perform activities of daily life.

For More Information, Contact:

Centers for Disease Control and Prevention
National Center for Chronic Disease Prevention and Health Promotion
Division of Nutrition and Physical Activity, MS K–46
4770 Buford Highway, NE
Atlanta, Georgia 30341
1-888-CDC-4NRG or 1-888-232-4674 (Toll Free)   http://www.cdc.gov

The President's Council on Physical Fitness and Sports
Box SG, Suite 250
701 Pennsylvania Avenue, NW
Washington, DE 20004

INDEX

Achilles tendonitis, 147-148
Adenosine triphosphate (ATP), 47
Aerobic dance, 141
Aerobic exercise, 44-48, 111, 124, 141-145, 177, 244-245
Aerobic intervals, 88
Aerobic-anaerobic interval training, 88
Airplane food, 197
Alcohol, 161, 168, 196-197, 245
Altitude sickness, 22
Amenorrhea, 210
American Heart Association program, 72
Amino acids, 178-179
Anabolic steroids, 21
Anaerobic exercise, 45
Anaerobic intervals, 88
Anemia, 189-190
Anorexia athletica, 210
Anorexia nervosa, 209
Antioxidants, 184-185
Association (as coping strategy), 51
Atherosclerosis, 175-176
Athlete's foot, 156
ATP. See Adenosine triphosphate.

Ballistic stretching, 111
Basal metabolic rate (BMR), 162
Base training, 82-86, 97
Behavior modification, 230-231
Bench step test, 68
Benefits of walking, jogging, and running, 51-52
Benson's training program, 87-88
Beta carotene, 184
Binge eating, 210
Blisters, 148
Blood pressure, 46-47
Body fat assessment, 214-223
    Bioelectrical impedance analysis, 215
    Body mass index (BMI), 214
    Circumferences, 218, 221
    Hydrostatic weighing, 214
    Mirror, 222
    Skinfold measurement, 215-218
Body weight, desirable, 211, 213
Bounding drills, 42
Breathing exercises, 43-44, 241
Bulimia nervosa, 210

Caffeine, 196
Calcium, 151, 187-188, 192
Calipers, 215-218
Calisthenics, 122, 123

Caloric expenditure, 225-226
Caloric intake, recommended, 166
Calorie, 161-162
Carbohydrate loading, 106-108
Carbohydrates, 166-170
Cardiorespiratory response (to exercise), 45-47
Cellulite, 222
Cholesterol, 175-178
Chondromalacia patella, 149-150
Clothing and equipment, 8-20
    Athletic bra/supporter, 18
    Body (rubberized) suits, 19, 229
    Hats/mittens/gloves, 18
    Heart monitors, 20
    Pedometers, 20
    Reflective materials, 19
    Shoes, 8-16
    Socks, 18
    Sunglasses, 20
    Sunscreens, 20
    Watches, 19
    Weights, 19-20
Clothing, cold weather, 17
Clothing, warm weather, 17
Clothing, wet weather, 18
Cool-down, 105
Cruise intervals, 90, 91
Cruise repetition workout, 90
Components of fitness, 2, 111
    Health-related, 2-3
    Skill-related, 2
Components of wellness, 4-5
Cooper programs, 73
Coronary heart disease, 176, 178
Costill's program, 88
Cross country skiing, 142, 144
Cross training, 141-145
    Activities, 141-145
    Programs, 144-145
    Values of, 142
Cycling workouts, 92-93, 142, 144

Daily values, 165
Daniel's program, 88-91
Dehydration, 106, 107, 194, 195
Dellinger's training system, 74, 79
Dietary Guidelines for Americans, 200-201
Diet. See Nutrition.
Diet aids, 228-229
Diets, fad, 227
Diets, low-calorie/liquid, 227-228

Index, Continued

Dissociation techniques, 51
Distress, 236
Downhill running, 42
Drugs, 21, 228, 245

Electrolytes, 192-193
  Drinks, 105-108
Endorphins, 52
Endurance training, 87
Eustress, 236
Exercise machines, passive, 229-230
Exercise prescription guidelines, 53, 56,
  57, 58

Fartleks, 85
Fast foods, 197-199
Fasting, 108, 227
Fat(s), 171-178
  Polyunsaturated, 173
  Saturated, 171, 172, 173
  Unsaturated, 171, 172-173

Fiber, 169-170
Finger-stick test (for cholesterol), 177
Fish oil capsules, 174-175
Fitness, components of, 2-3
Fitness-enhancing programs, 111-145
Fitness walking, 30-34
  Breathing, 33
  Increasing intensity, 33-34
  Mechanics, 30-32
  Practice suggestions, 33
Flexibility, 111-120. *See also* Stretching.
  Exercises for, 113-120
Fluids, 24, 25, 95, 96, 105-108
Food guide pyramid, 162-165
Foot shapes, 19, 20
Free weights, 122
Frequency (of training), 53, 57
Frostbite, 25-26

Galloway's training programs, 74, 79, 82-
  86, 94, 97, 98

Half-marathons. *See* Long-distance
  racing.
Hazards, 22-23
Heat, adjusting race pace for, 110
Heat application, 158
Heat cramps, 24
Heat exhaustion, 24
Heat-safety index, 24
Heatstroke, 25
Heart rate, monitoring, 53-56, 92-93

Target heart rate zone, 54-56
  Training zones, 92
Height-weight tables, 212, 213
Hill training workouts, 84-85, 93, 94, 96, 97
Hot weather exercise, 23-25
Hyperthermia, 25, 26
Hypoglycemia, 167
Hypothermia, 25, 26

Iliotibial band syndrome, 150
Injuries, 146-159
  Acute, 146
  Overuse, 146
  Prevention, 146-147
  Treatment of, 148, 150, 151, 152, 153,
    154, 156-158
Intensity (of training), 33-34, 53-56, 57, 108
Intervals, 85
Iron, 189-190
Isokinetic exercising, 122
Isometric muscle contraction, 112, 121
Isometric exercising, 121-122
Isotonic exercising, 233

Jogging and running, 37
  Breathing, 42-44
  Hand weights, 44
  Mechanics, 38-41
  Practice suggestions, 41-42
  Programs, 79-81
  Progression from jogging to running,
    44
  Progression from walking to jogging and
    running, 37-38

Labels (nutrition), 201-204
Lactate threshold-pace workouts, 90, 95,
  100
Lifetime activity recommendations, 53, 56,
  57, 58
Lipids. *See* Fat(s)
Lipoproteins, 176-178
Long-distance racing, 93-99
Lydiard's program, 87
Marathons. *See* Long-distance racing.
Massage, 244
Maximum heart rate, 56
Meditation, 241
Metabolism, 222, 223
METS, 53
Minerals, 185-191
Mitochondria, 47
Motivation (for exercise), 48-51
Muscle cramps, 150-151
Muscle fibers, 48

Index, Continued

Muscle soreness, 105, 151-152
Muscular response (to exercise), 47-48

Nutrients, 160-196
Nutrition (diet), 95, 96, 108, 160-205, 244
Nutrition label, 201-204

Obesity, 206-209, 211
  Theories of, 206-208
Omega-3 fatty acids, 173
Orthotics, 154
Osteoporosis, 187-189
Overhydration, 107
Overload principle, 58, 122-123
Overweight, 211, 212, 213
Oxygen uptake, 45. *See* VO$_2$ max.

Physical examination, 7
Plantar fascitis 152
Plyometrics, 138-140
  Pollution, 21-22
Prediction Time Chart for Half-Marathon
  and Marathon, 99
Pregnancy and walking, jogging, running,
  102-103
Preparation (for exercise), 7-29
Principles of training, 30-59
Programs (Fitness-enhancing), 111-145
Programs (Training), 69-110
  Based on fitness ratings, 69
  Cross training, 144-145
  Execution of, 104
  Introductory to beginner level, 69-70
  Jogging programs, 79-81
    High intermediate to advanced level,
      80
    Sample Advanced Beginner, 79
    Sample Intermediate, 79
  Long-distance running, 93-98
    Marathon, 98
    Sample Half-Marathon/Marathon, 97
  Racewalking programs, 100
  Running programs, 81
    Sample high intermediate, 81
    Ullyot Intermediate, 81
  Running and Racewalking programs
    for race competitors, 82-101
    Running programs, 82-99
      Benson's, 87-88
      Costill's, 88-90
      Daniels', 88-91
      Galloway's Pyramid, 82-86
      Lydiard's, 87
  Walking programs, 70-78
    American Heart Association, 72

Cooper Aerobic Exercise
Systems,
  73
  Reebok, 73
  Rockport Blue, 70
  Rockport Green, 71
  Rockport Orange, 78
  Rockport Red, 80
  Rockport Yellow, 77
  Sample beginner, 73
  Sample introductory, 72
Walking-Jogging Programs, 74-75
  Advanced beginner to
    intermediate, 76
  Sample beginner, 75
  Sample introductory, 75
Wheelchair workouts/racing, 104
Progression (of exercise), 58
Progressive relaxation, 241-243
Pronation, 13, 15
Proprioceptive neuromuscular
  facilitation (PNF), 112
Proteins, 178-181
Pulse, 53-54

Racewalking, 35-37
  Mechanics, 35-36
  Practice suggestions, 37
Reebok, 7
Repetition training, 42, 90
Repetitions, 123
Resting heart rate, 54-55
Retrogression, 59
R.I.C.E.S. formula, 156-157
RISKO, 60
Rockport programs, 69, 70-71, 76-78,
  80
Rockport Walking Test, 61-65
Rope-assisted stretching, 112
Rope skipping, 142, 144
Rosato's program, 74
Rowing, 142
Rubberized suits, 19
"Runner's knee," 149-150

Safety, 20-28
  Guidelines, 28
Salt. *See* Sodium.
Self-talk, 51, 246
Shin splints, 153-154
Shoes, 8-16, 147, 150, 154
  Running, 12, 13-16
  Walking, 10-11
Shopping (for food), 199

Index, Continued

Skating, in-line, 143, 144
Skinfold measurements, 215-218
Sleep, 241
Smoking, 178, 182
Sodium, 107, 192
Speedwork, 84, 87-88, 90, 94-95, 96, 97, 100-101
Sprains, 152-153
Stair climbing, 142
Stamina training, 87
Static stretching, 111
Step training, 143
Steroids, 21
Strains, 153
Strength training, 111, 121-138
    Exercises for, 124-138
Stress, 236-249
    Causes of, 238-240
    Defined, 236-237
    Management of, 237-248
    Symptoms of, 238, 239
Stress fractures, 152
Stretching exercises, 113-120
    Risky exercises, 120, 137-138
Sugar(s), 167
Supplements, 181, 190-191, 192
Swimming, 142-143, 144

Tapering (of training), 109
Target heart zone, 54-56
Tempo runs, 90
Testing (current level), 60-68
    1 Mile Run Test, 66
    1.5 Mile Test, 65-66
    One-Half Mile Test, 67
    RISKO, 60-61
    Rockport Walking Test, 61-65

3 Minute Bench Step Test, 68
Threshold-Pace Chart, 89
Time (duration of exercise session), 56, 57
Training principles (FITT), 52-59
    Children, 58
    Adolescents and young adults, 58
Training programs, 60-110. See also Programs.
Treadmills, 143, 144

Ullyot's training program, 74, 81
Uphill running, 42

Variable resistance machines, 122
Vegetarian food choices, 181
Visualization, 241
Vitamins, 181-185, 190-191
VO_2 max, 45, 92-93, 100-101

Walking programs, 70-78
Warm-up, 104, 146
Water, 105-108, 193-196. See also Fluids.
Water aerobics, 143
Water walking/jogging/running, 143, 144

Weight gain, 234
Weight loss, 222-233
    and exercise, 223-226
    and metabolism, 223
    and spot reduction, 226
Weight loss program guidelines, 231-232
Weight maintenance, 232-233
Weight management, 206-235
Weight training. See Strength training
Weights, hand or wrist, 19-20, 44
Wellness, 2, 4, 5, 248
    Components of, 4, 5
Wet test, 13
Wind-chill readings, 27